Musculoskeletal Health: Role of Nutrition

Musculoskeletal Health: Role of Nutrition

Editor: Josephine Ortiz

AMERICAN
MEDICAL PUBLISHERS
www.americanmedicalpublishers.com

AMERICAN
MEDICAL PUBLISHERS
www.americanmedicalpublishers.com

Cataloging-in-Publication Data

Musculoskeletal health : role of nutrition / edited by Josephine Ortiz.
p. cm.
Includes bibliographical references and index.
ISBN 978-1-63927-740-7
1. Musculoskeletal system--Diseases--Nutritional aspects. 2. Musculoskeletal system--Wounds and injuries--Nutritional aspects. 3. Musculoskeletal system--Diseases--Diet therapy. 4. Musculoskeletal system--Wounds and injuries--Diet therapy. 5. Musculoskeletal system--Physiology. 6. Muscles--Physiology. 7. Nutrition. I. Ortiz, Josephine.
RC925 .M87 2023
616.7--dc23

American Medical Publishers,
41 Flatbush Avenue,
1st Floor, New York,
NY 11217, USA

ISBN 978-1-63927-740-7 (Hardback)

Contents

Preface

The purpose of the book is to provide a glimpse into the dynamics and to present opinions and studies of some of the scientists engaged in the development of new ideas in the field from very different standpoints. This book will prove useful to students and researchers owing to its high content quality.

Musculoskeletal health refers to a condition of being healthy without any musculoskeletal conditions. These conditions can include numerous diseases, such as sarcopenia, osteoporosis, osteoarthritis, fibromyalgia, rheumatoid arthritis, etc. Musculoskeletal health is considered good when the bones, muscles and joints work well together without any pain. People who have good musculoskeletal health are able to perform their desired activities easily and without pain. The consumption of a varied and balanced diet rich in nutrients is helpful in maintaining musculoskeletal health. In the absence of important nutrients the chance of developing bone, joint or muscle disease increases, which can result in symptoms like restricted movement, joint deformity, swelling, pain and stiffness. Nutrition can modulate the immune system, help in suppressing inflammation and pain, and provide specialized nutrients required for maintenance, growth and repair. This book traces the progress of research on musculoskeletal health. It aims to shed light on the role of nutrition for improving musculoskeletal health. Researchers and students engaged in this area of study will be assisted by this book.

At the end, I would like to appreciate all the efforts made by the authors in completing their chapters professionally. I express my deepest gratitude to all of them for contributing to this book by sharing their valuable works. A special thanks to my family and friends for their constant support in this journey.

Editor

1

Distribution of Constituents and Metabolites of Maritime Pine Bark Extract (Pycnogenol®) into Serum, Blood Cells and Synovial Fluid of Patients with Severe Osteoarthritis

Melanie Mülek [1], Lothar Seefried [2], Franca Genest [2] and Petra Högger [1,*]

[1] Institut für Pharmazie und Lebensmittelchemie, Universität Würzburg, 97074 Würzburg, Germany; melanie.muelek@pharmazie.uni-wuerzburg.de

[2] Department of Orthopedics, Orthopedic Center for Musculoskeletal Research, 97074 Würzburg, Germany; l-seefried.klh@uni-wuerzburg.de (L.S.); f-genest.klh@uni-wuerzburg.de (F.G.)

* Correspondence: petra.hoegger@uni-wuerzburg.de

Abstract: The present randomized controlled study aimed to investigate the in vivo distribution of constituents or metabolites of the standardized maritime pine bark extract Pycnogenol®. Thirty-three patients with severe osteoarthritis scheduled for a knee arthroplasty were randomized to receive either 200 mg per day Pycnogenol® (P+) or no treatment (Co) over three weeks before surgery. Serum, blood cells, and synovial fluid samples were analyzed using liquid chromatography coupled to tandem mass spectrometry with electrospray ionization (LC-ESI/MS/MS). Considerable interindividual differences were observed indicating pronounced variability of the polyphenol pharmacokinetics. Notably, the highest polyphenol concentrations were not detected in serum. Catechin and taxifolin primarily resided within the blood cells while the microbial catechin metabolite δ-(3,4-dihydroxy-phenyl)-γ-valerolactone, ferulic, and caffeic acid were mainly present in synovial fluid samples. Taxifolin was detected in serum and synovial fluid exclusively in the P+ group. Likewise, no ferulic acid was found in serum samples of the Co group. Calculating ratios of analyte distribution in individual patients revealed a simultaneous presence of some polyphenols in serum, blood cells, and/or synovial fluid only in the P+ group. This is the first evidence that polyphenols distribute into the synovial fluid of patients with osteoarthritis which supports rationalizing the results of clinical efficacy studies.

Keywords: pine bark extract; LC-ESI/MS/MS; randomized controlled study; osteoarthritis; human; polyphenols

---

1. Introduction

Dietary polyphenols have been associated with numerous beneficial effects on human health. Studies investigating the absorption of polyphenols from the gastrointestinal tract revealed that blood concentrations of individual polyphenols are often very low [1]. Moreover, polyphenolic compounds are often subjected to an extensive metabolism [2]. Some metabolites generated by gut microbial metabolism obviously contribute to health effects [3].

One of those bioactive metabolites is δ-(3,4-dihydroxy-phenyl)-γ-valerolactone (M1) which is formed by the human intestinal flora from the procyanidins' catechin units [2]. It has been detected in urine and plasma samples after intake of Pycnogenol® [4,5]. The dietary supplement Pycnogenol® is a standardized extract of the French maritime pine, which conforms to the monograph "*Maritime pine extract*" in the United States Pharmacopeia (USP). It contains 65%–75% oligomeric procyanidins and polyphenolic monomers, phenolic, or cinnamic acids and their glycosides [6].

In numerous clinical studies Pycnogenol® demonstrated effects in different chronic diseases of, for example, inflammatory or cardiovascular origin [6,7].

Another chronic disease with high pharmacoeconomic burden and significant impact on the patients' quality of life is osteoarthritis (OA). OA is a chronic degenerative joint disease which is characterized by progressive cartilage destruction and it is the leading cause of pain and disability [8]. Treatment of OA includes pharmacological and non-pharmacological interventions and aims at pain relief and improvement of function. Severe OA might also require surgical interventions such as knee or hip arthroplasty [9]. Dietary factors or supplements have been discussed as options in the management or prevention of OA [10].

In clinical studies OA symptoms such as pain and joint stiffness have been shown to improve upon intake of Pycnogenol® [11,12]. While this clinical observation is consistent with a previously shown inhibition of nuclear factor κB (NF-κB) activation and inhibition of various matrix metalloproteinases by constituents or metabolites of this pine bark extract [13,14], it is not clear yet whether bioactive polyphenols would actually be present at the site of disease (e.g., in the joints affected by OA). After an oral intake of multiple doses of Pycnogenol® concentrations in the nanomolar range of catechin, taxifolin, caffeic acid, ferulic acid, and of a bioactive metabolite M1 have been detected in human plasma [5]. Moreover, an uptake of M1 into erythrocytes, monocytes, and endothelial cells has been observed in vitro [15,16]. The purpose of the current study was to investigate the in vivo distribution of constituents or metabolites of Pycnogenol® in serum, blood cells, and synovial fluid of patients with severe OA scheduled for a knee replacement surgery.

2. Materials and Methods

2.1. Clinical Study Design

The present study was a randomized controlled clinical trial involving patients with severe osteoarthritis (OA) according to the Western Ontario and McMaster Universities Arthritis Index (WOMAC) score, who were scheduled for an elective knee replacement surgery (Kellgren-Lawrence grade III–IV). Patients were not eligible if they regularly took non-steroidal anti-inflammatory drugs (NSAIDs) or glucocorticoids perorally within the past four weeks, if they currently received a therapy with anti-coagulants, or if they tested positive for the human immunodeficiency virus (HIV), hepatitis B or C, or if they had a previous or current infection of the affected knee joint. As rescue medication acetaminophen (paracetamol), tramadol, or a combination of tilidine and naloxone was allowed. The study was conducted in accordance with the Declaration of Helsinki, and the protocol was approved by the local Ethics Committee of the Medical Faculty of the University Würzburg (Project identification code 248/11).

A total of 33 OA patients were recruited for the study and gave informed written consent before they participated in the study. The chosen number of patients was based on a previous pharmacokinetic study with healthy volunteers receiving the pine bark extract [5]. Patients were randomized into two groups using a computer-generated randomization list which was not accessible to the physicians and nurses who were involved in the patient care and management. Study participants ($n = 16$) were assigned to the treatment group receiving 200 mg of the French maritime pine bark extract Pycnogenol® (Horphag Research Ltd., Geneva, Switzerland) per day (twice daily two capsules with each 50 mg) over three weeks prior to the planned surgery. The control group was comprised of 17 patients who did not receive Pycnogenol®. All patients were asked to comply with a polyphenol-free nutrition, especially two days before each blood sampling. For this purpose, they were provided with nutritional check-lists specifying food/beverages they should avoid and for recording what they ingested within the last two days before blood sampling. Adherence to the study medication was estimated based on the number of returned Pycnogenol® capsules upon hospitalization for the knee replacement surgery.

Blood samples from each study participant were collected (BD Vacutainer® SST II Advance; Becton Dickinson GmbH, Heidelberg, Germany) before oral intake of Pycnogenol® (V1, basal value);

during the intake, approximately 1–2 days before the surgery (V2); and during or shortly before knee surgery (V3), about 12 h after the last dose of Pycnogenol®. Immediately after blood sampling the serum and cellular fraction were separated under sterile conditions. On the day of the surgery residual knee cartilage and synovial fluid were also collected. All samples were shock-frozen immediately and stored at −80 °C. The outcome measure was the concentration of pine bark extract-derived polyphenols in serum, blood cells, and synovial fluid as determined by liquid chromatography coupled to tandem mass spectrometry with electrospray ionization (LC-ESI/MS/MS).

All medical procedures including enrollment of participants, surgery, patient care, and sample collection took place at the orthopedic center (Orthopädie und Orthopädische Klinik König-Ludwig-Haus, Universität Würzburg) between September 2012 and September 2014. The generation of the random allocation sequence, assignment of participants to the intervention or control group, and analysis of all patient samples took place at the Institut für Pharmazie und Lebensmittelchemie. Since the study primarily focused on pharmacokinetic/bioanalytical aspects, specifically on the analysis of polyphenols in various human specimen, an early registration was overlooked and the study was registered retroactively.

2.2. *Chemicals, Reagents, and Special Materials*

Analytical standards of (+)-catechin, taxifolin, ferulic acid, caffeic acid, and the internal standard (IS) 3,4-dihydroxyhydrocinnamic acid (hydrocaffeic acid) were all obtained from Sigma-Aldrich (Taufkirchen, Germany). The metabolite M1 (δ-(3.4-dihydroxy-phenyl)-γ-valerolactone) was synthesized by M. Rappold as part of his diploma thesis. Methanol (MeOH, LC-MS analyzed) from J.T.Baker Mallinckrodt and water (HiPerSolv CHROMANORM® for LC-MS) were obtained from VWR (Darmstadt, Germany). Ammonium formate (AF) and formic acid (FA) were purchased from Sigma-Aldrich. An enzymatic mixture of β-glucuronidase/sulfatase (β-Gln/Sulfa) from *Helix pomatia* (Type HP-2; Sigma-Aldrich) was used for enzymatic hydrolysis. Ethyl acetate, *tert*-butyl methyl ether (MTBE), and phosphate buffered saline (PBS, pH 7.4) were obtained from Sigma-Aldrich.

2.3. *Standard Solutions*

Stock solutions (1 mg/mL) of each standard substance ((+)-catechin, taxifolin, ferulic acid, caffeic acid, and M1) and of the internal standard (IS; hydrocaffeic acid) were prepared in 100% methanol and stored at −80 °C. They were diluted with methanol to yield working standards which were aliquoted and stored at −20 °C.

2.4. *Human Specimen for Calibration Curves*

Packed cells and serum were obtained from a blood bank (Bayerisches Rotes Kreuz (BRK), München, Germany) and handled as previously described [17,18]. Synovial fluid was collected from patients with intra-articular fluid accumulation who needed punctuation of the effusion for medical reasons. Synovial fluid samples were pooled to obtain a single batch for preparation of calibration standards for quantification of the clinical study samples.

2.5. *Liquid Chromatography (LC)*

Details of the LC method have been reported before [18,19]. Briefly, for the LC analysis an Agilent 1260 system was used. The chromatographic separation was carried out using a Pursuit PFP-C18 column (4.6 × 150 mm, particle size 3 μm) at 20 °C (all from Agilent Technologies, Santa Clara, CA, USA). The mobile phase consisted of 5 mM ammonium formate with 0.065% (*v/v*) formic acid (pH = 3.2; A) and methanol with 0.1% formic acid (B). The flow rate was set to 0.6 mL/min and the sample injection volume was 5 μL. The gradient elution was conducted starting at 60% B (0 min) to 95% B (2.50 min) and maintained to 95% B to 5.50 min followed by re-equilibration at 60% B. The total run time was 10.00 min with a post time of 3 min.

2.6. Mass Spectrometry (MS/MS)

Details of the MS/MS method using a G 6460 TripleQuad LC/MS with turbo electrospray ionization (ESI; Agilent Technologies, Santa Clara, CA, USA) have been previously reported [17,18]. The optimized MS/MS transitions and mass spectrometric parameters of the compounds to be quantified in human blood cell and serum samples were recently reported [18,19]; optimized parameters of additionally determined M1 metabolites in blood cells are listed in Table S1 in the electronic supplementary material. Optimized MS/MS transitions and mass spectrometric parameters of the compounds to be quantified in human synovial fluid samples are listed in Table S2.

2.7. Preparation of Human Serum Samples

Serum samples (1.5 mL) were prepared by liquid-liquid extraction with prior enzymatic incubation containing β-Gln/Sulfa to hydrolyze conjugated analytes [5], as previously described [18,19]. Additionally, 1.5 mL of serum was analyzed without prior enzymatic hydrolysis to calculate the degree of conjugation with sulfate and glucuronic acid.

2.8. Preparation of Human Blood Cell Samples

Human blood cell samples were prepared as previously detailed [18]. Therefore, 2.0 mL blood cells of each study volunteer were processed with prior enzymatic hydrolysis to determine the total concentration of the analytes.

2.9. Preparation of Human Synovial Fluid Samples

Synovial fluid samples were prepared with a newly developed and optimized liquid-liquid extraction method. Therefore, 40 μL 4% o-phosphoric acid was added to 1.0 mL human synovial fluid (pH 5.0). Afterwards, the samples were incubated with an enzyme mixture containing β-Gln/Sulfa (1500 U β-Gln and 2 U Sulfatase per mL synovial fluid) for 45 min at 37 °C on a horizontal shaker (100 rpm) to hydrolyze conjugated analytes [5]. Then, 60 μL 4% o-phosphoric acid (pH 3.2), 25 μL IS (24.85 ng/mL), and 3.0 mL extraction solvent containing ethyl acetate and *tert*-butyl methyl ether (1:1; *v/v*) were added, vortexed for 1 min (Multi-Vortex, VWR, Darmstadt, Germany), and centrifuged for 5 min at 3300× *g* (4 °C). Thereafter, 2.0 mL of the upper organic layer was evaporated to dryness under nitrogen. The residue was reconstituted in 75 μL of 100% MeOH and centrifuged at 18,000× *g* for 15 min at 4 °C before LC-MS/MS analysis.

A full validation was performed for the quantification of the analytes in human synovial fluid with the optimized liquid-liquid extraction method and prior enzymatic hydrolysis. The validation included the selectivity, linearity, lower limit of quantification (LLOQ), accuracy and precision (intra- and interday), recovery, process efficiency, matrix effects (quantitative), carry over, cross talk, and post-preparative stability. Also, the freeze- and thaw-, short-term-, and long-term stability of the analytes in human serum were investigated.

2.10. Quantification of the Samples of the Study Participants

For each patient, specimen human pooled matrix-matched calibration standards with an internal standard (structural) were used for quantification of the study samples. In case of a basal presence of an analyte in the blank matrix, the calibration curve was shifted along the y axis by the response of the zero-sample (containing the IS) [20].

2.11. Statistical Analysis

Data were analyzed using descriptive statistics. Typically, mean and standard deviation (SD) were calculated. For comparison of the study participants' basic demographic characteristics a Student's *t*-test was used to compare the patients of the treatment and control group.

3. Results

3.1. Patients and Protocol Adherence

A total of 33 patients were enrolled into the study and randomized to receive either Pycnogenol® ($n = 16$) or no treatment ($n = 17$). One patient of the control group decided against the scheduled knee replacement surgery and was excluded. During the surgical procedure, there was a failure to collect blood, synovial fluid, and cartilage samples for one patient in both the control group and the Pycnogenol® group. These patients were excluded from the analysis (Figure 1). Thus, 30 patients (66.7% female) underwent analysis after receiving Pycnogenol® ("P+"; 9 females, 6 males) or no treatment as the control group ("Co"; 11 females, 4 males). There was no statistically significant difference between the groups in any of the basic demographic characteristics (Student's t-test, $p > 0.05$), the mean age (± standard deviation SD) was 64.3 ± 8.2 years, height 1.69 ± 0.10 m, body weight 87.33 ± 15.66 kg (BMI 30.74 ± 5.29 kg/m^2).

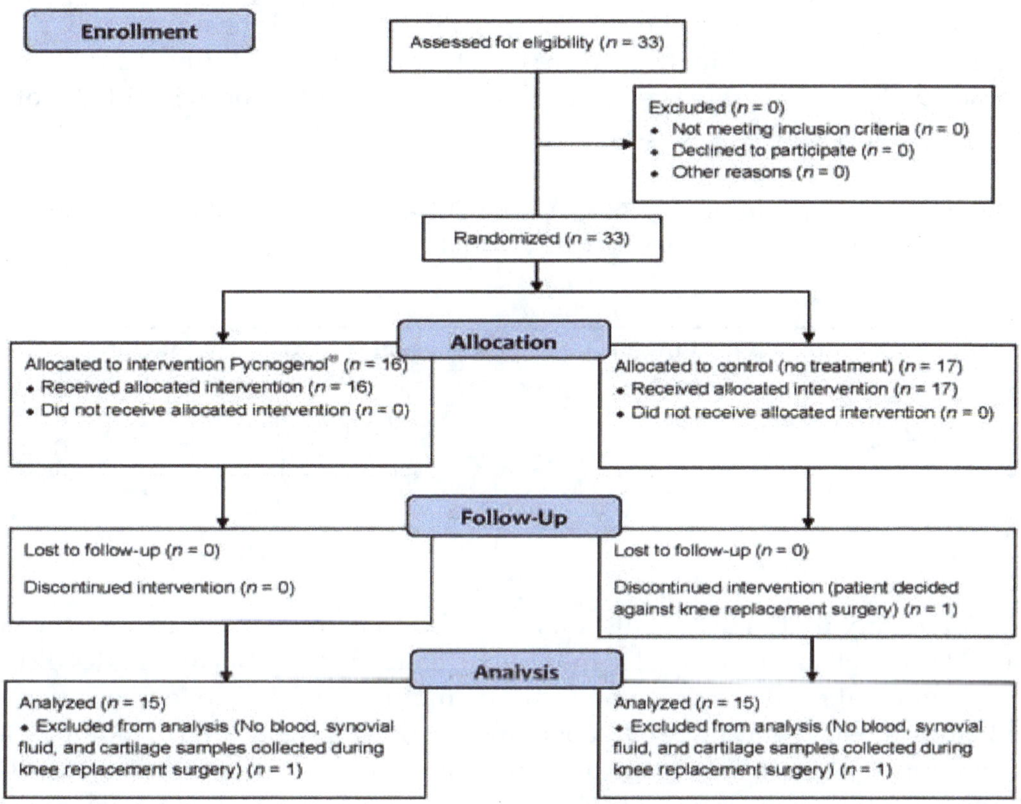

Figure 1. CONSORT (Consolidated Standards of Reporting Trials; www.consort-statement.org) 2010 Flow diagram of the study.

All study participants were requested to avoid polyphenol-rich food/beverages (e.g., coffee, green tea, wine, chocolate, some fruits and vegetables) within the last two days before the blood samplings. Analysis of the nutrition protocols revealed that the nutritional advice was not followed well and dietary violations were admitted before collecting 42% of the blood samples. Thus, concentrations of common polyphenols such as catechin or caffeic acid from other sources than Pycnogenol® were to be expected in the blood samples.

In contrast, the adherence to the study medication was excellent based on the pill count-back on returned medication containers. In the Pycnogenol® group the average adherence was 99.4% (range 96%–100%) for all but one study participant who apparently took only 76% of the capsules.

No treatment-associated adverse effects were reported except for one patient of the Pycnogenol® group who experienced flatulence.

3.2. Method for Analysis of Polyphenols in Human Synovial Fluid Samples

To the best of our knowledge, this is the first study describing the detection and quantification of polyphenols in human synovial fluid. Since concentrations in synovial fluid samples were possibly lower than in blood and based on the fact that a previous pharmacokinetic study revealed plasma concentrations of polyphenolic compounds in the nanomolar range after intake of Pycnogenol® [5], a highly sensitive method was required. In the course of method development, the main focus was the optimal detection and quantification of the metabolite M1.

Analogous to previously developed methods for analysis of Pycnogenol® polyphenols in serum and blood cells [18,19], various sample preparation techniques were compared and a liquid-liquid extraction method was chosen. For the analytes of highest interests, the lower limits of quantification (LLOQs) in synovial fluid were 0.080 ng/mL for taxifolin and 0.117 ng/mL for M1 (Table 1 and Table S9). The method was slightly less sensitive for ferulic acid (LLOQ of 1.53 ng/mL), catechin (2.14 ng/mL), and caffeic acid (3.07 ng/mL).

Table 1. Lower limits of quantification (LLOQs) of polyphenolic analytes of highest interest. Data for serum and blood cells was derived from previous work [18,19].

Analyte	LLOQ Synovial Fluid (ng/mL)	LLOQ Serum (ng/mL)	LLOQ Blood Cells (ng/mL)
Catechin	2.14	5.86	28.90
M1	0.12	0.16	0.12
Taxifolin	0.08	0.06	0.12
Caffeic Acid	3.07	8.22	48.40
Ferulic Acid	1.53	2.74	0.97

In the supplementary materials, details about the recovery, matrix effects, and process efficiency (Tables S10 and S11), as well as the internal standard normalized matrix factor (Table S12) in pooled and individual lots of synovial fluid are documented. The method was validated based on current EMA (European Medicines Agency) and FDA (US Food and Drug Administration) guidelines and complied with the requirements for selectivity, linearity (Table S3), precision and accuracy (Tables S6 and S7), robustness (Table S6), carry-over, cross-talk, and post-preparative stability (Tables S9 and S10).

Representative chromatograms of all three specimens of an individual study participant after multiple dosing of 200 mg/day Pycnogenol® over the course of three weeks (P+, V3) revealed total concentrations of 23.17 ng/mL catechin, 3.70 ng/mL ferulic acid, 0.19 ng/mL taxifolin, 0.16 ng/mL M1 in serum, 74.31 ng/mL catechin, 1.93 ng/mL ferulic acid, and 0.57 ng/mL taxifolin in blood cells, and 3.19 ng/mL ferulic acid, 0.18 ng/mL taxifolin, and 0.17 ng/mL M1 in synovial fluid (Figure 2).

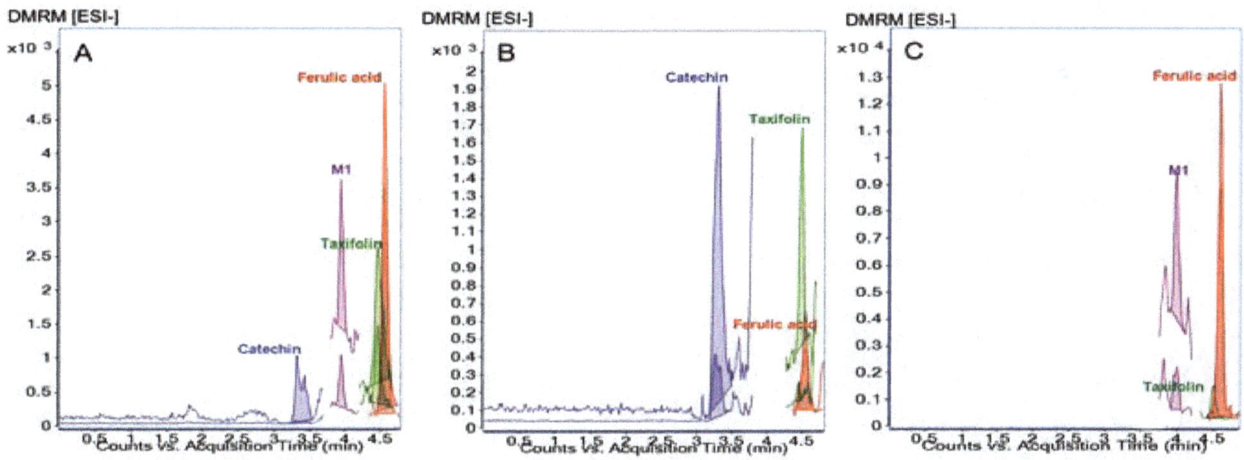

Figure 2. Example chromatograms for quantification in the three different sample matrices of one individual study participant after multiple dosing of 200 mg/day Pycnogenol® over the course of three weeks (P+, V3). (**A**) Serum; (**B**) Blood cells; (**C**) Synovial fluid.

3.3. Pycnogenol® Constituents and Metabolites in Serum Samples

In the basal serum samples (V1) the mean total concentrations (free and conjugated) of all study participants were 27.07 ± 16.39 ng/mL catechin (mean and standard deviation), 1.80 ± 2.63 ng/mL for M1, 0.07 ng/mL (n = 1) for taxifolin, 6.40 ± 2.58 ng/mL for ferulic acid, and 18.58 ± 6.32 ng/mL for caffeic acid. For example, catechin was detectable in 29 out of 30 V1 samples, and in 24 samples the concentrations were above 10 ng/mL. Thereby, catechin was primarily present as glucuronide-/sulfate-conjugate. When only the free concentrations were regarded, catechin was detectable in 20 out of 30 V1 samples, and in 11 samples the concentrations were above 10 ng/mL. There were no apparent differences in the basal concentrations between the participants assigned to the P+ or Co group. Even when disregarding those patients who admitted a violation of the dietary restrictions there were still considerable basal concentrations present in serum.

The analysis of serum samples obtained after three weeks (V3) of Pycnogenol® intake revealed the highest concentrations for catechin, followed by caffeic acid, ferulic acid, M1, and taxifolin (Table 2, panel A). Although there was a tendency of higher concentrations of catechin in the P+ compared to the control group, the serum concentrations of M1 and caffeic acid in the control group exceeded those in the P+ group (Table 2, panel A). When patients who admitted intake of, for example, coffee, green tea, or chocolate were excluded from the analysis the trend of higher catechin levels as well as clearly higher concentrations of M1 in the P+ group became obvious and caffeic acid was not even detectable in the control group (Table 2, panel B).

Table 2. Results of the sample analysis in serum, blood cells, and synovial fluid of patients taking Pycnogenol® 200 mg/day (P+) and control patients (Co) receiving no supplement. The population numbers (*n*) indicate the number of patients with detectable concentrations of the respective polyphenol. **A**: Total mean concentrations and standard deviations (SD) determined after three weeks (V3) without exclusion of patients who admitted violations of the dietary restrictions; **B**: Total mean concentrations and SD determined after three weeks (V3). Patients who admitted violations of the dietary restrictions in their nutritional protocols were excluded. n.d.: not detected; Conc.: concentration.

A		Catechin Conc. (ng/mL) ± SD		M1 Conc. (ng/mL) ± SD		Taxifolin Conc. (ng/mL) ± SD		Ferulic Acid Conc. (ng/mL) ± SD		Caffeic Acid Conc. (ng/mL) ± SD	
Serum	P+	52.53 ± 18.40	$n = 15$	0.54 ± 0.84	$n = 9$	0.20 ± 0.12	$n = 5$	3.02 ± 0.39	$n = 7$	9.28 ± 0.51	$n = 3$
	Co	45.85 ± 39.59	$n = 15$	1.07 ± 1.09	$n = 5$	n.d.	-	n.d.	-	14.84 ± 1.92	$n = 3$
Blood Cells	P+	71.18 ± 27.34	$n = 14$	0.19 ± 0.07	$n = 12$	0.52 ± 0.23	$n = 15$	1.86 ± 0.36	$n = 10$	n.d.	-
	Co	70.48 ± 36.22	$n = 13$	0.21 ± 0.05	$n = 5$	0.48 ± 0.32	$n = 15$	1.80 ± 0.85	$n = 7$	n.d.	-
Synovial Fluid	P+	2.99 ± 0.43	$n = 4$	0.62 ± 0.77	$n = 5$	0.21 ± 0.03	$n = 2$	4.29 ± 1.83	$n = 8$	10.32 ± 3.96	$n = 7$
	Co	3.94 ± 1.83	$n = 2$	0.78 ± 0.74	$n = 4$	n.d.	-	3.04 ± 0.79	$n = 6$	12.83 ± 8.95	$n = 10$

B		Catechin Conc. (ng/mL) ± SD		M1 Conc. (ng/mL) ± SD		Taxifolin Conc. (ng/mL) ± SD		Ferulic Acid Conc. (ng/mL) ± SD		Caffeic Acid Conc. (ng/mL) ± SD	
Serum	P+	48.41 ± 18.61	$n = 11$	0.70 ± 1.02	$n = 6$	0.20 ± 0.12	$n = 5$	3.09 ± 0.46	$n = 5$	9.78	$n = 1$
	Co	32.24 ± 17.38	$n = 8$	0.25 ± 0.05	$n = 2$	n.d.	-	n.d.		n.d.	-
Blood Cells	P+	73.75 ± 29.25	$n = 11$	0.20 ± 0.07	$n = 9$	0.56 ± 0.19	$n = 11$	1.85 ± 0.38	$n = 9$	n.d.	-
	Co	63.31 ± 31.28	$n = 7$	0.18 ± 0.05	$n = 2$	0.39 ± 0.16	$n = 8$	1.69 ± 0.10	$n = 3$	n.d.	-
Synovial Fluid	P+	3.00 ± 0.58	$n = 2$	0.92 ± 0.93	$n = 3$	0.21 ± 0.03	$n = 2$	4.31 ± 2.10	$n = 6$	10.63 ± 3.86	$n = 4$
	Co	2.65	$n = 1$	0.17 ± 0.03	$n = 2$	n.d.	-	3.16 ± 0.22	$n = 3$	10.99 ± 5.79	$n = 4$

The degree of analyte conjugation with sulfate and glucuronic acid in serum was determined for all samples (V1 and V3) and ranged from 54.29% ± 26.77% for catechin (n = 51) to 98.34% ± 4.40% for M1 (n = 30; Table 3).

Table 3. Mean and standard deviation (SD) of the conjugation degree in serum samples (both P+ and Co group; V1, V2, and V3 blood samples; in total n = 90 samples). Results were compared with former investigations [5].

Analytes	Conjugation Degree (%)					
	Current Study			Former Investigation		
	Mean	± SD	Sample Size	Mean	± SD	Sample Size
Catechin	54.29	26.77	n = 51	56.50	27.90	n = 5
M1	98.34	4.40	n = 30	100 *		
Taxifolin	96.75	7.23	n = 11	100 *		
Ferulic Acid	90.32	16.58	n = 24	100 *		
Caffeic Acid	80.95	17.95	n = 10	69.40	11.80	n = 3

* A conjugation degree of 100% was assumed because no free concentrations were detectable.

3.4. *Pycnogenol® Constituents and Metabolites in Blood Cell Samples*

As seen with the serum samples before, basal total concentrations of the analytes with the exception of caffeic acid were detectable at V1, with no differences between the participants assigned to the P+ or Co group. Mean concentrations of 61.38 ± 40.25 ng/mL catechin (mean ± SD), 1.68 ± 0.55 ng/mL ferulic acid, 0.40 ± 0.18 ng/mL taxifolin, and 0.19 ± 0.08 ng/mL M1 were determined.

The analysis of blood cell samples obtained after three weeks (V3) of intake of Pycnogenol® revealed the highest concentrations for catechin, followed by ferulic acid, M1, and taxifolin (Table 2, panel A). No caffeic acid was detectable in any of the samples. There were no clear differences in the concentrations determined in the P+ or Co group. When patients who admitted non-adherence to the dietary restrictions were excluded from the analysis there was a slight trend towards higher catechin, taxifolin, and ferulic acid levels in the P+ group compared to the control group (Table 2, panel B).

In the V3 samples of the P+ group, the open-chained ester form of M1 (M1-COOH; n = 5; Figure S1A) was identified as well as the glutathione conjugate of M1 (M1-GSH; n = 1; Figure S1B). In the V3 samples of the Co group, only the M1-COOH was detected in one patient sample.

3.5. *Pycnogenol® Constituents and Metabolites in Synovial Fluid Samples*

In the present study, synovial fluid samples were obtained at the time of knee surgery. The analysis revealed the highest concentrations for caffeic acid, followed by ferulic acid, catechin, M1, and taxifolin (Table 2, panel A). With the exception of taxifolin, there were no vast differences in the concentrations of the other polyphenols.

3.6. *Distribution of Pycnogenol® Constituents and Metabolites between Specimen*

To exclude the chance that individual trends in distribution of the analytes were overlooked if only group mean concentrations were considered, the individual ratios of the analyte concentrations in the different specimen of single patients were calculated and summarized (Figure 3).

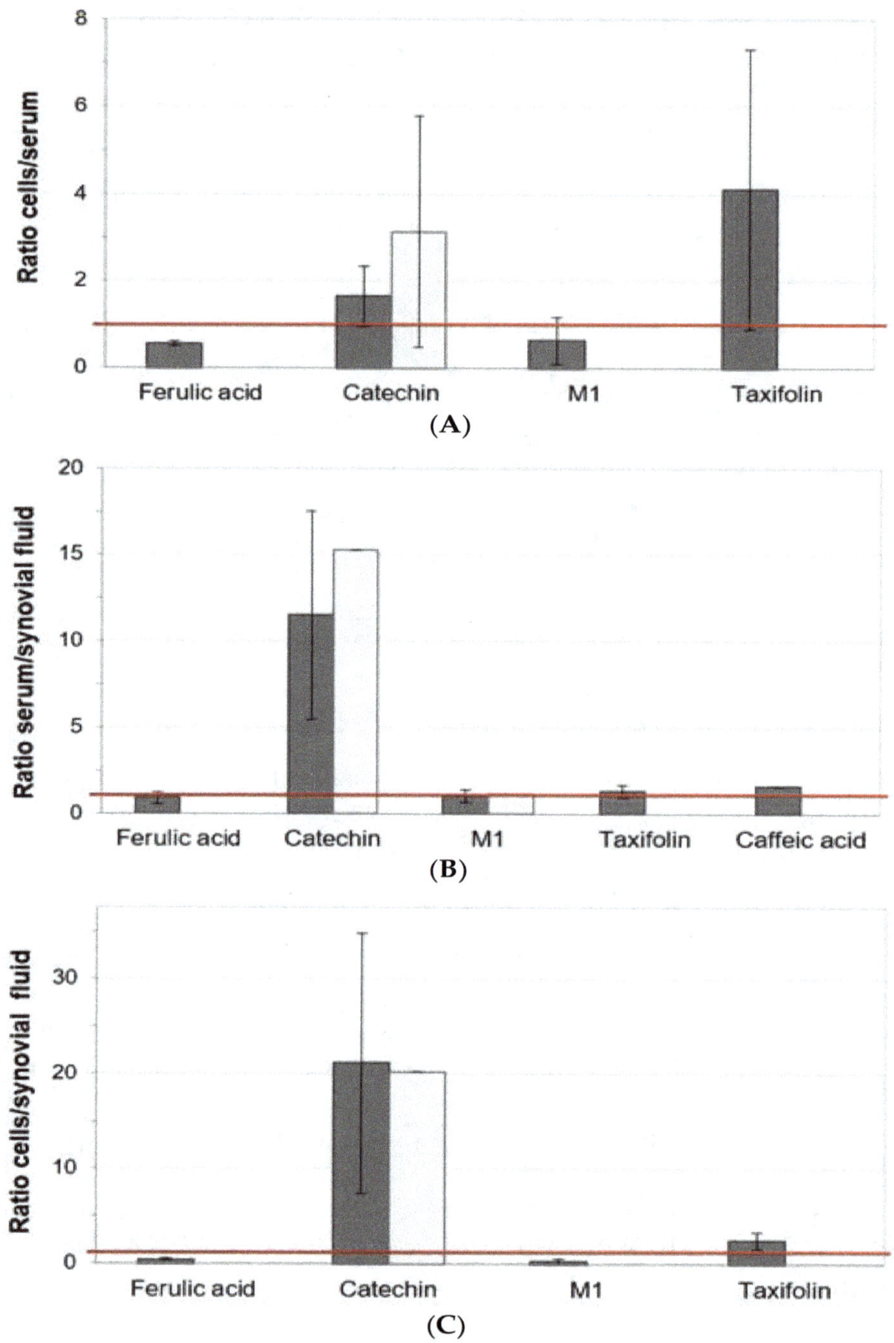

Figure 3. Summarized individual ratios of the analyte concentrations in different specimens of single study participants. Columns of the intervention (P+; dark gray) and control (Co; light grey) group represent the mean and standard deviation of the individual calculated ratios. (**A**) Ratio cells/serum. (**B**) Ratio serum/synovial fluid. (**C**) Ratio cells/synovial fluid.

The mean and standard deviations of the individual concentration ratios of the analytes in blood cells and serum (total concentrations, V3) showed that ferulic acid (0.56 ± 0.06; n = 4), M1 (0.64 ± 0.54; n = 5), and taxifolin (4.11 ± 3.21; n = 5) were detected in both matrices exclusively in the P+ group (Figure 3, panel A). With ratios above 1.0, taxifolin and catechin were clearly more present in blood cells compared to serum. In the patient group receiving 200 mg/day Pycnogenol®, the catechin distribution into blood cells (1.65 ± 0.69; n = 11) was less pronounced than in the control group (3.14 ± 2.65; n = 7).

The individual concentration ratios of analytes in serum and synovial fluid revealed that in both patient groups catechin was primarily distributed into serum compared to the synovial fluid

(P+: 11.51 ± 6.04; n = 4 and Co: 15.27; n = 1; Figure 3, panel B). Caffeic acid (1.60; n = 1), taxifolin (1.33 ± 0.38; n = 2), and ferulic acid (0.89 ± 0.32; n = 4) were present in both matrices only after intake of Pycnogenol® and not in the control group. Ferulic acid preferentially resided in the synovial fluid, while taxifolin and caffeic acid showed the opposite tendency. The metabolite M1 was detected both in the P+ (1.01 ± 0.37; n = 3) and Co group (1.14; n = 1) and it appeared to be almost in equilibrium between serum and synovial fluid.

The individual analyte distribution between blood cells and synovial fluid revealed a strong tendency of catechin for localization within blood cells compared to the synovial fluid (Figure 3, panel C). This was observed in both groups of the study participants (P+: 21.11 ± 13.70; n = 2 and Co: 20.15; n = 1). Taxifolin (2.48 ± 0.90; n = 2), M1 (0.27 ± 0.27; n = 2), and ferulic acid (0.45 ± 0.15; n = 5)) were present in both matrices exclusively in the P+ group. With a distribution ratio higher than 1.0, taxifolin was more present in blood cells compared to synovial fluid, while M1 and ferulic acid preferentially resided in the synovial fluid.

4. Discussion

In the present study, the in vivo distribution of constituents and metabolites of the maritime pine extract Pycnogenol® between human serum, blood cells, and synovial fluid was investigated for the first time. A newly developed and validated highly sensitive LC-ESI/MS/MS method allowed for the detection and quantification of various polyphenolic compounds in synovial fluid and thereby facilitated the proof that polyphenols are actually distributed into joints.

Analysis of samples obtained before the start of the intervention (V1) revealed that catechin and other polyphenols were ubiquitously present in human serum samples at measurable basal levels. Similar observations have been reported by others [21]. Based on the fact that the most controlled condition (lifestyle/diet, timely intake of Pycnogenol® capsules) the patients were subjected to was after their hospitalization (V3) when they were under observation of a study nurse, data analysis focused on V3 samples comparing the intervention (P+) with the control group (Co).

As already observed in an earlier pharmacokinetic study [5], not all polyphenols were discovered in biofluid samples of all participants, which reflected the high interindividual variability of absorption, distribution, metabolism, and/or elimination of plant constituents. The fact that the time between the last intake of Pycnogenol® and the collection of the specimen slightly varied around 12 h might have also contributed to the variability of measured compound concentrations. Although the mean polyphenol concentrations in serum, blood cells, and synovial fluid were similar in the P+ and Co group, due to non-adherence to the dietary restrictions, distinctive observations were made in the P+ group.

In serum samples, taxifolin and ferulic acid were only detectable in the P+, not in the Co group. In a previous pharmacokinetic study with healthy volunteers, taxifolin was not detectable under steady state conditions, which was most probably due to the less sensitive analytical method [5]. This is consistent with the very low concentrations of taxifolin found in the present study. Ferulic acid has been suggested to be a marker of consumption of maritime pine bark extract. In healthy volunteers adhering to a low polyphenol diet, both free and conjugated ferulic acid were determined in urine samples [22].

The conjugation degree of the investigated polyphenols in serum was high and ranged from 54.29% ± 26.77% for catechin to 98.34% ± 4.40% for M1. This is consistent with the data determined in a former investigation [5]. However, as observed before and reported by others [22], the interindividual variability of the conjugation degree of the analytes was high. Even in the individual person the degree of conjugation cannot be regarded as a constant since it apparently also depends on the current analyte concentration in the specimen [23].

Blood cells and erythrocytes represent a significant pharmacological compartment for distribution of xenobiotics [24,25]. Individual polyphenols have been shown to accumulate in human blood cells, macrophage-derived foam, or endothelial cells [15,16,25,26]. Notably, only low concentrations of

M1 were found in the cellular fraction of the blood samples. This apparently contradicts previous results showing an enhanced cellular uptake of M1, possibly via the GLUT-1 transporter, into human erythrocytes [16]. However, M1 is subsequently subjected to an extensive intracellular metabolism [17] which would explain the low remaining intracellular levels of M1 under steady state conditions. Consequently, the blood cells samples of the present study were also screened for the presence of any of the previously detected cellular M1 metabolites [17]. Indeed, in the P+ group, the open-chained ester form of M1 (M1-COOH) and the glutathione conjugate of M1 (M1-GSH) were identified, though not quantified. In the Co group, only M1-COOH was detected.

Sampling of synovial fluid is typically practiced for diagnostic reasons (e.g., for detection of a septic arthritis). In research, there is great interest in osteoarthritis biomarkers such as cytokines that might assist diagnosis or prognosis [27]. In contrast, drug concentrations are rarely reported for synovial fluid samples. To the best of our knowledge, this is the first study investigating polyphenol concentrations in human synovial fluid samples of patients with osteoarthritis. Similar to the results of serum analysis, mean polyphenol concentrations were similar in the P+ and Co groups, but taxifolin was only detectable in the P+ group. Thus, it might be a marker of Pycnogenol® consumption.

Comparing mean concentrations of the constituents and metabolites in serum, blood cells, and synovial fluid revealed that the individual compounds did not distribute equally between the specimen. Notably, the highest concentrations of the polyphenols were not detected in serum. Catechin and taxifolin primarily resided within the blood cells, while M1, ferulic, and caffeic acid were mainly present in synovial fluid samples. Generally, data on distribution of polyphenols in humans is scarce. Although numerous investigations focus on absorption, metabolism, and elimination of polyphenols [1,28], only a few studies investigate the distribution, for example, into human tissues [29,30]. Distribution into or accumulation in certain body compartments might help with understanding the effects of polyphenols despite the typically low plasma/serum concentrations that are usually observed [1,29].

Although there were some trends towards higher analyte concentrations in the specimen of the patients who received Pycnogenol® in the present study, the mean concentrations were similar for both groups and were subject to high interindividual variability. It was possible that individual trends in distribution of the analytes could have been overlooked if only group mean concentrations were considered. Therefore, the individual ratios of the analyte concentrations in the different specimens of single patients were calculated and summarized. Since ratios higher than 1 indicate that the analyte is primarily distributed into, for example, blood cells compared to serum, it can be concluded that higher concentrations of taxifolin and catechin were present in blood cells while ferulic acid and M1 preferentially resided in serum. This observation confirms the differential distribution of polyphenolic compounds between serum, blood cells, and synovial fluid that was already seen when mean concentrations were examined. On an individual level, a simultaneous presence of ferulic acid, M1, and taxifolin in blood cells and serum or cells and synovial fluid was only observed after intake of the pine bark extract. Also, ferulic acid, taxifolin, and caffeic acid were only detected in both serum and synovial fluid in the P+ group.

The fact that the control group received no placebo capsules to conceal the allocation to the intervention group could be seen as a potential study limitation. However, the primary interest was the bioanalysis of polyphenols in different specimens, and it is highly unlikely that any of the analyte concentrations were deliberately influenced by the patients' knowledge of group allocation. All analytical procedures were fully validated and left no room for subjective data interpretation. A study limitation was the small group size. Since not all polyphenols were present in the biofluid samples of all patients due to interindividual pharmacokinetic differences and also as a result of the non-adherence of the participants to the dietary restrictions, a statistical differentiation between the groups was not feasible. However, the results of the present study provide a basis for sample size calculations in future studies. Those studies would then be sufficiently powered for statistical analysis and could reliably uncover significant differences between treatment and control groups. The fact that the study participants of the present study did not follow the dietary suggestions improves the generalizability of the results since they mirror real life conditions under which foods or beverages rich in polyphenols are occasionally or regularly consumed.

5. Conclusion

The results of this study provide the first evidence that polyphenols distribute into the synovial fluid of patients with osteoarthritis, which supports rationalizing the results of clinical efficacy studies.

Supplementary Materials:
Figure S1: Example chromatograms for identification of intracellular metabolites of M1 in blood cells of study participants after multiple dosing of 200 mg/day Pycnogenol® over the course of three weeks (P+, V3), Table S1: Additional optimized transitions and parameters in dynamic multiple reaction monitoring (DMRM) mode for identification of compounds in human blood cells, Table S2: Optimized transitions and parameters in dynamic multiple reaction monitoring (DMRM) employing negative ESI ionization mode for LC-MS/MS analysis of prepared synovial fluid samples, Table S3: Calibration range, calibration function and correlation coefficients of the five analytes extracted from human pooled synovial fluid, Table S4: Intraday accuracy and precision of the analytes in human pooled synovial fluid, Table S5: Interday accuracy and precision of the analytes in human pooled synovial fluid, Table S6: Robustness of the developed method at two concentrations with human pooled synovial fluid which was intentionally contaminated with 1% human whole blood, Table S7: Post-preparative stability: autosampler stability of the analytes after 6 h and 12 h at room temperature after previous LC/MS/MS analysis, Table S8: Post-preparative stability: stability of the analytes after one freeze-thaw cycle, Table S9: Lower limit of quantification (LLOQ) and related accuracy of the five analytes extracted from human pooled synovial fluid, Table S10: Recovery, matrix effects and process efficiency of the five analytes extracted from human pooled synovial fluid at three concentrations, Table S11: Recovery, matrix effects and process efficiency of the five analytes extracted from three lots of synovial fluid at two concentrations, Table S12: Internal standard (hydrocaffeic acid) normalized matrix factor at human pooled synovial fluid in three concentrations and in three lots of synovial fluid at two concentrations.

Acknowledgments: We gratefully acknowledge the excellent assistance of Jasmin Bauman and Ursula Hellwich (Orthopedic Center for Musculoskeletal Research, Würzburg) in patient management. We would like to thank Bruno Pasurka, Würzburg, for help with the collection of synovial fluid samples used for calibration standard preparation. We are grateful for an unrestricted educational grant from Horphag Research Ltd. The study sponsor was not involved in the study design, collection, analysis and interpretation of data, in writing the manuscript or in the decision to submit the manuscript for publication. This publication was funded by the German Research Foundation (DFG) and the University of Würzburg in the funding program Open Access Publishing.

Author Contributions: M.M. planned and performed the experiments and contributed to drafting of the manuscript; L.S. and F.G. were involved in patient management, recording of clinical data, and contributed to drafting of the manuscript; P.H. conceived of and planned the study and contributed to drafting of the manuscript.

References

1. Manach, C.; Williamson, G.; Morand, C.; Scalbert, A.; Remesy, C. Bioavailability and bioefficacy of polyphenols in humans. I. Review of 97 bioavailability studies. *Am. J. Clin. Nutr.* **2005**, *81*, 230S–242S. [PubMed]
2. Monagas, M.; Urpi-Sarda, M.; Sanchez-Patan, F.; Llorach, R.; Garrido, I.; Gomez-Cordoves, C.; Andres-Lacueva, C.; Bartolome, B. Insights into the metabolism and microbial biotransformation of dietary flavan-3-ols and the bioactivity of their metabolites. *Food Funct.* **2010**, *1*, 233–253. [CrossRef] [PubMed]
3. Högger, P. Nutrition-derived bioactive metabolites produced by gut microbiota and their potential impact on human health. *Nutr. Med. (NUME)* **2013**, *1*, 1.
4. Düweler, K.G.; Rohdewald, P. Urinary metabolites of French maritime pine bark extract in humans. *Pharmazie* **2000**, *55*, 364–368. [PubMed]
5. Grimm, T.; Skrabala, R.; Chovanova, Z.; Muchova, J.; Sumegova, K.; Liptakova, A.; Durackova, Z.; Högger, P. Single and multiple dose pharmacokinetics of maritime pine bark extract (Pycnogenol) after oral administration to healthy volunteers. *BMC Clin. Pharmacol.* **2006**, *6*, 4. [CrossRef] [PubMed]
6. Rohdewald, P. A review of the French maritime pine bark extract (Pycnogenol), a herbal medication with a diverse clinical pharmacology. *Int. J. Clin. Pharmacol. Ther.* **2002**, *40*, 158–168. [CrossRef] [PubMed]

7. Maimoona, A.; Naeem, I.; Saddiqe, Z.; Jameel, K. A review on biological, nutraceutical and clinical aspects of French maritime pine bark extract. *J. Ethnopharmacol.* **2011**, *133*, 261–277. [CrossRef] [PubMed]
8. Silverwood, V.; Blagojevic-Bucknall, M.; Jinks, C.; Jordan, J.L.; Protheroe, J.; Jordan, K.P. Current evidence on risk factors for knee osteoarthritis in older adults: A systematic review and meta-analysis. *Osteoarthr Cartil.* **2015**, *23*, 507–515. [CrossRef] [PubMed]
9. McAlindon, T.E.; Bannuru, R.R.; Sullivan, M.C.; Arden, N.K.; Berenbaum, F.; Bierma-Zeinstra, S.M.; Hawker, G.A.; Henrotin, Y.; Hunter, D.J.; Kawaguchi, H.; et al. Oarsi guidelines for the non-surgical management of knee osteoarthritis. *Osteoarthr Cartil.* **2014**, *22*, 363–388. [CrossRef] [PubMed]
10. Green, J.A.; Hirst-Jones, K.L.; Davidson, R.K.; Jupp, O.; Bao, Y.; MacGregor, A.J.; Donell, S.T.; Cassidy, A.; Clark, I.M. The potential for dietary factors to prevent or treat osteoarthritis. *Proc. Nutr. Soc.* **2014**, *73*, 278–288. [CrossRef] [PubMed]
11. Belcaro, G.; Cesarone, M.R.; Errichi, S.; Zulli, C.; Errichi, B.M.; Vinciguerra, G.; Ledda, A.; Di Renzo, A.; Stuard, S.; Dugall, M.; et al. Treatment of osteoarthritis with Pycnogenol. The SVOS (San Valentino Osteo-arthrosis Study). Evaluation of signs, symptoms, physical performance and vascular aspects. *Phytother. Res.* **2008**, *22*, 518–523. [CrossRef] [PubMed]
12. Cisar, P.; Jany, R.; Waczulikova, I.; Sumegova, K.; Muchova, J.; Vojtassak, J.; Durackova, Z.; Lisy, M.; Rohdewald, P. Effect of pine bark extract (Pycnogenol) on symptoms of knee osteoarthritis. *Phytother. Res.* **2008**, *22*, 1087–1092. [CrossRef] [PubMed]
13. Grimm, T.; Schäfer, A.; Högger, P. Antioxidant activity and inhibition of matrix metalloproteinases by metabolites of maritime pine bark extract (Pycnogenol). *Free Radic. Biol. Med.* **2004**, *36*, 811–822. [CrossRef] [PubMed]
14. Grimm, T.; Chovanova, Z.; Muchova, J.; Sumegova, K.; Liptakova, A.; Durackova, Z.; Högger, P. Inhibition of NF-κb activation and MMP-9 secretion by plasma of human volunteers after ingestion of maritime pine bark extract (Pycnogenol). *J. Inflamm. (Lond.)* **2006**, *3*, 1. [CrossRef] [PubMed]
15. Uhlenhut, K.; Högger, P. Facilitated cellular uptake and suppression of inducible nitric oxide synthase by a metabolite of maritime pine bark extract (Pycnogenol). *Free Radic. Biol. Med.* **2012**, *53*, 305–313. [CrossRef] [PubMed]
16. Kurlbaum, M.; Mülek, M.; Högger, P. Facilitated uptake of a bioactive metabolite of maritime pine bark extract (Pycnogenol) into human erythrocytes. *PLoS ONE* **2013**, *8*, e63197. [CrossRef] [PubMed]
17. Mülek, M.; Fekete, A.; Wiest, J.; Holzgrabe, U.; Mueller, M.J.; Högger, P. Profiling a gut microbiota-generated catechin metabolite's fate in human blood cells using a metabolomic approach. *J. Pharm. Biomed. Anal.* **2015**, *114*, 71–81. [CrossRef] [PubMed]
18. Mülek, M.; Högger, P. Highly sensitive analysis of polyphenols and their metabolites in human blood cells using dispersive SPE extraction and LC-MS/MS. *Anal. Bioanal. Chem.* **2015**, *407*, 1885–1899. [CrossRef] [PubMed]
19. Mülek, M. Distribution and Metabolism of Constituents and Metabolites of a Standardized Maritime Pine Bark Extract (Pycnogenol®) in Human Serum, Blood Cells and Synovial Fluid of Patients with Severe Osteoarthritis. Ph.D. Thesis, Julius Maximilians-Universität, Würzburg, Germany, 2015.
20. Cavaliere, C.; Foglia, P.; Gubbiotti, R.; Sacchetti, P.; Samperi, R.; Lagana, A. Rapid-resolution liquid chromatography/mass spectrometry for determination and quantitation of polyphenols in grape berries. *Rapid Commun. Mass Spectrom.* **2008**, *22*, 3089–3099. [CrossRef] [PubMed]
21. Henning, S.M.; Wang, P.; Abgaryan, N.; Vicinanza, R.; de Oliveira, D.M.; Zhang, Y.; Lee, R.P.; Carpenter, C.L.; Aronson, W.J.; Heber, D. Phenolic acid concentrations in plasma and urine from men consuming green or black tea and potential chemopreventive properties for colon cancer. *Mol. Nutr. Food Res.* **2013**, *57*, 483–493. [CrossRef] [PubMed]
22. Virgili, F.; Pagana, G.; Bourne, L.; Rimbach, G.; Natella, F.; Rice-Evans, C.; Packer, L. Ferulic acid excretion as a marker of consumption of a French maritime pine (*Pinus maritima*) bark extract. *Free Radic. Biol. Med.* **2000**, *28*, 1249–1256. [CrossRef]
23. Soleas, G.J.; Yan, J.; Goldberg, D.M. Ultrasensitive assay for three polyphenols (catechin, quercetin and resveratrol) and their conjugates in biological fluids utilizing gas chromatography with mass selective detection. *J. Chromatogr. B Biomed. Sci. Appl.* **2001**, *757*, 161–172. [CrossRef]
24. Highley, M.S.; de Bruijn, E.A. Erythrocytes and the transport of drugs and endogenous compounds. *Pharm. Res.* **1996**, *13*, 186–195. [CrossRef] [PubMed]

25. Biasutto, L.; Marotta, E.; Hgarbisa, S.; Zoratti, M.; Paradisi, C. Determination of quercetin and resveratrol in whole blood—Implications for bioavailability studies. *Molecules* **2010**, *15*, 6570–6579. [CrossRef] [PubMed]
26. Kawai, Y.; Tanaka, H.; Murota, K.; Naito, M.; Terao, J. (−)-epicatechin gallate accumulates in foamy macrophages in human atherosclerotic aorta: Implication in the anti-atherosclerotic actions of tea catechins. *Biochem. Biophys. Res. Commun.* **2008**, *374*, 527–532. [CrossRef] [PubMed]
27. Mabey, T.; Honsawek, S. Cytokines as biochemical markers for knee osteoarthritis. *World J. Orthop.* **2015**, *6*, 95–105. [CrossRef] [PubMed]
28. Clifford, M.N.; van der Hooft, J.J.; Crozier, A. Human studies on the absorption, distribution, metabolism, and excretion of tea polyphenols. *Am. J. Clin. Nutr.* **2013**, *98*, 1619S–1630S. [CrossRef] [PubMed]
29. Henning, S.M.; Aronson, W.; Niu, Y.; Conde, F.; Lee, N.H.; Seeram, N.P.; Lee, R.P.; Lu, J.; Harris, D.M.; Moro, A.; et al. Tea polyphenols and theaflavins are present in prostate tissue of humans and mice after green and black tea consumption. *J. Nutr.* **2006**, *136*, 1839–1843. [PubMed]
30. Del Rio, D.; Borges, G.; Crozier, A. Berry flavonoids and phenolics: Bioavailability and evidence of protective effects. *Br. J. Nutr.* **2010**, *104* (Suppl. 3), S67–S90. [CrossRef] [PubMed]

2

Gut Microbial, Inflammatory and Metabolic Signatures in Older People with Physical Frailty and Sarcopenia: Results from the BIOSPHERE Study

Anna Picca [1,2], Francesca Romana Ponziani [2], Riccardo Calvani [1,2,*], Federico Marini [3], Alessandra Biancolillo [3,4], Hélio José Coelho-Júnior [5], Jacopo Gervasoni [1,2], Aniello Primiano [1,2], Lorenza Putignani [6], Federica Del Chierico [7], Sofia Reddel [7], Antonio Gasbarrini [1,2], Francesco Landi [1,2], Roberto Bernabei [1,2,*] and Emanuele Marzetti [1,2]

1 Institute of Internal Medicine and Geriatrics, Università Cattolica del Sacro Cuore, 00168 Rome, Italy; anna.picca1@gmail.com (A.P.); jacopo.gervasoni@policlinicogemelli.it (J.G.); aniello.primiano@unicatt.it (A.P.); antonio.gasbarrini@unicatt.it (A.G.); francesco.landi@unicatt.it (F.L.); emanuele.marzetti@policlinicogemelli.it (E.M.)

2 Fondazione Policlinico Universitario "Agostino Gemelli" IRCCS, 00168 Rome, Italy; francesca.ponziani@gmail.com

3 Department of Chemistry, Sapienza Università di Roma, 00185 Rome, Italy; federico.marini@uniroma1.it (F.M.); alessandra.biancolillo@univaq.it (A.B.)

4 Department of Physical and Chemical Sciences, University of L'Aquila, 67100 Coppito, Italy

5 Applied Kinesiology Laboratory–LCA, School of Physical Education, University of Campinas, 13.083-851 Campinas-SP, Brazil; coelhojunior@hotmail.com.br

6 Unit of Parasitology and Unit of Human Microbiome, Bambino Gesù Children's Hospital IRCCS, 00168 Rome, Italy; lorenza.putignani@opbg.net

7 Unit of Human Microbiome, Bambino Gesù Children's Hospital IRCCS, 00168 Rome, Italy; federica.delchierico@opbg.net (F.D.C.); sofia.reddel@opbg.net (S.R.)

* Correspondence: riccardo.calvani@gmail.com (R.C.); roberto.bernabei@unicatt.it (R.B.);

Abstract: Physical frailty and sarcopenia (PF&S) share multisystem derangements, including variations in circulating amino acids and chronic low-grade inflammation. Gut microbiota balances inflammatory responses in several conditions and according to nutritional status. Therefore, an altered gut-muscle crosstalk has been hypothesized in PF&S. We analyzed the gut microbial taxa, systemic inflammation, and metabolic characteristics of older adults with and without PF&S. An innovative multi-marker analytical approach was applied to explore the classification performance of potential biomarkers for PF&S. Thirty-five community dwellers aged 70+, 18 with PF&S, and 17 nonPF&S controls were enrolled. Sequential and Orthogonalized Covariance Selection (SO-CovSel), a multi-platform regression method developed to handle highly correlated variables, was applied. The SO-CovSel model with the best prediction ability using the smallest number of variables was built using seven mediators. The model correctly classified 91.7% participants with PF&S and 87.5% nonPF&S controls. Compared with the latter group, PF&S participants showed higher serum concentrations of aspartic acid, lower circulating levels of concentrations of threonine and macrophage inflammatory protein 1α, increased abundance of *Oscillospira* and *Ruminococcus* microbial taxa, and decreased abundance of Barnesiellaceae and Christensenellaceae. Future investigations are warranted to determine whether these biomediators are involved in PF&S pathophysiology and may, therefore, provide new targets for interventions.

Keywords: aging; muscle; amino acids; metabolism; systemic inflammation; profiling; biomarkers; multi-marker; physical performance; gut microbiota

1. Introduction

Sarcopenia, the progressive age-related decline in muscle mass and strength/function, is a major determinant of negative health-related outcomes, including disability, loss of independence, institutionalization, and mortality [1,2].

When focusing on the physical domain, sarcopenia shows remarkable clinical overlap with frailty, a geriatric "multidimensional syndrome characterized by decreased reserve and diminished resistance to stressors", often envisioned as a pre-disability condition [3]. As such, sarcopenia can be considered to be the biological substratum for the development of physical frailty (PF) and the pathophysiologic foundation of adverse PF-related health outcomes [4,5].

Due to the described commonalities, the two conditions have recently been merged into a new entity (i.e., PF & sarcopenia—PF&S) [6] that was operationalized in the context of the "Sarcopenia and Physical fRailty IN older people: multi-componenT Treatment strategies" (SPRINTT) project [7,8].

Multisystem derangements contribute to muscle loss and may ultimately lead to the development of PF&S [9]. Anabolic resistance, chronic low-grade inflammation, and oxidative stress are advocated among the factors contributing to PF&S [10,11]. These mechanisms are enhanced in the setting of physical inactivity and poor nutrition [12,13]. In this scenario, multi-component interventions encompassing physical activity and adapted nutrition are pillars for the prevention of adverse outcomes associated with PF&S [14].

As recently shown by our group, older adults with PF&S are commonly overweight or obese [15], a feature that has been incorporated in the concept of sarcopenic obesity [16]. Compelling evidence indicates that excessive adiposity contributes to physical frailty and functional limitations in advanced age [17,18]. Adipose tissue is metabolically active and promotes systemic inflammation and oxidative stress [19]. In addition, obesity exacerbates fat infiltration within muscles (i.e., myosteatosis), which, in turn, contributes to muscle dysfunction and physical frailty [20,21].

Gut microbiota is a major player in balancing pro- and anti-inflammatory responses in various disease conditions and in relation to nutritional status [22]. Indeed, the existence of a gut-muscle axis has been hypothesized in the context of PF&S [23]. However, the mechanisms whereby changes in gut microbes–host interactions may influence AA availability, systemic inflammation, and muscle homeostasis in PF&S are yet unexplored.

To address this research question, we used data from the "BIOmarkers associated with Sarcopenia and Physical frailty in EldeRly pErsons" (BIOSPHERE) and the Gut-Liver (GuLiver) Axis studies. BIOSPHERE was designed to determine and validate a panel of PF&S biomarkers pertaining to several pathophysiologic domains (i.e., inflammation, oxidative stress, muscle remodeling, neuromuscular junction dysfunction, and AA metabolism) through multivariate statistical modeling [10,11,24]. The GuLiver Axis study was designed to analyze the relationship among gut microbiota, inflammation, and nutritional and metabolic status in people with and without liver disease [25,26].

The availability of these well-characterized cohorts of older adults enabled us to explore the association among gut microbial profiles, systemic inflammation, and metabolic characteristics in PF&S.

2. Materials and Methods

2.1. Participants

Participants were recruited among enrollees of BIOSPHERE and GuLiver Axis studies. Both studies were approved by the Ethics Committee of the Università Cattolica del Sacro Cuore (Rome, Italy; protocol number BIOSPHERE: 8498/15; protocol number GuLiver Axis: 741). Study procedures and criteria for participant selection have been previously described [24,25].

In both studies, community-dwellers aged 70+ were recruited after signing written informed consent. The presence of PF&S was established according to the operational definition elaborated in the SPRINTT project [7,27]: (a) physical frailty, based on a summary score on the Short Physical Performance Battery (SPPB) [28] between 3 and 9; (b) low appendicular muscle mass (aLM), according to the cutpoints of the Foundation for the National Institutes of Health (FNIH) sarcopenia project [29]; and (c) absence of mobility disability (i.e., ability to complete the 400-m walk test) [30]. The present investigation involved 35 participants, 18 with PF&S, and 17 nonsarcopenic nonfrail (nonPF&S) controls. Gut microbial profiles, circulating inflammatory mediators, and serum AAs and derivatives were assessed.

2.2. *Measurement of Appendicular Lean Mass by Dual X-ray Absorptiometry (DXA)*

aLM was quantified through whole-body DXA scans on a Hologic Discovery A densitometer (Hologic, Inc., Bedford, MA, USA) according to the manufacturer's procedures. Criteria for low aLM were as follows: (a) aLM to body mass index (BMI) ratio (aLM_{BMI}) <0.789 and <0.512 in men and women; or (b) crude aLM <19.75 kg in men and <15.02 kg in women when the aLM/BMI criterion was not met [29].

2.3. *Blood Sample and Stool Collection*

Blood samples were collected in the morning by venipuncture of the median cubital vein after overnight fasting, using commercial collection tubes (BD Vacutainer®; Becton, Dickinson and Co., Franklin Lakes, NJ, USA). Serum separation was obtained after 30 min of clotting at room temperature and subsequent centrifugation at 1000× *g* for 15 min at 4 °C. The upper clear fraction (serum) was collected in 0.5 mL aliquots and stored at −80 °C until analysis.

Participants were carefully instructed on the procedures for fecal sample collection. Stool samples were collected at home in a commercial sterile, dry screw-top container. Upon collection, stool samples were delivered to the Human Microbiome Unit at the Bambino Gesù Children's Hospital (Rome, Italy) and immediately frozen at −80 °C until further processing.

2.4. *Measurement of Circulating Inflammatory Mediators*

A multi-marker immunoassay was used to measure circulating levels of a panel of inflammatory markers [11,25,26,31]. Briefly, a set of 27 pro- and anti-inflammatory mediators, including cytokines, chemokines, and growth factors, were assayed in duplicate in serum samples using the Bio-Plex Pro Human Cytokine 27-plex Assay kit (#M500KCAF0Y, Bio-Rad, Hercules, CA, USA) on a Bio-Plex® System with Luminex xMap Technology (Bio-Rad) (Table 1). Data acquisition was performed with the Bio-Plex Manager Software 6.1 (Bio-Rad) using instrument default settings. Optimization of standard curves across all of the assayed analytes was carried out to remove outliers. Results were obtained as concentrations (pg/mL).

Table 1. List of serum inflammatory biomarkers assayed by multiplex immunoassay.

Cytokines	IFNγ, IL1β, IL1Ra, IL2, IL4, IL5, IL6, IL7, IL8, IL9, IL10, IL12, IL13, IL15, IL17, TNF-α
Chemokines	CCL5, CCL11, IP-10, MCP-1, MIP-1α, MIP-1β
Growth factors	FGF-β, G-CSF, GM-CSF, PDGF-BB

Abbreviations: CCL, C-C motif chemokine ligand; FGF, fibroblast growth factor; G-CSF, granulocyte colony-stimulating factor; GM-CSF, granulocyte macrophage colony-stimulating factor; IFN, interferon; IL, interleukin; IL1Ra, interleukin 1 receptor agonist; IP: interferon-induced protein; MCP-1: monocyte chemoattractant protein 1; MIP: macrophage inflammatory protein; PDGFBB, platelet derived growth factor BB; TNF, tumor necrosis factor.

2.5. *Determination of Circulating Amino Acids*

Serum concentrations of 37 AAs and derivatives were determined by ultraperformance liquid chromatography/mass spectrometry (UPLC/MS), as described previously [10]. Briefly, 50 μL of sample was added to 100 μL 10% (w/v) sulfosalicylic acid containing an internal standard mix (50 μM) (Cambridge Isotope Laboratories, Inc., Tewksbury, MA, USA) and subsequently centrifuged at 1000× *g* for 15 min. The supernatant was collected, and 10 μL was mixed with 70 μL of borate buffer and

20 μL of AccQ Tag reagents (Waters Corporation, Milford, MA, USA). The mixture was subsequently heated at 55 °C for 10 min. Samples were eventually loaded onto a CORTECS UPLC C18 column 1.6 μm 2.1 × 150 mm (Waters Corporation) for chromatographic separation (ACQUITY H-Class, Waters Corporation) and eluted at a flow rate of 500 μL/min with a linear gradient (9 min) from 99:1 to 1:99 water 0.1% formic acid/acetonitrile 0.1% formic acid. Analyte detection was performed on an ACQUITY QDa single quadrupole mass spectrometer equipped with electrospray source operating in positive mode (Waters Corporation). AA controls (level 1 and level 2) manufactured by the MCA laboratory of the Queen Beatrix Hospital (Winterswijk, The Netherlands) were used to monitor the analytic process.

2.6. Gut Microbiota DNA Extraction, 16S rRNA Amplification, and Sequencing

Total genome DNA was extracted from fecal samples using the QIAmp Fast DNA Stool mini kit (Qiagen, Germany), according to the manufacturer's instructions.

The V3-V4 region of the 16S rRNA gene (~460 bp) was amplified using the primer pairs 16S_F (5′-TCG TCG GCA GCG TCA GAT GTG TAT AAG AGA CAG CCT ACG GGN GGC WGC AG-3′) and 16S_R (5′-GTC TCG TGG GCT CGG AGA TGT GTA TAA GAG ACA GGA CTA CHV GGG TAT CTA ATC C–3′), reported in the MiSeq rRNA Amplicon Sequencing protocol (Illumina, San Diego, CA, USA). Amplification reactions were set up using a 2× KAPA HiFi HotStart Ready Mix (KAPA Biosystems Inc., Wilmington, MA, USA). AMPure XP beads (Beckman Coulter Inc., Beverly, MA, USA) were employed to clean-up the DNA amplicons. To obtain a unique combination of bar-code sequences, a second amplification step was performed using the Illumina Nextera forward and reverse adaptor-primers (Illumina, San Diego, CA, USA). The final library was quantified after a clean-up step using a Quant-iT™ PicoGreen® dsDNA Assay Kit (Thermo Fisher Scientific, Waltham, MA, USA) and diluted in an equimolar concentration (4 nM).

Samples were sequenced using an Illumina MiSeqTM platform, following the manufacturer's specifications, generating 300 base-length paired-end reads. Bacterial 16S rRNA amplicon data were analyzed using a combination of the QIIME 1.9.1 software pipeline and the VSEARCH v1.1 pipeline. Fastq-join was used to merge paired-end raw sequences, followed by a split library step (QIIME). After dereplication and chimera checking (VSEARCH), reads were then clustered into operational taxonomic units (OTUs) at 97% identity. Taxonomy of each of 16S rRNA gene sequence was assigned using the UCLUST against the Greengenes 13.8 database (97% sequence similarity).

2.7. Statistical Analysis

Analyses were performed using the freely available software environment for statistical computing and graphics R statistics program (version 3.4.0). Sequential and Orthogonalized Covariance Selection (SO-CovSel) statistics were run under Matlab R2015b environment by means of in-house written functions (freely available at www.chem.uniroma1.it/romechemometrics/research/algorithms/).

Descriptive statistics were run on all data. Differences in demographic, anthropometric, clinical, functional characteristics, and inflammatory and metabolic markers between PF&S and nonPF&S participants were assessed via *t*-test statistics and χ^2 or Fisher exact tests, for continuous and categorical variables, respectively. All tests were two-sided, with statistical significance set at $p < 0.05$.

To compare the gut microbiota alpha diversity between PF&S and nonPF&S participants, Chao1 index was calculated on raw data and differences were assessed by Wilcoxon test.

Data were then preprocessed removing OTUs not seen more than three times in at least 20% of the samples and were normalized using a regularized logarithm transformation (rlog). Differential abundance analysis between PF&S and nonPF&S groups at the phylum, family, and genus levels was carried out using a negative binomial distribution on data normalized by "size factors", taking into account sequencing depth between samples. Differences in bacterial abundance were reported as $\log_2$ fold change ($\log_2$FC). Only comparisons with a $\log_2$FC > or <±1.5 and an adjusted (Benjamini–Hochberg method) p value < 0.05 were considered significant.

After import into MatLab, serum concentrations of inflammatory and metabolic markers and the abundance of gut microbial OTUs were organized into three matrices (Table 2), to be further processed through a multi-block approach. Given its ability to provide accurate predictions and, at the same time, to identify a parsimonious number of relevant variables (putative markers), the analysis was carried out through the recently developed SO-CovSel algorithm [32].

Table 2. Composition of the multi-block dataset used for Sequential and Orthogonalized Covariance Selection (SO-CovSel) analysis.

Data Block	Biological Pathway	Variables
Matrix 1	Inflammation	CCL5, CCL11, IFN-γ, FGF-β, G-CSF, GM-CSF, IL1β, IL1ra, IL2, IL4, IL5, IL6, IL7, IL8, IL9, IL10, IL12, IL13, IL15, IL17, IP-10, MCP-1, MIP-1α, MIP-1β, PDGF-BB, TNF-α
Matrix 2	Protein/amino acid metabolism	1-methylhistidine, 3-methylhistidine, 4-hydroxyproline, α-aminobutyric acid, β-alanine, β-aminobutyric acid, γ-aminobutyric acid, alanine, aminoadipic acid, anserine, arginine, asparagine, aspartic acid, carnosine, citrulline, cystathionine, cystine, ethanolamine, glutamic acid, glycine, histidine, isoleucine, leucine, lysine, methionine, ornithine, phenylalanine, phosphoethanolamine, phosphoserine, proline, sarcosine, serine, taurine, threonine, tryptophan, tyrosine, valine
Matrix 3	Gut microbiota	*Actinobacteria, Adlercreutzia, Aerostipes, Aerotruncus, Akkermansia, Alcaligenaceae, Atopobium, Bacteroidaceae, Bacteroides, Bacteroidetes, Barnesiellaceae, Bifidobacteriaceae, Bifidobacterium, Bilophila, Blautia, Carnobacteriaceae, Christensenella, Christensenellaceae, Clostridiaceae, Collinsella, Coprococcus, Coriobacteriaceae, Cyanobacteria, Dehalobacteriaceae, Dehalobacterium, Desulfovibrionaceae, Dethiosulfovibrionaceae, Dialister, Dorea, Eggerthella, Enterobacteriaceae, Enterococcaceae, Enterococcus, Erysipelotrichaceae, EtOH8, Eubacterium, Euryarchaeota, Faecalibacterium, Firmicutes, Granulicatella, Haemophilus, Lachnobacterium, Lachnospira, Lachnospiraceae, Lactobacillaceae, Lactobacillus, Methanobacteriaceae, Methanobrevibacter, Mogibacteriacea, Oscillospira, Parabacteroides, Paraprevotella, Paraprevotellaceae, Pasteurellaceae, Peptostreptococcaceae, Phascolarctobacterium, Porphyromonadaceae, Prevotella, Prevotellaceae, Proteobacteria, Pyramidobacter, Rikenellaceae, Roseburia, Ruminococcaceae, Ruminococcus, Ruminococcus, S24-7, Slackia, Streptococcaceae, Streptococcus, Sutterella, Synergistetes, Tenericutes, TM7, Veillonella, Veillonellaceae, Verrucomicrobia, Verrucomicrobiaceae*

SO-CovSel is a predictive method that couples variable selection (through the CovSel approach) with sequential multiblock modeling, and it can be used to deal with both quantitative and qualitative responses. According to the method, the response(s) to be predicted can be expressed as a linear combination of variables from the different blocks, as described by the following equation:

$$Y = X_1B_1 + X_2B_2 + X_3B_3$$

The matrices B_1, B_2, and B_3 collect the regression coefficients relating the individual blocks to the response(s). Within the multiblock linear regression framework summarized by the previous equation, one of the main peculiarities of the SO-CovSel methods is that not all the variables from the various blocks are used as predictors, but only the most relevant ones, which are selected according to the CovSel algorithm [33]. In CovSel, the first variable is selected as the one having the maximum covariance with the response. The subsequent variables are selected according to the same criterion, but after having orthogonalized both the X and the Y with respect to the contribution of the previously selected predictors, to avoid redundancy. The other main characteristic of the SO-CovSel method, which derives from its analogy with sequential and orthogonalized partial least squares regression (SO-PLS) [34,35], is that the different blocks are sequentially modeled, after having been orthogonalized with respect to the contribution of the previous ones. This avoids scaling issues and allows evaluating whether the block adds new information or it is redundant.

Based on these considerations, for a problem involving three blocks of predictors, as the one addressed in the present study, the SO-CovSel algorithm can be schematically summarized by the following steps:

1. CovSel algorithm is used to select relevant variables and calculate a regression model between the first block and the responses

$$Y = X_{1sel}B_1 + E_1$$

2. The second block is orthogonalized with respect to the variables selected in the first block

$$X_{2orth} = \left[I - X_{1sel}\left(X_{1sel}^T X_{1sel}\right)X_{1sel}^T\right]X_2$$

3. CovSel algorithm is used to select relevant variables and calculate a regression model between the orthogonalized second block and the residuals from the first fit

$$E_1 = X_{2selorth}B_{2orth} + E_2$$

4. The third block is orthogonalized with respect to the variables selected in the first and second blocks

$$X_{3orth} = \left[I - X_{12sel}\left(X_{12sel}^T X_{12sel}\right)X_{12sel}^T\right]X_3$$

   where

$$X_{12sel} = \left[X_{1sel}X_{2orthsel}\right]$$

5. CovSel algorithm is used to select relevant variables and calculate a regression model between the orthogonalized third block and the residuals from the second fit

$$E_2 = X_{3selorth}B_{3orth} + E_3$$

6. An overall prediction model is built as

$$Y = \hat{Y} + E_3 = X_{1sel}B_1 + X_{2selorth}B_{2orth} + X_{3selorth}B_{3orth} + E_3$$

   where the predicted response $\hat{Y}$ is calculated as

$$\hat{Y} = X_{1sel}B_1 + X_{2selorth}B_{2orth} + X_{3selorth}B_{3orth}$$

The algorithm, described in the steps above for regression (i.e., for the prediction of a quantitative response) can easily be adapted for classification problems, such as the one addressed in the present study. Indeed, by suitably coding the response matrix Y, a classification problem can be straightforwardly turned into a regression one. In particular, for a problem involving two classes, Y is a binary coded vector that takes the value 1 for PF&S participants and 0 for nonPF&S controls. The classification is then accomplished by properly thresholding the value of the predicted response.

3. Results

3.1. Characteristics of the Study Population

Thirty-five participants were included in the study: 18 older adults with PF&S (mean age 75.5 ± 3.9 years; 56.0% women) and 17 nonPF&S controls (mean age 73.9 ± 3.2 years; 29.0% women). Clinical and demographic characteristics of study participants are presented in Table 3. Age, sex distribution, and number of co-morbid conditions and medications did not differ between groups. Participants with PF&S showed higher BMI than nonPF&S controls.

Table 3. Main characteristics of study participants according to the presence of physical frailty & sarcopenia (PF&S).

	PF&S (n = 18)	NonPF&S (n = 17)	p
Age, years (mean ± SD)	75.5 ± 3.9	73.9 ± 3.2	0.2204
Gender (female), n (%)	10 (56)	5 (29)	0.2223
BMI, kg/m^2 (mean ± SD)	32.14 ± 6.02	26.27 ± 2.55	0.0008
SPPB (mean ± SD)	7.19 ± 1.22	11.24 ± 0.97	<0.0001
aLM, kg (mean ± SD)	17.75 ± 3.17	22.50 ± 2.93	<0.0001
aLM_{BMI} (mean ± SD)	0.55 ± 0.11	0.87 ± 0.15	<0.0001
Number of disease conditions * (mean ± SD)	3.2 ± 1.7	3.0 ± 2.1	0.8046
Number of medications ** (mean ± SD)	3.4 ± 1.2	2.9 ± 1.6	0.1034

Abbreviations: aLM: appendicular lean mass; BMI: body mass index; PF&S: physical frailty & sarcopenia; nonPF&S: nonphysically frail, nonsarcopenic; SD: standard deviation; SPPB: short physical performance battery. * Includes hypertension, coronary artery disease, prior stroke, peripheral vascular disease, diabetes, chronic obstructive pulmonary disease, and osteoarthritis. ** Includes prescription and over-the-counter medications.

3.2. Features of Gut Microbiota According to the Presence of PF&S

No differences in microbial alpha diversity were determined between PF&S and nonPF&S participants (Figure 1).

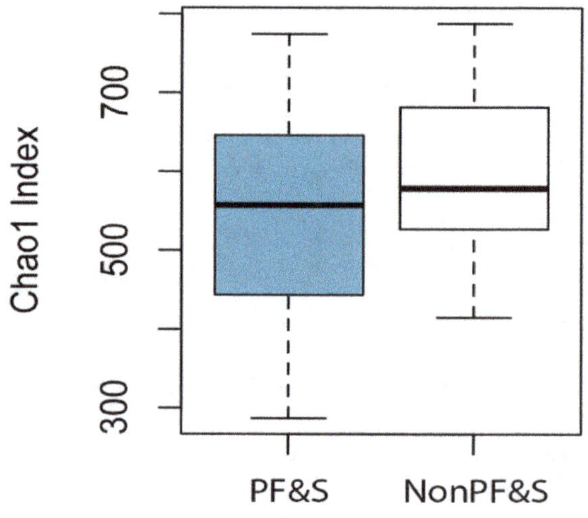

Figure 1. Chao1 index of gut microbial alpha diversity in participants with PF&S and in nonPF&S controls.

The analysis of the differential abundance of microbial taxa between PF&S and nonPF&S groups at the phylum, family, and genus levels showed an increase in Peptostreptococcaceae (p = 0.008 Table S1) and Bifidobacteriaceae (p = 0.013) at the family level and of *Dialister* (p = 0.028), *Pyramidobacter* (p = 0.043), and *Eggerthella* (p = 0.05) at the genus level, and a depletion in *Slackia* (p < 0.0001) and *Eubacterium* (p = 0.028) in PF&S participants (Figure 2). No significant differences in the relative abundance of intestinal bacteria phyla were found between groups.

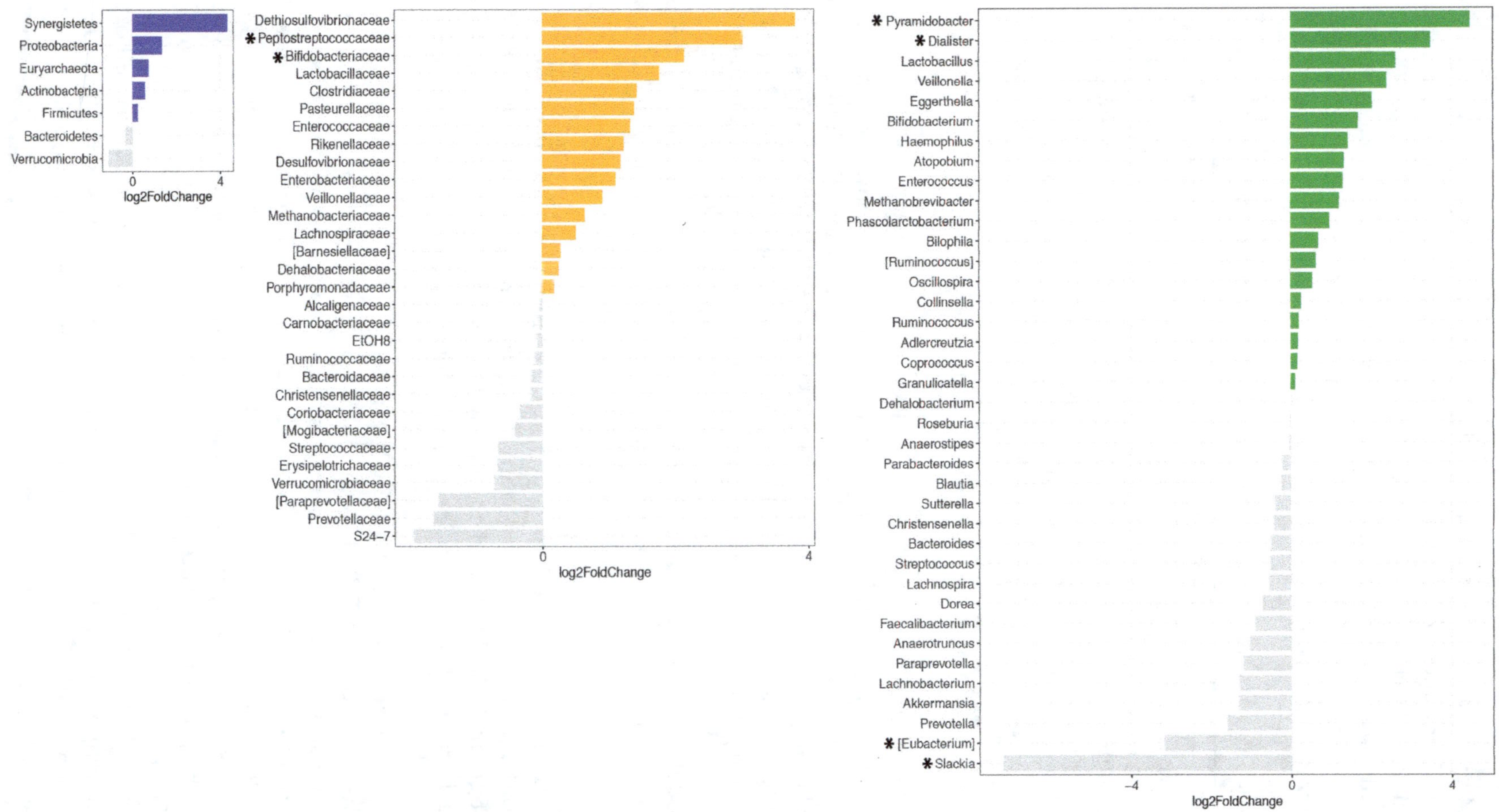

Figure 2. Comparison of gut microbiota relative abundance at the phylum (left panel, blue), family (middle panel, orange), and genus (right panel, green) levels between participants with PF&S and nonPF&S controls. Comparisons with a negative $\log_2$ fold change (log2FC) are represented in grey. Only comparisons with a log2FC higher or lower than ± 1.5 and an adjusted p value < 0.05 are considered significant (*).

3.3. SO-CovSel Analysis

Serum levels of 64 biomolecules, including cytokines, chemokines, growth factors, amino acids, and derivatives, and the abundance of 77 gut microbial taxa, were assayed through multiple analytical platforms. Concentrations of serum mediators are reported in Table S2. Several SO-CovSel models were built using the multimatrix dataset. Among all of the tested models, the one that allowed the best classification of PF&S and nonPF&S participants with the smallest number of variables was selected. This latter was built using only seven analytes (Table 4).

Table 4. Levels of relevant analytes as resulted from SO-CovSel analysis.

	PF&S (n = 18)	nonPF&S (n = 17)
MIP-1α (pg/mL)	2.98 (11.04)	10.64 (11.15)
Aspartic acid (μmol/L)	26.95 (9.33)	16.10 (9.28)
Threonine (μmol/L)	109.90 (33.60)	125.80 (55.60)
Barnesiellaceae (log2FC)	0.0010 (0.007)	0.0030 (0.003)
Christensenellaceae (log2FC)	0.0004 (0.005)	0.0023 (0.004)
Oscillospira (log2FC)	0.0147 (0.227)	0.0109 (0.009)
Ruminococcus (log2FC)	0.0674 (0.091)	0.0620 (0.058)

Data are shown as median and interquartile range.

The rate of correct classification was 91.7% for PF&S participants and 87.5% for the nonPF&S group (90.0% in the whole study population), with an average area under the receiver operating characteristic (AUROC) curve very close to 1. When compared with their distributions under the null hypothesis, all of the classification figures of merit were statistically significant ($p < 0.0001$). Among the discriminant analytes selected by the SO-CovSel model, participants with PF&S showed lower levels of MIP-1β. As for the metabolic signature, the level of the aspartic acid was higher in PF&S participants, while that of threonine was higher in the nonPF&S group. Among the gut microbes contributing to the model, *Oscillospira* and *Ruminococcus* were more abundant in PF&S participants, while Barnesiellaceae *and* Christensenellaceae were higher in the nonPF&S group (Table 4).

4. Discussion

In this study, we profiled the gut microbiota and determined the levels of inflammatory and metabolic markers in older adults with and without PF&S to investigate whether PF&S is associated with specific profiles of gut microbial taxa and circulating biomolecules. We also applied an innovative multi-marker analytical approach to determine the classification performance of a set of potential biomarkers for PF&S.

Findings from the present study highlight the possibility that changes in gut microbiota composition may be associated with PF&S. Although no differences in microbial alpha diversity were found between PF&S and nonPF&S groups, results from the analysis of the differential abundance of gut microbial taxa showed increased Peptostreptococcaceae and Bifidobacteriaceae at the family level and *Dialister*, *Pyramidobacter*, and *Eggerthella* at the genus level, and depletion of *Slackia* and *Eubacterium* in participants with PF&S. The taxa involved in the association between gut microbiota and PF&S identified in the present study are in-keeping with those previously associated with frailty and biological aging [36–42].

The application of the SO-CovSel-based analytical strategy by incorporating all of the assayed variables into three different matrices allowed distinguishing participants with PF&S from nonPF&S controls by using only seven markers, among which gut microbes were the most represented (Table 4).

The existence of a gut microbiota profile associated with sarcopenia and involving changes in the abundance of health-related *Bifidobacteria* has previously been shown in rats [43]. While very little is known about a possible functional link between *Oscillospira* and PF&S, the existence of a trait for butyrate-producing bacteria *Ruminococcus* is in-keeping with previously reported associations between *Ruminococcus* abundance and frailty [40]. Indeed, *Oscillospira* represents a more enigmatic and under-studied anaerobic butyrate producer (*Clostridium* clusters IV) often associated with leanness [44], with a metabolism and physiology not fully understood [44,45]. However, the overall apparent dysbiotic shift of gut microbiota towards a greater abundance of butyrate-producing bacteria in PF&S similar to what was observed in higher functioning people may indicate a positive role for these microbes in muscle function. Indeed, butyrate, by reinforcing tight junction assembly and enhancing intestinal barrier function [46], may prevent endotoxin translocation and reduce systemic inflammation [47]. Short-chain fatty acids (SCFAs), including butyrate, also promote fatty acid oxidation, thereby improving muscle bioenergetics [48] and limiting myosteatosis [49,50]. On the other hand, reduced SCFA production may trigger insulin resistance and result in increased fatty acid deposition within the muscle. The ensuing lower muscle quality may further promote insulin resistance, feeding a vicious circle that contributes to the onset and progression of PF&S [51,52]. Whether and how *Ruminococcus* and *Oscillospira* abundance impacts muscle metabolism and function in the context of PF&S warrants further investigation. In this regard, it is noteworthy that the abundance of *Bacteroides* was increased by aerobic training in healthy older women, which was associated with improved cardiorespiratory fitness [53]. Variations in *Ruminococcus* in association with *Eubacterium* and *Eggerthella* were also identified in frail nursing-home residents compared with fit matched community-dwellers [36,37]. This finding was attributed to different dietary patterns and, in particular, to long-term protein supplementation among nursing-home residents [40]. Indeed, diet influences gut microbiota composition and functionality, which may ultimately impact skeletal muscle. While high protein intake has been endorsed as a strategy against sarcopenia [54], protein-enriched diets may shift bacterial metabolism towards AA degradation and fermentation [55]. Hence, the role of gut microbes as transducers of nutrient signaling to the host implies the need of monitoring the composition and function of gut microbiota during nutritional interventions for sarcopenia.

This view is strengthened by the presence of the AAs aspartic acid and threonine among the most relevant mediators in the SO-CovSel model.

Aspartic acid, together with asparagine and glutamic acid is among the AAs providing amino groups and ammonia for the synthesis of glutamine and alanine, whose carbon skeletons can solely be used for the de novo synthesis of Kreb's cycle intermediates and glutamine [56]. Notably, we previously showed that higher serum levels of aspartic acid, asparagine, and glutamic acid were among the descriptors of the AA signature of older persons with PF&S [10].

Threonine is an essential AA (EAA) that must be provided with the diet to meet nutritional requirements and is relevant for muscle protein turnover and overall metabolism [57]. The finding of threonine as a contributor to the SO-CovSel model in discriminating PF&S participants is in-keeping with a recent work reporting levels of several EAAs, including threonine, as inversely associated with sarcopenia in community-dwelling older adults [58]. Low plasma levels of EAAs were also found in severely frail older people [59]. These findings may be associated to malnutrition (both quantitative and qualitative), a common underlying factor of frailty and sarcopenia [60].

Finally, the relationship observed between the abundance of specific intestinal bacteria, metabolic markers, and serum levels of distinct inflammatory biomolecules suggests the existence of an additional pathway through which changes in gut microbiota may impinge on PF&S pathophysiology. A relationship among gut microbiota composition, chronic inflammation, and age-related conditions was shown in pre-clinical models [61] but not in humans. Furthermore, altered gut microbiota composition has been hypothesized to contribute to anabolic resistance and muscle wasting through promoting chronic inflammation [62,63]. Age-associated alterations in intestinal mucosa permeability (i.e., "leaky gut") and the resulting systemic absorption of bacterial products may further ignite systemic inflammation [64–66]. Although our investigation does not provide mechanistic elements to support such a hypothesis, the relevance of systemic inflammation to PF&S has previously been shown [11]. From this perspective, systemic inflammation would represent one of the effectors of the "gut-muscle axis" that has recently been proposed to contribute to the development of PF&S [23,63,67].

Hence, untangling the relationship among gut microbiota, metabolic changes and muscle homeostasis in advanced age represents a highly promising research area to devise new interventions against PF&S.

Although reporting novel findings, our study presents some limitations that need to be acknowledged. Participants with PF&S had higher BMI than controls, indicative of a sarcopenic obesity phenotype. Because this body composition profile is intrinsic to the PF&S condition [27], the relative contribution of low muscle and excessive adiposity to systemic inflammation, metabolic changes, and gut microbiota composition could not be discerned. The cross-sectional design of the present investigation does not allow inferring causality about changes in gut microbiota and the development of PF&S. Nevertheless, the presence of a gut-muscle axis actively involved in the genesis of frailty and sarcopenia is supported by other studies (reviewed in [67]). Here, for the first time, we show that specific relationships exist among gut microbiota, systemic inflammatory mediators, and metabolic alterations in older adults with PF&S. The relatively small size of the study population comprising only Caucasian people calls for a cautious interpretation of results and impedes generalization of findings to other ethnic groups. Because of the limited sample size, the possible influence of numerous factors, including diet, physical activity, co-morbid conditions, and medications, could not be taken into account in the analysis. Finally, although a fairly large number of metabolic and inflammatory biomolecules were assayed, it cannot be excluded that more robust associations between gut microbiota composition and PF&S might have been obtained through the analysis of a larger range of biomediators.

Supplementary Materials:
Table S1: Differential abundance analysis of bacterial taxa at phylum, family, and genus level in participants with physical frailty and sarcopenia (PF&S) and nonPF&S. Table S2: Serum concentrations of nonsignificant inflammatory mediators, amino acids, and derivatives in participants with and without physical frailty & sarcopenia (PF&S).

Author Contributions: Conceptualization, A.P. (Anna Picca), E.M., and F.R.P.; methodology, A.P. (Aniello Primiano), F.D.C., J.G., and S.R.; software, A.B. and F.M.; validation, A.P. (Anna Picca), E.M., F.R.P., H.J.C.-J., and R.C.; formal analysis, A.B. and F.M.; investigation, A.P. (Anna Picca), E.M., and R.C.; resources, A.G., F.L., L.P., and R.B.; data curation, A.P. (Anna Picca), F.R.P., and R.C.; writing—original draft preparation, A.P. (Anna Picca) and E.M.; writing—review and editing, F.M., H.J.C.-J., J.G., and R.C.; visualization, A.P. (Aniello Primiano), F.D.C., J.G., and S.R.; supervision, A.G., F.L., L.P., and R.B.; funding acquisition, R.B. All authors have read and agreed to the published version of the manuscript.

Acknowledgments: The authors would like to thank all participants for their involvement in this study.

References

1. Hirani, V.; Blyth, F.; Naganathan, V.; Le Couteur, D.G.; Seibel, M.J.; Waite, L.M.; Handelsman, D.J.; Cumming, R.G. Sarcopenia is associated with incident disability, institutionalization, and mortality in community-dwelling older men: The Concord Health and Ageing in Men Project. *J. Am. Med. Dir. Assoc.* **2015**, *16*, 607–613. [CrossRef] [PubMed]
2. Marzetti, E.; Calvani, R.; Tosato, M.; Cesari, M.; Di Bari, M.; Cherubini, A.; Collamati, A.; D'Angelo, E.; Pahor, M.; Bernabei, R.; et al. SPRINTT Consortium. Sarcopenia: An overview. *Aging Clin. Exp. Res.* **2017**, *29*, 11–17. [CrossRef] [PubMed]
3. Cesari, M.; Calvani, R.; Marzetti, E. Frailty in older persons. *Clin. Geriatr. Med.* **2017**, *33*, 293–303. [CrossRef] [PubMed]
4. Landi, F.; Calvani, R.; Cesari, M.; Tosato, M.; Martone, A.M.; Bernabei, R.; Onder, G.; Marzetti, E. Sarcopenia as the biological substrate of physical frailty. *Clin. Geriatr. Med.* **2015**, *31*, 367–374. [CrossRef] [PubMed]

5. Cesari, M.; Landi, F.; Vellas, B.; Bernabei, R.; Marzetti, E. Sarcopenia and physical frailty: Two sides of the same coin. *Front. Aging Neurosci.* **2014**, *6*, 192. [CrossRef]
6. Cesari, M.; Landi, F.; Calvani, R.; Cherubini, A.; Di Bari, M.; Kortebein, P.; Del Signore, S.; Le Lain, R.; Vellas, B.; Pahor, M.; et al. SPRINTT Consortium. Rationale for a preliminary operational definition of physical frailty and sarcopenia in the SPRINTT trial. *Aging Clin. Exp. Res.* **2017**, *29*, 81–88. [CrossRef]
7. Marzetti, E.; Calvani, R.; Landi, F.; Hoogendijk, E.O.; Fougère, B.; Vellas, B.; Pahor, M.; Bernabei, R.; Cesari, M. SPRINTT Consortium. Innovative Medicines Initiative: The SPRINTT project. *J. Frailty Aging* **2015**, *4*, 207–208. [CrossRef]
8. Calvani, R.; Marini, F.; Cesari, M.; Tosato, M.; Anker, S.D.; von Haehling, S.; Miller, R.R.; Bernabei, R.; Landi, F.; Marzetti, E. SPRINTT consortium. Biomarkers for physical frailty and sarcopenia: State of the science and future developments. *J. Cachexia Sarcopenia Muscle* **2015**, *6*, 278–286. [CrossRef]
9. Picca, A.; Calvani, R.; Bossola, M.; Allocca, E.; Menghi, A.; Pesce, V.; Lezza, A.M.S.; Bernabei, R.; Landi, F.; Marzetti, E. Update on mitochondria and muscle aging: All wrong roads lead to sarcopenia. *Biol. Chem.* **2018**, *399*, 421–436. [CrossRef]
10. Calvani, R.; Picca, A.; Marini, F.; Biancolillo, A.; Gervasoni, J.; Persichilli, S.; Primiano, A.; Coelho-Junior, H.J.; Bossola, M.; Urbani, A.; et al. A distinct pattern of circulating amino acids characterizes older persons with physical frailty and sarcopenia: Results from the BIOSPHERE study. *Nutrients* **2018**, *10*, 1691. [CrossRef]
11. Marzetti, E.; Picca, A.; Marini, F.; Biancolillo, A.; Coelho-Junior, H.J.; Gervasoni, J.; Bossola, M.; Cesari, M.; Onder, G.; Landi, F.; et al. Inflammatory signatures in older persons with physical frailty and sarcopenia: The frailty "cytokinome" at its core. *Exp. Gerontol.* **2019**, *122*, 129–138. [CrossRef] [PubMed]
12. Landi, F.; Calvani, R.; Tosato, M.; Martone, A.M.; Ortolani, E.; Savera, G.; Sisto, A.; Marzetti, E. Anorexia of aging: Risk factors, consequences, and potential treatments. *Nutrients* **2016**, *8*, 69. [CrossRef] [PubMed]
13. Landi, F.; Calvani, R.; Tosato, M.; Martone, A.M.; Ortolani, E.; Savera, G.; D'Angelo, E.; Sisto, A.; Marzetti, E. Protein intake and muscle health in old age: From biological plausibility to clinical evidence. *Nutrients* **2016**, *8*, 295. [CrossRef] [PubMed]
14. Landi, F.; Cesari, M.; Calvani, R.; Cherubini, A.; Di Bari, M.; Bejuit, R.; Mshid, J.; Andrieu, S.; Sinclair, A.J.; Sieber, C.C.; et al. SPRINTT Consortium. The "Sarcopenia and Physical fRailty IN older people: Multi-componenT Treatment strategies" (SPRINTT) randomized controlled trial: Design and methods. *Aging Clin. Exp. Res.* **2017**, *29*, 89–100. [CrossRef]
15. Chen, H.; Rejeski, W.J.; Gill, T.M.; Guralnik, J.; King, A.C.; Newman, A.; Blair, S.N.; Conroy, D.; Liu, C.; Manini, T.M.; et al. LIFE Study. A comparison of self-report indices of major mobility disability to failure on the 400-m walk test: The LIFE study. *J. Gerontol. A Biol. Sci. Med. Sci.* **2018**, *73*, 513–518. [CrossRef]
16. Roubenoff, R. Sarcopenic obesity: Does muscle loss cause fat gain? Lessons from rheumatoid arthritis and osteoarthritis. *Ann. N. Y. Acad. Sci.* **2006**, *904*, 553–557. [CrossRef]
17. Binkley, N.; Krueger, D.; Buehring, B. What's in a name revisited: Should osteoporosis and sarcopenia be considered components of "dysmobility syndrome?". *Osteoporos. Int.* **2013**, *24*, 2955–2959. [CrossRef]
18. Porter Starr, K.N.; McDonald, S.R.; Bales, C.W. Obesity and physical frailty in older adults: A scoping review of lifestyle intervention trials. *J. Am. Med. Dir. Assoc.* **2014**, *15*, 240–250. [CrossRef]
19. Hulsegge, G.; Herber-Gast, G.-C.M.; Spijkerman, A.M.W.; Susan, H.; Picavet, J.; van der Schouw, Y.T.; Bakker, S.J.L.; Gansevoort, R.T.; Dollé, M.E.T.; Smit, H.A.; et al. Obesity and age-related changes in markers of oxidative stress and inflammation across four generations. *Obesity* **2016**, *24*, 1389–1396. [CrossRef]
20. Goodpaster, B.H.; Carlson, C.L.; Visser, M.; Kelley, D.E.; Scherzinger, A.; Harris, T.B.; Stamm, E.; Newman, A.B. Attenuation of skeletal muscle and strength in the elderly: The health ABC study. *J. Appl. Physiol.* **2001**, *90*, 2157–2165. [CrossRef]
21. Visser, M.; Goodpaster, B.H.; Kritchevsky, S.B.; Newman, A.B.; Nevitt, M.; Rubin, S.M.; Simonsick, E.M.; Harris, T.B. Muscle mass, muscle strength, and muscle fat infiltration as predictors of incident mobility limitations in well-functioning older persons. *J. Gerontol. A Biol. Sci. Med. Sci.* **2005**, *60*, 324–333. [CrossRef] [PubMed]
22. O'Connor, E.M. The role of gut microbiota in nutritional status. *Curr. Opin. Clin. Nutr. Metab. Care* **2013**, *16*, 509–516. [CrossRef] [PubMed]
23. Picca, A.; Fanelli, F.; Calvani, R.; Mulè, G.; Pesce, V.; Sisto, A.; Pantanelli, C.; Bernabei, R.; Landi, F.; Marzetti, E. Gut dysbiosis and muscle aging: Searching for novel targets against sarcopenia. *Mediat. Inflamm.* **2018**, *2018*. [CrossRef] [PubMed]

24. Calvani, R.; Picca, A.; Marini, F.; Biancolillo, A.; Cesari, M.; Pesce, V.; Lezza, A.M.S.; Bossola, M.; Leeuwenburgh, C.; Bernabei, R.; et al. The "BIOmarkers associated with Sarcopenia and PHysical frailty in EldeRly pErsons" (BIOSPHERE) study: Rationale, design and methods. *Eur. J. Intern. Med.* **2018**, *56*, 19–25. [CrossRef]
25. Ponziani, F.R.; Putignani, L.; Paroni Sterbini, F.; Petito, V.; Picca, A.; Del Chierico, F.; Reddel, S.; Calvani, R.; Marzetti, E.; Sanguinetti, M.; et al. Influence of hepatitis C virus eradication with direct-acting antivirals on the gut microbiota in patients with cirrhosis. *Aliment. Pharmacol. Ther.* **2018**, *48*, 1301–1311. [CrossRef]
26. Ponziani, F.R.; Bhoori, S.; Castelli, C.; Putignani, L.; Rivoltini, L.; Del Chierico, F.; Sanguinetti, M.; Morelli, D.; Paroni Sterbini, F.; Petito, V.; et al. Hepatocellular carcinoma is associated with gut microbiota profile and inflammation in nonalcoholic fatty liver disease. *Hepatology* **2019**, *69*, 107–120. [CrossRef]
27. Marzetti, E.; Cesari, M.; Calvani, R.; Msihid, J.; Tosato, M.; Rodriguez-Mañas, L.; Lattanzio, F.; Cherubini, A.; Bejuit, R.; Di Bari, M.; et al. SPRINTT Consortium. The "Sarcopenia and Physical fRailty IN older people: Multi-componenT Treatment strategies" (SPRINTT) randomized controlled trial: Case finding, screening and characteristics of eligible participants. *Exp. Gerontol.* **2018**, *113*, 48–57. [CrossRef]
28. Guralnik, J.M.; Simonsick, E.M.; Ferrucci, L.; Glynn, R.J.; Berkman, L.F.; Blazer, D.G.; Scherr, P.A.; Wallace, R.B. A short physical performance battery assessing lower extremity function: Association with self-reported disability and prediction of mortality and nursing home admission. *J. Gerontol.* **1994**, *49*, M85–M94. [CrossRef]
29. Studenski, S.A.; Peters, K.W.; Alley, D.E.; Cawthon, P.M.; McLean, R.R.; Harris, T.B.; Ferrucci, L.; Guralnik, J.M.; Fragala, M.S.; Kenny, A.M.; et al. The FNIH sarcopenia project: Rationale, study description, conference recommendations, and final estimates. *J. Gerontol. A Biol. Sci. Med. Sci.* **2014**, *69*, 547–558. [CrossRef]
30. Newman, A.B.; Simonsick, E.M.; Naydeck, B.L.; Boudreau, R.M.; Kritchevsky, S.B.; Nevitt, M.C.; Pahor, M.; Satterfield, S.; Brach, J.S.; Studenski, S.A.; et al. Association of long-distance corridor walk performance with mortality, cardiovascular disease, mobility limitation, and disability. *JAMA* **2006**, *295*, 2018–2026. [CrossRef]
31. Picca, A.; Guerra, F.; Calvani, R.; Bucci, C.; Lo Monaco, M.R.; Bentivoglio, A.R.; Landi, F.; Bernabei, R.; Marzetti, E. Mitochondrial-derived vesicles as candidate biomarkers in Parkinson's disease: Rationale, design and methods of the EXosomes in PArkiNson Disease (EXPAND) study. *Int. J. Mol. Sci.* **2019**, *20*, 2373. [CrossRef] [PubMed]
32. Biancolillo, A.; Marini, F.; Roger, J. SO-CovSel: A novel method for variable selection in a multiblock framework. *J. Chemom.* **2019**, e3120. [CrossRef]
33. Roger, J.M.; Palagos, B.; Bertrand, D.; Fernandez-Ahumada, E. CovSel: Variable selection for highly multivariate and multi-response calibration. Application to IR spectroscopy. *Chemom. Intell. Lab. Syst.* **2011**, *106*, 216–223. [CrossRef]
34. Naes, T.; Tomic, O.; Mevik, B.-H.; Martens, H. Path modelling by sequential PLS regression. *J. Chemom.* **2011**, *25*, 28–40. [CrossRef]
35. Biancolillo, A.; Naes, T. The Sequential and Orthogonalized PLS Regression for Multiblock Regression: Theory, Examples, and Extensions. In *Data Fusion Methodology and Applications*; Cocchi, M., Ed.; Elsevier: Oxford, UK, 2019; Volume 31, pp. 157–177.
36. Claesson, M.J.; Jeffery, I.B.; Conde, S.; Power, S.E.; O'connor, E.M.; Cusack, S.; Harris, H.M.B.; Coakley, M.; Lakshminarayanan, B.; O'sullivan, O.; et al. Gut microbiota composition correlates with diet and health in the elderly. *Nature* **2012**, *488*, 178–184. [CrossRef]
37. Jackson, M.A.; Jackson, M.; Jeffery, I.B.; Beaumont, M.; Bell, J.T.; Clark, A.G.; Ley, R.E.; O'Toole, P.W.; Spector, T.D.; Steves, C.J. Signatures of early frailty in the gut microbiota. *Genome Med.* **2016**, *8*, 8. [CrossRef]
38. Maffei, V.J.; Kim, S.; Blanchard, E.; Luo, M.; Jazwinski, S.M.; Taylor, C.M.; Welsh, D.A. Biological Aging and the Human Gut Microbiota. *J. Gerontol. A Biol. Sci. Med. Sci.* **2017**, *72*, 1474–1482. [CrossRef]
39. Ticinesi, A.; Milani, C.; Lauretani, F.; Nouvenne, A.; Mancabelli, L.; Lugli, G.A.; Turroni, F.; Duranti, S.; Mangifesta, M.; Viappiani, A.; et al. Gut microbiota composition is associated with polypharmacy in elderly hospitalized patients. *Sci. Rep.* **2017**, *7*, 11102. [CrossRef]
40. Haran, J.P.; Bucci, V.; Dutta, P.; Ward, D.; McCormick, B. The nursing home elder microbiome stability and associations with age, frailty, nutrition and physical location. *J. Med. Microbiol.* **2018**, *67*, 40–51. [CrossRef]
41. Verdi, S.; Jackson, M.A.; Beaumont, M.; Bowyer, R.C.E.; Bell, J.T.; Spector, T.D.; Steves, C.J. An investigation into physical frailty as a link between the gut microbiome and cognitive health. *Front. Aging Neurosci.* **2018**, *10*, 398. [CrossRef]

42. Ogawa, T.; Hirose, Y.; Honda-Ogawa, M.; Sugimoto, M.; Sasaki, S.; Kibi, M.; Kawabata, S.; Ikebe, K.; Maeda, Y. Composition of salivary microbiota in elderly subjects. *Sci. Rep.* **2018**, *8*, 414. [CrossRef] [PubMed]
43. Siddharth, J.; Chakrabarti, A.; Pannérec, A.; Karaz, S.; Morin-Rivron, D.; Masoodi, M.; Feige, J.N.; Parkinson, S.J. Aging and sarcopenia associate with specific interactions between gut microbes, serum biomarkers and host physiology in rats. *Aging* **2017**, *9*, 1698–1720. [CrossRef] [PubMed]
44. Gophna, U.; Konikoff, T.; Nielsen, H.B. Oscillospira and related bacteria—From metagenomic species to metabolic features. *Environ. Microbiol.* **2017**, *19*, 835–841. [CrossRef] [PubMed]
45. Konikoff, T.; Gophna, U. Oscillospira: A central, enigmatic component of the human gut microbiota. *Trends Microbiol.* **2016**, *24*, 523–524. [CrossRef] [PubMed]
46. Peng, L.; Li, Z.-R.; Green, R.S.; Holzman, I.R.; Lin, J. Butyrate enhances the intestinal barrier by facilitating tight junction assembly via activation of AMP-activated protein kinase in Caco-2 cell monolayers. *J. Nutr.* **2009**, *139*, 1619–1625. [CrossRef] [PubMed]
47. Cox, M.A.; Jackson, J.; Stanton, M.; Rojas-Triana, A.; Bober, L.; Laverty, M.; Yang, X.; Zhu, F.; Liu, J.; Wang, S.; et al. Short-chain fatty acids act as antiinflammatory mediators by regulating prostaglandin E2 and cytokines. *World J. Gastroenterol.* **2009**, *15*, 5549–5557. [CrossRef]
48. Saint-Georges-Chaumet, Y.; Edeas, M. Microbiota-mitochondria inter-talk: Consequence for microbiota-host interaction. *Pathog. Dis.* **2016**, *74*, ftv096. [CrossRef]
49. Hénique, C.; Mansouri, A.; Vavrova, E.; Lenoir, V.; Ferry, A.; Esnous, C.; Ramond, E.; Girard, J.; Bouillaud, F.; Prip-Buus, C.; et al. Increasing mitochondrial muscle fatty acid oxidation induces skeletal muscle remodeling toward an oxidative phenotype. *FASEB J.* **2015**, *29*, 2473–2483. [CrossRef]
50. Gumucio, J.P.; Qasawa, A.H.; Ferrara, P.J.; Malik, A.N.; Funai, K.; McDonagh, B.; Mendias, C.L. Reduced mitochondrial lipid oxidation leads to fat accumulation in myosteatosis. *FASEB J.* **2019**, *33*, 7863–7881. [CrossRef]
51. Poggiogalle, E.; Lubrano, C.; Gnessi, L.; Mariani, S.; Di Martino, M.; Catalano, C.; Lenzi, A.; Donini, L.M. The decline in muscle strength and muscle quality in relation to metabolic derangements in adult women with obesity. *Clin. Nutr.* **2019**, *38*, 2430–2435. [CrossRef]
52. Sachs, S.; Zarini, S.; Kahn, D.E.; Harrison, K.A.; Perreault, L.; Phang, T.; Newsom, S.A.; Strauss, A.; Kerege, A.; Schoen, J.A.; et al. Intermuscular adipose tissue directly modulates skeletal muscle insulin sensitivity in humans. *Am. J. Physiol. Endocrinol. Metab.* **2019**, *316*, E866–E879. [CrossRef] [PubMed]
53. Morita, E.; Yokoyama, H.; Imai, D.; Takeda, R.; Ota, A.; Kawai, E.; Hisada, T.; Emoto, M.; Suzuki, Y.; Okazaki, K. Aerobic exercise training with brisk walking increases intestinal bacteroides in healthy elderly women. *Nutrients* **2019**, *11*, 868. [CrossRef] [PubMed]
54. Landi, F.; Calvani, R.; Tosato, M.; Martone, A.M.; Picca, A.; Ortolani, E.; Savera, G.; Salini, S.; Ramaschi, M.; Bernabei, R.; et al. Animal-derived protein consumption is associated with muscle mass and strength in community-dwellers: Results from the Milan EXPO survey. *J. Nutr. Health Aging* **2017**, *21*, 1050–1056. [CrossRef] [PubMed]
55. Beaumont, M.; Portune, K.J.; Steuer, N.; Lan, A.; Cerrudo, V.; Audebert, M.; Dumont, F.; Mancano, G.; Khodorova, N.; Andriamihaja, M.; et al. Quantity and source of dietary protein influence metabolite production by gut microbiota and rectal mucosa gene expression: A randomized, parallel, double-blind trial in overweight humans. *Am. J. Clin. Nutr.* **2017**, *106*, 1005–1019. [CrossRef] [PubMed]
56. Wagenmakers, A.J.M. Protein and amino acid metabolism in human muscle. *Adv. Exp. Med. Biol.* **1998**, *441*, 307–319. [CrossRef]
57. Wu, G. Amino acids: Metabolism, functions, and nutrition. *Amino Acids* **2009**, *37*, 1–17. [CrossRef]
58. Lu, Y.; Karagounis, L.G.; Ng, T.P.; Carre, C.; Narang, V.; Wong, G.; Ying Tan, C.T.; Zin Nyunt, M.S.; Gao, Q.; Abel, B.; et al. Systemic and metabolic signature of sarcopenia in community-dwelling older adults. *J. Gerontol. A Biol. Sci. Med. Sci.* **2019**. [CrossRef]
59. Adachi, Y.; Ono, N.; Imaizumi, A.; Muramatsu, T.; Andou, T.; Shimodaira, Y.; Nagao, K.; Kageyama, Y.; Mori, M.; Noguchi, Y.; et al. Plasma amino acid profile in severely frail elderly patients in Japan. *Int. J. Gerontol.* **2018**, *12*, 290–293. [CrossRef]
60. Cruz-Jentoft, A.J.; Kiesswetter, E.; Drey, M.; Sieber, C.C. Nutrition, frailty, and sarcopenia. *Aging Clin. Exp. Res.* **2017**, *29*, 43–48. [CrossRef]

61. Thevaranjan, N.; Puchta, A.; Schulz, C.; Naidoo, A.; Szamosi, J.C.; Verschoor, C.P.; Loukov, D.; Schenck, L.P.; Jury, J.; Foley, K.P.; et al. Age-associated microbial dysbiosis promotes intestinal permeability, systemic inflammation, and macrophage dysfunction. *Cell Host Microbe* **2017**, *21*, 455–466. [CrossRef]
62. Grosicki, G.J.; Fielding, R.A.; Lustgarten, M.S. Gut microbiota contribute to age-related changes in skeletal muscle size, composition, and function: Biological basis for a gut-muscle axis. *Calcif. Tissue Int.* **2018**, *102*, 433–442. [CrossRef] [PubMed]
63. Ticinesi, A.; Lauretani, F.; Milani, C.; Nouvenne, A.; Tana, C.; Del Rio, D.; Maggio, M.; Ventura, M.; Meschi, T. Aging gut microbiota at the cross-road between nutrition, physical frailty, and sarcopenia: Is there a gut–muscle axis? *Nutrients* **2017**, *9*, 1303. [CrossRef] [PubMed]
64. Ferrucci, L.; Fabbri, E. Inflammageing: Chronic inflammation in ageing, cardiovascular disease, and frailty. *Nat. Rev. Cardiol.* **2018**, *15*, 505–522. [CrossRef] [PubMed]
65. Sovran, B.; Hugenholtz, F.; Elderman, M.; Van Beek, A.A.; Graversen, K.; Huijskes, M.; Boekschoten, M.V.; Savelkoul, H.F.J.; De Vos, P.; Dekker, J.; et al. Age-associated impairment of the mucus barrier function is associated with profound changes in microbiota and immunity. *Sci. Rep.* **2019**, *9*, 1437. [CrossRef]
66. Ticinesi, A.; Lauretani, F.; Tana, C.; Nouvenne, A.; Ridolo, E.; Meschi, T. Exercise and immune system as modulators of intestinal microbiome: Implications for the gut-muscle axis hypothesis. *Exerc. Immunol. Rev.* **2019**, *25*, 84–95.
67. Ticinesi, A.; Nouvenne, A.; Cerundolo, N.; Catania, P.; Prati, B.; Tana, C.; Meschi, T. Gut microbiota, muscle mass and function in aging: A focus on physical frailty and sarcopenia. *Nutrients* **2019**, *11*, 1633. [CrossRef]

3

Influence of Diets with Varying Essential/Nonessential Amino Acid Ratios on Mouse Lifespan

Claudia Romano [1,†], Giovanni Corsetti [1,*,†], Vincenzo Flati [2,†], Evasio Pasini [3], Anna Picca [4,5], Riccardo Calvani [4,5], Emanuele Marzetti [4] and Francesco Saverio Dioguardi [6,*]

1 Division of Human Anatomy and Physiopathology, Department of Clinical and Experimental Sciences, University of Brescia, 25124 Brescia, Italy; cla300482@gmail.com

2 Department of Biotechnological and Applied Clinical Sciences, University of L'Aquila, 67100 L'Aquila, Italy; vincenzo.flati@univaq.it

3 Istituti Clinici Scientifici Maugeri - IRCCS Lumezzane - Cardiac Rehabilitation Division, 25065 Lumezzane (Brescia), Italy; evpasini@gmail.com

4 Fondazione Policlinico Universitario "Agostino Gemelli" IRCCS, 00168 Rome, Italy; anna.picca1@gmail.com (A.P.); riccardo.calvani@gmail.com (R.C.); emarzetti@live.com (E.M.)

5 Institute of Internal Medicine and Geriatrics, Università Cattolica del Sacro Cuore, 00168 Rome, Italy

6 Department of Internal Medicine, University of Cagliari, 09042 Monserrato (Cagliari), Italy

* Correspondence: giovanni.corsetti@unibs.it (G.C.); fsdioguardi@gmail.com (F.S.D.)

† These authors contributed equally to this work.

Abstract: An adequate intake of essential (EAA) and non-essential amino acids (NEAA) is crucial to preserve cell integrity and whole-body metabolism. EAA introduced with diet may be insufficient to meet the organismal needs, especially under increased physiological requirements or in pathological conditions, and may condition lifespan. We therefore examined the effects of iso-caloric and providing the same nitrogenous content diets, any diet containing different stoichiometric blends of EAA/NEAA, on mouse lifespan. Three groups of just-weaned male Balb/C mice were fed exclusively with special diets with varying EAA/NEAA ratios, ranging from 100%/0% to 0%/100%. Three additional groups of mice were fed with different diets, two based on casein as alimentary proteins, one providing the said protein, one reproducing the amino acidic composition of casein, and the third one, the control group, was fed by a standard laboratory diet. Mouse lifespan was inversely correlated with the percentage of NEAA introduced with each diet. Either limiting EAA, or exceeding NEAA, induced rapid and permanent structural modifications on muscle and adipose tissue, independently of caloric intake. These changes significantly affected food and water intake, body weight, and lifespan. Dietary intake of varying EAA/NEAA ratios induced changes in several organs and profoundly influenced murine lifespan. The balanced content of EAA provided by dietary proteins should be considered as the preferable means for "optimal" nutrition and the elevated or unbalanced intake of NEAA provided by food proteins may negatively affect the health and lifespan of mice.

Keywords: amino acids intake; essential amino acids; diet; extended lifespan; mice

1. Introduction

Proteins are macromolecules serving a vast array of functions within the cell, and a balanced protein synthesis and degradation is crucial for preserving cell homeostasis. Hence, increased proteolysis and reduced protein synthesis have been associated with the severe depletion of body protein reserves, eventually resulting in malnutrition. This may impact the progression of several disease-associated conditions [1]. For example, muscle wasting in people aged over 65 years old, hospitalized for a variety of chronic disease conditions, has been related with the disarrangement of protein balance [2].

Therefore, an adequate nutritional supply of protein may represent a relevant means for the management of patients who are malnourished as a consequence of reduced food intake or increased metabolic demand (i.e., chronic and acute diseases).

Dietary proteins with their various compositions of amino acids (AAs) are nitrogen (N) sources for almost all organisms. From a nutritional point of view, AAs can be classified as non-essential (NEAA) or essential (EAA), depending on their potential to be synthesized endogenously or not [3,4], although the original definitions of the two terms focused on their efficiency in promoting protein deposition [5,6].

Adequate dietary provision of AAs is essential for the growth, development, health, and survival of animals and humans [7]. It is also established that the administration of an adequate EAA+NEAA mix favors an increase in rat body weight, which is considered an appropriate parameter to evaluate the success of the animal in terms of growth and wellness [3,7–9]. However, this concept should be profoundly reconsidered if associated to lifespan. Indeed, caloric restriction and short-term caloric deficit improve the efficiency of mitochondria in humans just as in rodents, which might have the potential to increase their longevity [10].

Previous work by our group showed that the supplementation of a laboratory standard diet, containing special EAA formulations, increased rodents' lifespan in older mice [11]. At the molecular level, such a dietary regimen was able to promote mitochondrial biogenesis and to induce organelle ultrastructural changes in the heart, skeletal muscle and adipose tissue [12–14]. In addition, an EAA-rich diet prevented liver damage induced by chronic ethanol consumption [15,16], boosted the effects of rosuvastatin on the kidneys [17] and accelerated wound healing in late middle-aged rats, by promoting collagen integrity [18]. Furthermore, in vitro data showed that variations in the EAA/NEAA ratio might be crucial for the fate of cancer cells via the induction of apoptosis [19]. Taken as a whole, these findings indicate that varying dietary EAA/NEAA ratios may affect cell metabolism.

While dietary proteins are the major source of AAs, the exact amounts of EAA contained in animal and vegetable proteins, introduced daily with diet, are difficult to establish. Indeed, the EAA content varies considerably depending on the source. However, any dietary protein has an EAA/NEAA ratio $\leq$0.9 at best. In other words, we introduce a very large amount of NEAA to meet the need for EAA and the excess of NEAA must be eliminated through complex metabolic pathways [20].

Many individual AAs have been tested by dietary exclusion studies in rodents, in order to demonstrate their influence on metabolism and health. For example, the restriction of methionine increases the expression of FGF21 with fall-out effects on insulin-dependent glucose uptake [21]. Other studies have been carried out in rodents with the restriction of branched-chain-AAs [22] or leucine alone [23], assessing their effects on various metabolic aspects (e.g., improving glucose tolerance or white and brown adipose tissue remodeling, respectively). The effects of caloric, protein and carbohydrate restriction on animal survival and welfare have also been studied [24–26]. While the restriction of individual AAs and groups of AAs has been looked at extensively in terms of metabolism and ageing, no studies have been performed specifically about EAA/NEAA ratio in the context of longevity.

Recent data from our studies on late middle-aged animals, fed for one month with iso-caloric and iso-nitrogenous diets containing different EAA/NEAA ratios, showed significant changes in body mass and blood parameters [27]. We therefore investigated the lifelong effects on male mice of iso-caloric and iso-nitrogenous special diets containing five specific EAA/NEAA ratios, compared to a standard laboratory rodent diet.

2. Materials and methods

2.1. Animals

Three-week old outbred male Balb/C mice (Envigo, Holland) were housed in plastic cages with white wood chips for bedding, in a quiet room under controlled lighting (12 h day/night cycle) and temperature (22 ± 1°C) conditions. Animals were regularly examined by veterinary doctors for their health, the maintenance of normal daily and nocturnal behavioral activities, and for criteria of increased disease burden, according to ethics standards for animal studies. The experimental protocol was conducted in accordance with the directives of the Italian Ministry of Health and complied with 'The National Animal Protection Guidelines'. The Ethics Committee for animal experiments of IZSLER (Brescia, Italy) (the "National Reference Centre for Animal Welfare" (http://www.izsler.it)), and the Italian Ministry of Health approved all of the procedures.

2.2. Diet Composition

We used three specific diets with different EAA/NEAA ratios ranging from 100%/0% to 0%/100%, as previously described [27]. A summary of diet composition and EAA/NEAA ratios is shown in Table 1.

(1) EAA-100% diet contained exclusively EAA as the source of nitrogen [11,17,18,28].
(2) EAA-30% diet (EAA-poor diet) and thus NEAA-rich diet (70% of NEAA).
(3) NEAA-100% diet contained exclusively NEAA as the source of nitrogen (thus 0% of EAA).
(4) Casein-Prot diet contained only whole casein protein of highest quality.
(5) Casein-AA (casein-like) diet contained free AAs equivalent to the composition of casein (EAA/NEAA = 49/51).
(6) A commercial standard rodent laboratory diet (StD) (Mucedola srl, Milan, Italy) was also used.

The Casein-Prot and Casein-AA diets were used as special test diets, since no composition of AAs in StD proteins was available even for the producer, and we needed to test the safety of life-long nutrition by free AAs.

All special diets provided quantitatively equal amounts of lipids, carbohydrate and micronutrients. All diets were thus iso-caloric and provided the same amounts of nitrogen, although nitrogen content was provided by different formulations of AAs or proteins, according to those presented in Table 1. All special diets were prepared for Nutriresearch s.r.l. (Milan, Italy) by Dottori Piccioni (Milan, Italy) in accordance with AIN76-A/NIH-7 rules [29].

Animals were randomly assigned to one of the six groups. Each group was fed exclusively with a specific diet [i.e., EAA-100% diet (n = 30), Casein-AA diet (n = 30), Casein-Prot (n = 30), StD (n = 40), EAA-30% diet (n = 30), or NEAA-100% diet (n = 30)]. All animals had free access to food and water.

Table 1. Diet composition.

Nutrients	EAA-100%	Casein-AA	Casein-Prot	StD	EAA-30%	NEAA-100%
KCal/Kg	3995	3995	3995	3952	3995	3995
Carbohydrates %	61.76	61.76	61.76	54.61	61.76	61.76
Lipids %	6.12	6.12	6.12	7.5	6.12	6.12
Nitrogen %	20 *	20 *	20 ^	21.8 °	20 *	20 *
Proteins: % of total nitrogen content	0	0	100	95.93	0	0
Free AAs: % of total nitrogen content	100	100	0	4.07	100	100
EAA/NEAA (% in grams)	100/0	49/51	-	-	30/70	0/100
Free AAs composition (%)						
L-Leucine *(bcaa)*	31.25	9.5	–	–	9.4	–
L-Isoleucine *(bcaa)*	15.62	6	–	–	4.7	–
L-Valine *(bcaa)*	15.62	6.5	–	–	4.7	–
L-Lysine	16.25	7	–	0.97	6.24	–
L-Threonine	8.75	4	–	–	2.7	–
L-Hystidine	3.75	2.8	–	–	1.1	–
L-Phenylalanine	2.5	5	–	–	0.8	–
L-Cysteine	–	0.8	–	–	–	–
L-Cystine	3.75	–	–	0.39	1.1	–
L-Methionine	1.25	2.5	–	0.45	0.4	–
L-Tyrosine	0.75	5	–	–	2.6	1.0
L-Triptophan	0.5	1.3	–	0.28	0.01	–
L-Alanine	–	3.2	–	–	24.0	35.0
L-Glycine	–	2.4	–	0.88	10.39	15.0
L-Arginine	–	3.4	–	1.1	13.5	14.0
L-Proline	–	9.5	–	–	8.2	12.0
L-Glutamine	–	9.5	–	–	3.0	12.0
L-Serine	–	5.1	–	–	4.1	6.0
L-Glutamic Acid	–	9.5	–	–	2.5	2.0
L-Asparagine	–	3.5	–	–	0.79	2.0
L-Aspartic Acid	–	3.5	–	–	1.1	1.0

* Nitrogen (%) from free amino acids (AAs) only. ° Nitrogen (%) from vegetable and animal proteins and added AAs. ^ whole casein protein. EAA-100% = free essential amino acid-exclusive diet; Casein-AA = Casein-like free AAs diet; Casein-Prot = Casein whole protein diet; StD = Standard diet; EAA-30% = free essential amino acid-poor diet; NEAA-100% = non-essential free amino acid-exclusive diet. The black line represents the limit between EAA (above) and NEAA (below). *bcaa* = branched-chain amino acids.

2.3. Data and Sample Collections

Body weight (BW), mean food and water consumption (g/days and mL/day, respectively) were calculated weekly in all groups. Mortality was monitored daily.

Animals from the two groups fed with NEAA-100% and EAA-30% had a mortality > 70% at the 7th week, and all those still surviving were euthanized for ethical reasons linked to a drop in weight, as discussed in results. Five animals from each of the other groups were euthanized after 12 and 18 months to check their morphometric and clinical parameters. Specifically, BW and nose–tail length (body length, BL) were measured. Blood samples from the hearts and urine from the bladders were immediately collected for further analysis. Glycaemia was also measured by a glucometer in venous blood samples collected from tail veins. Subsequently, the heart, kidneys, liver, spleen, *triceps surae*, retroperitoneal white adipose tissue (rpWAT) pad and brown adipose tissue (BAT) were quickly removed and weighed [30].

2.4. Blood and Urine Analysis

Blood samples were collected either in tubes containing the K3-EDTA anti-coagulant for cell count analysis, or in tubes without anti-coagulants for serum separation. The blood cell count was performed with a Cell-Dyn 3700 laser-impedance cell counter (Abbott Diagnostics Division, Abbott Laboratories, IL, USA). Serum and urine levels of albumin and creatinine were assessed with an ILab Aries (Instrumentation Laboratory, Lexington, MA, USA) automatic analyzer. Serum levels of haptoglobin (Hpg) [31] and the neutrophils to lymphocytes ratio (NLR) [32,33] were also assessed as inflammatory markers. These analyses were carried out by personnel of the "Division of Laboratory Animals" of IZSLER (Brescia, Italy).

2.5. Statistical Analysis

Differences between experimental groups were evaluated by one-way analysis of variance (ANOVA) followed by a Bonferroni test or Student t-test when appropriate. All analyses were performed using the Primer of Biostatistics software, with statistical significance set at $p < 0.05$.

Spearman (r) regression values were calculated and reported where appropriate. A Mantel–Cox test (z) was used to test survival differences between diets [34].

3. Results

The average survival time was markedly reduced in animals fed with the two diets where EAA were absent or deficient. Indeed, NEAA-100% diet allowed a lifespan of 44.56 ± 3.85 days, while the lifespan of EAA-30%-fed animals was slightly prolonged at 53 ± 1.97 days, on average <20%. Animals fed with Casein-Prot and Casein-AA diets survived for maximum 14 and 16 months, respectively. StD-fed animals survived for maximum 22 months. The longest survival time (25 months) was observed for the EAA-100%-fed animals (Figure 1). The percentage of EAA in the diet is correlated with survival ($r = 0.901$, $p < 0.001$).

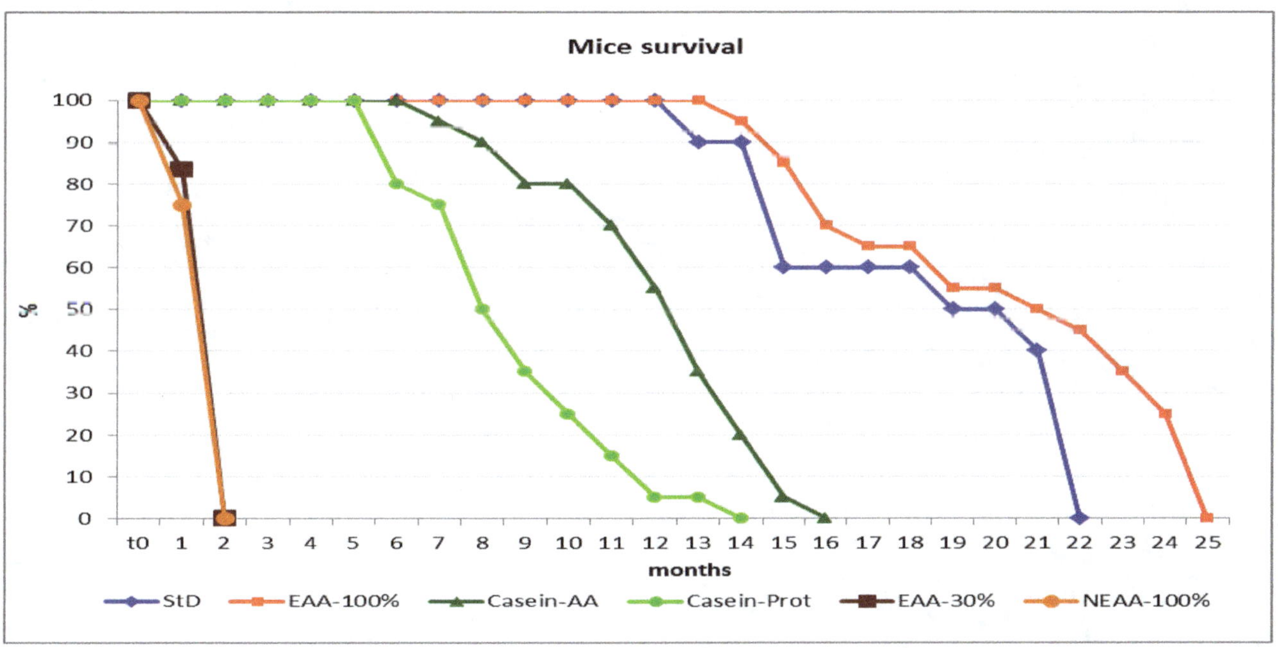

Figure 1. Percentage of mice's survival according to diet. Animals fed with NEAA-100% and EAA-30% diets (orange and brown lines) had shorter lifespans when compared to StD (blue line). It is interesting to observe the different survival curves between the animals fed with the diet containing casein whole protein (light-green line) and those fed with free AAs of casein (dark-green line). In addition, note the longest survival of the mice fed with EAA-100% diet (red line). Mantel–Cox test: Casein-AA vs. Casein-Prot, z = 3.95, p < 0.001; Casein-AA vs. StD, z = 5.17, $p < 0.001$; EAA-100% vs. StD, z = 2.28, p = 0.0226; EAA-30% vs. NEAA-100%, z = 0.21, p = 0.83.

3.1. Parameters Evaluation after 2 Months

3.1.1. Body Weight (BW) and Length (BL)

BW and BL are determined by the quality of nitrogen intake. For the diets poorest in EAA, NEAA-100% and EAA-30% diets, there is a rapid mortality correlating with BW loss ($r = 0.92$, $p < 0.000$) and also BL ($r = 0.99$, $p < 0.000$) when compared to all diets. A relatively modest increase in EAA provided by Casein-AA or Casein-Prot diet (which each contain about 19% more EAA than EAA-30% diet), drives a BL increase comparable to those observed in EAA-100% diet and StD. On the contrary, BW is most increased by StD and either Casein-Prot or Casein-AA diet. Instead, EAA-100% diet allows a growth in BL comparable to StD, Casein-Prot and Casein-AA.

EAA-100% diet induced the smallest BW increase among animals fed all diets compatible with prolonged lifespan. That is, the BW of EAA-100%-fed animals, while increasing if compared with the diets poorest in EAA (NEAA-100% and EAA-30%), is significantly less increased ($p < 0.001$) when compared to both StD and either Casein-Prot or Casein-AA diets.

The BW and BL of mice fed with Casein-Prot and Casein-AA diets were comparable to those of animals fed StD (see Table 2).

Table 2. Body weight (BW), body length (BL) and organ weight after 2, 12 and 18 months (mean ± sd).

	NEAA-100%	EAA-30%	EAA-100%	StD	Casein-Prot	Casein-AA		
2 months							*F*	*p*
Body W. (g)	7.09 ± 0.41 *^	7.31 ± 0.52 *^	14.93 ± 0.62 *	22.35 ± 1.9	22.02 ± 1.2	21.84 ± 0.9	238.26	0.000
Body L. (cm)	6.61 ± 0.1 *^	6.63 ± 0.12 *^	9.15 ± 0.13 *	9.66 ± 0.1	9.62 ± 0.2	9.47 ± 0.17	1024.88	0.000
Heart (g)	0.08 ± 0.015 *	0.08 ± 0.01 *	0.08 ± 0.03 *	0.13 ± 0.006	-	-	9.75	0.000
Kidneys (g)	0.12 ± 0.008 *^	0.12 ± 0.009 *^	0.24 ± 0.028 *	0.40 ± 0.05	-	-	105.71	0.000
Liver (g)	0.32 ± 0.049 *^	0.34 ± 0.61 *^	0.75 ± 0.066 *	1.10 ± 0.17	-	-	70.95	0.000
Spleen (g)	0.02 ± 0.004 *	0.02 ± 0.003 *	0.05 ± 0.008 *	0.11 ± 0.032	-	-	32.35	0.000
rpWAT (g)	0 *	0 *	0.02 ± 0.002 *	0.11 ± 0.02	-	-	123.97	0.000
BAT (g)	0.02 ± 0.01 *^	0.02 ± 0.009 *^	0.09 ± 0.01 *	0.13 ± 0.015	-	-	112.59	0.000
Triceps (g)	0.07 ± 0.01 *^	0.06 ± 0.002 *^	0.10 ± 0.011 *	0.19 ± 0.01	-	-	215.38	0.000
12 months							*F*	*p*
Body W. (g)	-	-	24.51 ± 1.9 *	31.78 ± 1.69	30.39 ± 2.79 ^	29.56 ± 1.0 ^	12.95	0.000
Body L. (cm)	-	-	9.82 ± 0.12	10.0 ± 0.13	10.01 ± 0.14	9.87 ± 0.13	2.65	0.085
Heart (g)	-	-	0.15 ± 0.02 *°	0.23 ± 0.03	0.18 ± 0.02	0.22 ± 0.05	6.51	0.000
Kidneys (g)	-	-	0.46 ± 0.06 *°§	0.8 ± 0.1	0.7 ± 0.05	0.69 ± 0.06	21.0	0.000
Liver (g)	-	-	1.36 ± 0.13 *°	1.79 ± 0.2	1.56 ± 0.2	1.7 ± 0.2	5.13	0.011
Spleen (g)	-	-	0.12 ± 0.03	0.15 ± 0.06	0.18 ± 0.02	0.15 ± 0.04	1.85	0.179
rpWAT (g)	-	-	0.07 ± 0.02 *§	0.17 ± 0.01	0.16 ± 0.08	0.09 ± 0.03 *	6.39	0.005
BAT (g)	-	-	0.13 ± 0.02 §	0.2 ± 0.04	0.23 ± 0.06	0.17 ± 0.03	5.62	0.008
Triceps (g)	-	-	0.18 ± 0.01 *°§	0.26 ± 0.02	0.31 ± 0.02 *	0.34 ± 0.03 *	54.35	0.000
18 months							*t*	*p*
Body W. (g)	-	-	23.67 ± 1.15 *	28.31 ± 1.04	-	-	6.692	0.000
Body L. (cm)	-	-	9.79 ± 0.11	9.95 ± 0.13	-	-	2.101	0.069
Heart (g)	-	-	0.15 ± 0.01 *	0.2 ± 0.01	-	-	7.906	0.000
Kidneys (g)	-	-	0.47 ± 0.04 *	0.68 ± 0.07	-	-	5.824	0.000
Liver (g)	-	-	1.18 ± 0.09 *	1.6 ± 0.15	-	-	5.369	0.000
Spleen (g)	-	-	0.08 ± 0.03 *	0.13 ± 0.04	-	-	2.236	0.000
rpWAT (g)	-	-	0.07 ± 0.03 *	0.11 ± 0.02	-	-	2.481	0.038
BAT (g)	-	-	0.12 ± 0.01 *	0.17 ± 0.01	-	-	7.906	0.000
Triceps (g)	-	-	0.15 ± 0.01 *	0.21 ± 0.01	-	-	9.487	0.000
22 months							*t*	*p*
Body W. (g)	-	-	22.2 ± 1.56 *	25.01 ± 1.2	-	-	4.515	0.000
Body L. (cm)	-	-	9.75 ± 0.12	9.81 ± 0.14	-	-	0.794	0.444

Note the similar changes in organ weight in EAA-30% and NEAA-100%-fed animals compared to StD after 2 months. Furthermore, it should be noted that the EAA-100% diet causes a slowdown in the BW and OW at all times compared to StD. ANOVA and Bonferroni t-test: * $p < 0.05$ vs. StD, ^ $p < 0.05$ vs. EAA-100%, ° $p < 0.05$ vs. Casein-AA; § $p < 0.05$ vs. Casein-Prot. WAT, white adipose tissue. BAT, brown adipose tissue.

3.1.2. Food and Water Consumption

The amounts of food and water consumed daily were influenced markedly by different diets. NEAA-100%-fed groups rapidly stopped growing in BL and showed a dramatically rapid BW loss similar to that of EAA-30% (Figure 2A), although the food consumption and therefore caloric intake of NEAA-100% during the first two weeks was significantly higher than any other diet except StD. With the proceeding of BW loss, and particularly in the 80% animals surviving after the sixth week, food consumption also declined, and all animals died in the following two weeks (Figure 2A,B). In NEAA-100%-fed animals, a striking difference between the grams of daily food intake, and thus calories, and BW was evident. Indeed, NEAA-100% and EAA-30%-fed animals progressively decreased in BW although their caloric intake was similar to that of EAA-100%-fed animals. Indeed, the correlation (r) between NEAA-100% or EAA-30% food intake and BW was –0.3 or –0.5, respectively. On the contrary, there was a higher correlation between EAA-100% food intake and BW ($r = 0.9$, $p < 0.001$) (Figure 2A,B). Only in the case of the NEAA-100% group, water consumption increased significantly from the first week of treatment ($p < 0.001$, about six-fold), and then decreased progressively to around the average water intake in StD-fed animals, before dying (Figure 2C).

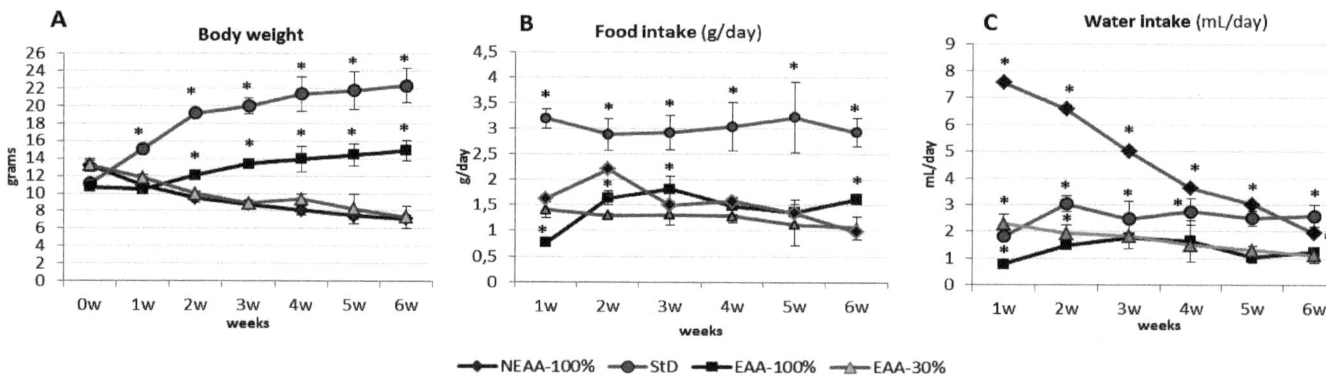

Figure 2. Comparison between BW (**A**), food (g/day) (**B**), and water (mL/day) consumption (**C**) (mean ± sd) of animals fed with NEAA-100% and EAA-30% diets, StD and EAA-100% diet after 6 weeks. NEAA-100% and EAA-30% diets drive rapid BW decrease, whereas EAA-100% diet slowly increases BW compared to StD (**A**). Note that EAA-100% diet was consumed in the same amount as NEAA-100% and EAA-30% diets (**B**). NEAA-100%-fed animals showed a higher water intake compared to StD, whereas EAA-30% and EAA-100%-fed animals had a lower water consumption than StD (**C**). Black square, EAA-100%; gray rhombus, NEAA-100%; gray triangle, EAA-30%; gray circle, StD. ANOVA and Bonferroni t-test, * $p < 0.05$ vs. all diets.

3.1.3. Organ Weights

The weights of specific organs (organ weight, OW) in animals fed with NEAA-100%, EAA-30% and EAA-100% diets were significantly lower than those in animals fed with StD. The weights of the kidneys, livers, BAT and *triceps surae* of the animals fed with NEAA-100% and EAA-30% diets were significantly less than those of the EAA-100%-fed animals. The OW of animals was similar in both NEAA-100% and EAA-30% diets but, interestingly, the rpWAT was near absent in those groups (Table 2).

3.1.4. Blood and Urinary Parameters

The two groups fed with NEAA-100% and EAA-30% diets had altered blood and urine parameters when compared to StD and EAA-100%-fed mice. This is especially evident in the reduction in blood concentration of hemoglobin and albumin, in the increase in neutrophils to lymphocytes ratio (NLR), and in the reduction of albumin and increase of creatinine in the urine. Blood and urine parameters from the EAA-100%-fed group did not differ from those of the StD-fed group, except for the Hpg value which was found to be lower (Table 3).

Table 3. Blood and urine data (mean ± sd) after 2, 12 and 18 months of treatment. See text for description.

	NEAA-100%	EAA-30%	EAA-100%	StD	Casein-Prot	Casein-AA		
Blood 2 months							F	p
Glucose (mg/dL)	108.3 ± 6.7 *^	111.7 ± 7.9 *	122.04 ± 8.1	127.3 ± 9.6	-	-	8.47	0.000
Erythrocytes (M/μL)	7.75 ± 1.93	8.01 ± 1.32	9.04 ± 0.58	9.13 ± 0.29	-	-	1.69	0.210
Hemoglobin (g/dL)	10.23 ± 2.37 *^	11.46 ± 2.15 *^	14.18 ± 1.16	14.8 ± 0.46	-	-	8.04	0.002
NLR	1.88 ± 1.02 *^	1.64 ± 0.93 *^	0.68 ± 0.26	0.67 ± 0.25	-	-	3.95	0.028
Albumin (g/L)	22.58 ± 1.68 *^	24.75 ± 1.56 *	26.8 ± 1.83	28.66 ± 2.57	-	-	9.03	0.000
Creatinine (μmol/L)	25.92 ± 4.54	24.95 ± 3.9	22.8 ± 1.75	23.82 ± 1.89	-	-	0.86	0.480
Haptoglobin (mg/mL)	0.02 ± 0.01 *^	0.04 ± 0.01 *^	0.13 ± 0.02 *	0.18 ± 0.02	-	-	113.83	0.000
Urine 3 months								
Albumin (g/L)	0.9 ± 0.4 *^	0.8 ± 0.6 *^	2.2 ± 0.4	1.8 ± 0.3	-	-	12.19	0.000
Creatinine (μmol/L)	5502 ± 443 *^	5653 ± 520 *^	3956 ± 824	4066 ± 1027	-	-	7.49	0.002
Blood 12 months							F	p
Glucose (mg/dL)	-	-	119.3 ± 11.4	124.3 ± 19.4	127.25 ± 14	113.25 ± 4.3	1.04	0.40
Erythrocytes (M/μL)	-	-	9.65 ± 0.62	9.93 ± 0.37	9.28 ± 0.33	9.8 ± 0.28	2.23	0.124
Hemoglobin (g/dL)	-	-	13.35 ± 1.02	14.4 ± 1.5	14.32 ± 0.3	14.4 ± 0.2	1.54	0.243
NLR	-	-	0.71 ± 0.1	0.72 ± 0.12	0.65 ± 0.07	0.67 ± 0.14	0.45	0.723
Albumin (g/L)	-	-	29.7 ± 1.7	30.88 ± 2.1	46.2 ± 8.03 *^	31.6 ± 6.6 ^	11.09	0.000
Creatinine (μmol/L)	-	-	46.9 ± 2.3	42.9 ± 5.7	72.33 ± 12.7 *^	57.0 ± 12.4	9.75	0.000
Haptoglobin (mg/mL)	-	-	0.10 ± 0.04 *	0.15 ± 0.07	4.53 ± 0.15 *^	4.97 ± 0.06 *^	3968	0.000
Urine 12 months								
Albumin (g/L)	-	-	2.13 ± 0.23	1.94 ± 0.21	1.3 ± 0.19 *^	1.02 ± 0.35 *^	21.46	0.000
Creatinine (μmol/L)	-	-	3581 ± 526	3832 ± 364	2934 ± 355 *^	2595 ± 222.7 *^	11.13	0.000
Blood 18 months							t	p
Glucose (mg/dL)	-	-	127.2 ± 8.3	133.4 ± 12.6	-	-	0.919	0.385
Erythrocytes (M/μL)	-	-	9.73 ± 0.25	9.97 ± 1.06	-	-	0.493	0.635
Hemoglobin (g/dL)	-	-	14.23 ± 0.15	14.87 ± 1.4	-	-	1.016	0.339
NLR	-	-	0.95 ± 0.2 *	1.44 ± 0.08	-	-	5.087	0.000
Albumin (g/L)	-	-	29.1 ± 0.7 *	27.4 ± 0.78	-	-	2.332	0.04
Creatinine (μmol/L)	-	-	38.3 ± 2.69	37.8 ± 1.45	-	-	0.366	0.724
Haptoglobin (mg/mL)	-	-	0.33 ± 0.15 *	0.56 ± 0.16	-	-	2.268	0.05
Urine 18 months								
Albumin (g/L)	-	-	1.58 ± 0.99 *	3.49 ± 0.87	-	-	3.241	0.01
Creatinine (μmol/L)	-	-	2954.9 ± 927	3421.7 ± 670	-	-	*0.913*	*0.388*

NLR = Neutrophils lymphocytes ratio. ANOVA and Bonferroni t-test: * $p < 0.05$ vs. StD, ^ $p < 0.05$ vs. EAA-100%.

3.2. *Parameter Evaluation after 12 Months.*

3.2.1. Body Weight and Length

After one year of follow-up, BW and length were still determined by the quality of nitrogen intake. The growth of mice on Casein-Prot-based diets did not differ from that of StD-fed mice. On the contrary, the EAA-100%-fed animals showed a more modest increase in BW, which remained significantly lower than the BW of the StD, Casein-Prot and EAA-100%-fed groups (Figure 3A, Table 2).

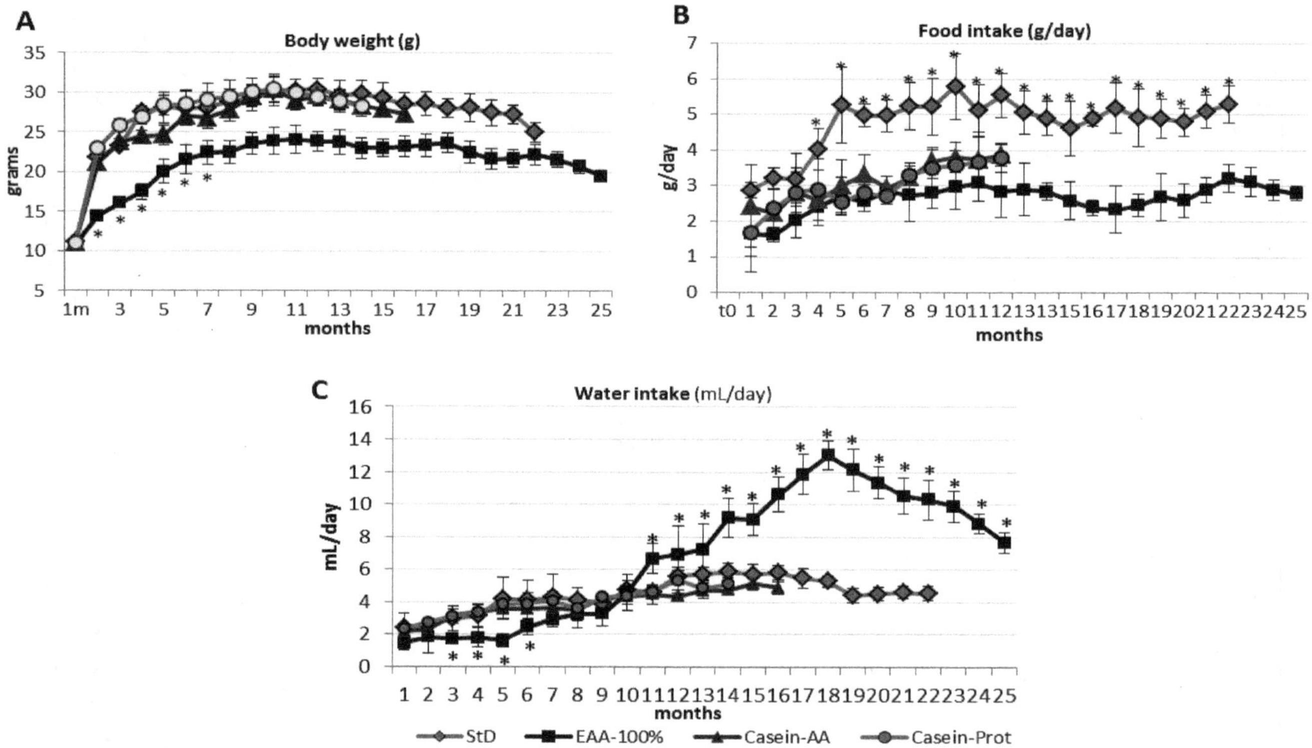

Figure 3. BW (**A**), food (**B**) and water (**C**) consumption (mean ± sd) according to StD, EAA-100%, Casein-Prot and Casein-AA diets during the whole survival period of mice. After about eight months, EAA-100%-fed mice significantly increase their water consumption (**C**), although food consumption (**B**) and BW (**A**) remain unchanged. See text for description. Black square, EAA-100%; gray rhombus, StD; gray triangle, Casein-AA; gray circle, Casein-Prot. ANOVA and Bonferroni t-test: * $p < 0.05$ vs. all diets.

3.2.2. Food and Water Consumption

The Casein-AA, Casein-Prot and EAA-100%-fed animals showed a substantially comparable daily food intake (g/day). All those groups registered a daily food consumption that was significantly reduced compared to that of the StD-fed animals, from the 4th month onwards. Water consumption (ml/day) was similar among StD, Casein-AA and Casein-Prot, whereas EAA-100%-fed mice showed a significantly increased water consumption starting from the eighth month and continuing all along the remaining follow-up (Figure 3C).

3.2.3. Organ Weights

Comparable to BW, mice from the EAA-100% group showed the lowest OW except for spleen. In particular, kidney and *triceps surae* weights were significantly lower than those recorded in all other groups. The heart weights of the EAA-100%-fed animals were significantly lower than in the StD and Casein-AA groups, whereas the rpWAT weights were lower in EAA-100% than in both StD and Casein-Prot groups. Liver weight was significantly higher in the StD and Casein-Prot and Casein-AA groups than in EAA-100%. BAT weight in EAA-100% was significantly lower than the Casein-Prot group, while animals fed with Casein-AA and Casein-Prot diets had a significantly increased *triceps surae* weight, when compared to the StD group. Interestingly, the Casein-AA diet induced a significant weight decrease for rpWAT, similar to that observed in EAA-100%-fed animals. On the other hand, rpWAT weights of mice fed Casein-Prot did not differ from those of mice fed with StD (Table 1).

3.2.4. Blood and Urinary Parameters

Serum concentrations of Hpg were markedly increased (about fifty times, $p < 0.001$) in animals fed with the Casein-AA and Casein-Prot diets as compared to StD-fed animals. In addition, mice fed with the Casein-AA and Casein-Prot diets had increased levels of serum and lowered levels of urinary albumin and creatinine. On the other hand, EAA-100%-fed animals had normal blood parameters and urinary concentrations of albumin and creatinine, and also showed a significantly lower Hpg level even compared to the StD-fed mice (Table 3).

3.3. Parameter Evaluation after 18 Months.

3.3.1. Body Weight and Length.

After 18 months, only animals fed with the StD and EAA-100% diets survived (Figure 1). EAA-100%-fed animals had lower BW than the StD-fed animals, whereas BL did not vary (Table 2). The fur appearance and spontaneous motor activity of EAA-100%-fed animals seemed to be preserved far better than in StD-fed ones. In fact, the animals fed with EAA-100% showed greater vitality than the others and often clung to the cage, keeping themselves suspended without difficulty.

3.3.2. Food and Water Consumption

The food consumption of EAA-fed animals was consistently lower than in StD-fed ones (Figure 3B). On the contrary, EAA-100%-fed animals showed a progressively and significantly increased water consumption (Figure 3C).

3.3.3. Organ Weights.

All OW of EAA-100%-fed animals were significantly smaller than StD-fed animals (Table 2).

3.3.4. Blood and Urinary Parameters

EAA-100%-fed mice had lower NLR, lower Hpg and higher serum albumin levels in comparison to StD-fed mice. Noticeably, urinary albumin losses were also the lowest in EAA-100%-fed animals (Table 3).

3.4. Parameter Evaluation after 22 Months

After 22 months, we were able to measure only BW and BL of the few surviving animals, i.e., four animals fed with StD and nine animals fed with the EAA-100% diet (Table 2). The four StD-fed mice died a few days after these last measurements. The EAA-100% fed mice, albeit showing lower BW, appeared vital, with thick and shiny furs (Figure 1). The last mouse died at the age of 25 months and belonged to the EAA-100% group.

4. Discussion

The main result of our study was the observation that the lifespan of mice was affected by the quality of the AAs content in the diets. Here, we have shown that the EAA-100%-fed animals lived the longest, although they had the lowest total energy (calories) intake, and the lowest BW compared to animals fed with the other diets, while growth in BL was unaffected. These observations confirm and extend previous studies in mice whose diets were supplemented with particular EAA blends, where a prolonged lifespan paralleled improved mitochondrial biogenesis and other parameters connected with healthy aging [11–13].

Furthermore, we also showed that the EAA-30% diet induced a progressive BW decrease by rapid loss of muscle mass and stopped growth in BL. This was followed by precocious death.

The diet without EAA (alias NEAA-100% diet) quickly arrested development and induced a rapid decay of animals' health, as the availability of EAA is, for instance, the main promoter of muscle protein anabolism [35]. However, the effects of NEAA-100% and EAA-30% diets were similar, suggesting that diets providing even a relatively modestly unbalanced lowering of the EAA/NEAA ratio, in our case a diet only about <20% poorer in EAA than the Casein-Prot and Casein-AA diets (common food proteins), may trigger a severe catabolic imbalance leading to body consumption and premature death. Since the animals fed with NEAA-100% and EAA-30% diets ate less than those fed with StD, at least in the last weeks of their short lives, this could lead to the obvious conclusion that the effects were due to quantitative (and thus caloric) malnutrition. However, the daily consumption of the NEAA-100% and EAA-30% diets was comparable to the consumption of the EAA-100% diet, but in this latter case, the'animals survived the longest and even longer than the StD-fed animals, albeit with reduced growth in weight (BW), but not length (BL). On this basis, we suggest that the EAA/NEAA ratio played a more prominent role than calories in ensuring animal well-being and survival.

Special NEAA-100% and EAA-30% (thus NEAA-70%) diets strongly reduced the mass of organs and determined a complete loss of rpWAT with a proportional decrease of BAT. This was unexpected, especially for the EAA-30% diet, suggesting again that a minor reduction in the EAA/NEAA ratio (EAA were <20% lower than in the Casein diets) can lead to extremely serious consequences for the whole body. In addition, we observed that malnutrition induced by NEAA-100% and EAA-30% diets led to a decrease in serum hemoglobin and albumin values. This was probably due to reduced protein synthesis and higher turnover, dependent on a poor EAA availability. However, direct and inhibitory effects exerted by elevated plasma NEAA on albumin synthesis cannot be excluded. In fact, this would be in agreement with previous observations in adult animals [27] and in undernourished patients [36,37].

Significant changes, induced by NEAA-100% and EAA-30% diets, were also observed for serum Hpg levels. Hpg is a hemoglobin-binding protein synthesized in the liver and released into the circulation, where it acts as an acute phase reactant protein. In fact, it increases during acute conditions such as infection, injury, tissue destruction, some cancers, burns, surgery or trauma, in response to inflammation. On the contrary, it decreases under other pathological conditions such as chronic liver disease, hematoma and hemolytic anemia. Because Hpg levels become depleted in the presence of large amounts of free hemoglobin, a decreased Hpg is considered a good marker of hemolysis [38,39]. In our experimental setup, the NEAA-100% and EAA-30% diets induced a sharp decrease in the serum Hpg level, but also induced higher NLR, with a concomitant decrease in hemoglobin concentration, red blood cell number and spleen mass. So, we believe that the very low level of Hpg observed in NEAA and EAA-30% diets was due not only to hemolytic events, but also to an impairment of Hpg synthesis by the liver. We also observed that the EAA-100% diet reduced Hpg level, but not NLR ratio, more than StD. This confirms that EAA have anti-inflammatory activity as observed previously [11,40].

All special diets were consumed in significantly lower quantities than StD, thus leading to a decreasing proportion of caloric intake. It is possible that StD has a more pleasing taste than other diets. However, in our recent work, we have observed that when mice can choose between special diets and StD, the StD is not the first choice [27]. Instead, previous studies have indicated an association between increased plasma AA concentration and decreased appetite [41]. So, the quick and free AAs availability provided by special diets can trigger satiety signals, thereby decreasing food intake. Interestingly, in the case of the diets containing casein, low intake did not influence BW and OW in comparison to StD. This suggests that caloric intake is not the only parameter that influenced BW. This agree with previous works showing that EAA/NEAAA ratio plays a pivotal role in changes in body composition [3,9,27]. In addition, according to previous authors, a difference in BW and OW between

EAA-100% diet and StD was observed, and we believe that this depends on the slowdown in growth caused by the EAA-100% diet.

Curiously, NEAA-100%-fed mice had an early and sharp increase in water intake without an increase in water retention. This finding agrees with previous observations in adult mice [27]. We believe that this may be related to enhanced muscle proteolysis and hyperosmolarity due to the increased release of different N-related products (such as creatinine) into the bloodstream. Indeed, all NEAA-100% and EAA-30%-fed mice had higher urinary creatinine levels compatible with muscular wasting induced by EAA deficiency. On this basis, we propose that animals fed with these diets could be used as an experimental model for muscle loss, since such a model would be inexpensive, easy to reproduce, and can be efficiently reversed by re-nutrition.

Besides StD, in line with previous studies [29,42], as a comparison we used two diets containing, respectively, casein in the form of the whole protein (Casein-Prot) or in the form of free AAs (Casein-AA) equivalent to the composition of casein, establishing a composition of reference (see Table 1). This was suitable for the purpose of comparing a whole protein needing digestion to its free AAs composition, which was more rapidly and completely available for absorption. Casein is a widely used protein in rodent pellets, but it has been shown not to provide sufficient amounts of sulphur-containing AAs, and therefore should be integrated with other proteins from animal sources in order to match the animals' needs for sulphur-providing AAs [29].

We compared two casein diets (-Prot and -AA) to evaluate possible biological differences between feeding proteins, which must be digested prior to absorption, and free AAs. Our choice was dictated by the fact that, unfortunately, an AAs composition of the commercially available StD was not available, since it contains 15% of unspecified "fish-based proteins" whose AAs composition is unknown to producers. On the contrary, casein-based diets were fully controlled in terms of AAs composition. Furthermore, an earlier study showed that the minimum concentration of casein which supports adequate growth, reproduction and lactation in mice was 13.6%, supplying 5.9 mg of total nitrogen/Cal [43]. Our Casein-Prot diet provided a 20% concentration of protein, thus ensuring adequate amounts of nitrogen to support growth, albeit with the cited and well known deficiencies in methionine and cisteine that identify this protein as not fully adequate to maintain a maximally prolonged life [29]. This is why we found that animals fed with Casein-Prot and Casein-AA diets had a drastically reduced survival in comparison to StD. Furthermore, Casein-Prot-fed animals lived shorter than Casein-AA-fed animals. These results might be interpreted on the basis of two main points: First, protein digestion was incomplete, since efficiency of protein digestion is <80% [44], indigested proteins contribute to fecal composition, and may thus have influenced both intestinal microbiota and promoted syntheses of some toxic metabolites [35,45]; second, the more efficient absorption of free AAs, coupled with the reduced metabolic costs of producing digestive enzymes [46] may have been responsible for survival differences. Thus, in line with previous clinical studies [47], we have shown here that the ingestion of EAA in a free form is a more efficient anabolic stimulus than the ingestion of a similar amount of AAs in the form of proteins, and that this kind of superior N intake can significantly affect life expectancy.

Animals fed with casein diets had no evident modifications of BW and BL, but lifespan was shorter compared to those on StD. However, although the animals ate significantly less calories and macronutrients than those on StD, their muscle mass increased significantly. This is in line with a previous work which has shown that casein protein intake could stimulate muscle protein synthesis without influencing lipid metabolism [48]. This observation opens some questions about the possible puzzling roles of methionine and cysteine in controlling protein syntheses and healthy life in humans and rodents. It is interesting to notice also that, by a different protocol, methionine restriction has been linked to improved lifespan in rodents, but administration of cisteine in a ratio suitable to match total sulphur containing amino acids needs, and also reducing methionine-linked toxicity, was not contemplated [20,49].

In any case, after 12 months, animals fed with casein diets had higher serum albumin (particularly in those fed with the Casein-Prot diet). High serum albumin, concomitantly with decreased urine albumin, suggests an improvement in both globular blood proteins synthesis and nephron function [50]. However, both casein diets also resulted in very high values of Hpg, suggesting that these diets provided some deficit-inducing high levels of chronic inflammation and potentially leading animals to their premature death when compared with StD or EAA-100% diet.

Indeed, after 12 months, the urinary creatinine excretion in the Casein-Prot-fed mice was lower, whereas the blood creatinine was higher than in the StD-fed animals. This finding would suggest an impairment of kidney function [51], although urinary albumin losses were unaffected. On the contrary, in Casein-AA-fed mice, although their urinary creatinine level reached lower values than in StD-fed mice, blood creatinine did not differ from that of StD-fed mice. This would suggest a more beneficial effect on the kidneys by the free AAs intake and absorption, when compared to feeding the whole proteins. Perhaps this unidentified mechanism also provides some effects connected to a potential advantage responsible for the longer lifespan observed in Casein-AA-fed animals when compared to the Casein-Prot-fed animals.

Animals fed with the EAA-100% diet survived longer than all other groups. This is in agreement with a previous study showing that this particular EAA-blend supplementation improves mitochondrial biogenesis, thus increasing lifespan [11]. However, we also observed that these mice had slower body growth and were always (at all times) smaller than those fed with control diets. However, since no significant difference in food consumption was observed between EAA-100% and other special diets, the weight difference was not attributable to the amount of calories introduced, but was very likely due to the quality of nitrogen (thus of AAs) present in the diet. This is in agreement with a recent work where animals fed with a special blend of EAA-100% diet for one month showed similar outcomes [27]. Furthermore, other studies have demonstrated that a prolonged life is correlated with a smaller body size, both in mice [52] and in humans [53], an effect also provided by caloric restriction, which also supports our thesis.

Unexpectedly, in animals fed with EAA-100% diet, we also observed a progressive increase in water intake after eight months on this diet, although hematologic and urinary parameters did not differ from StD-fed mice. Unfortunately, to our knowledge, there is no literature that can help us to explain this behavior which, however, had no adverse effect upon or even promoted animal health.

We also observed that the EAA-100% diet reduced inflammation, as suggested by the lower Hpg level found in animals on this diet, even when compared to StD. This is in agreement with the anti-inflammatory activity of EAA observed in previous experimental [11,40] and clinical settings [1,54,55]. Those effects on inflammation modulation could represent one of the mechanisms underpinning the longer lifespan reached by these animals.

The EAA-100% and Casein-AA diets induced a partial loss of rpWAT. rpWAT is a very plastic tissue capable of storing and releasing lipids in response to metabolic needs. A WAT decrease suggests a change in the balance of substrates used for energy production and/or an increased energy expenditure. However, it has been shown that mice fed with an L-leucine-deficient diet quickly reduced in their fat mass and lipogenic activity [56]. Our Casein-AA diet contained an adequate amount of L-leucine, whereas the EAA-Ex diet contained an even higher amount of L-leucine. Therefore, other factors besides leucine concentration are probably involved in fat loss. The reason why free AAs decreased rpWAT, and through which mechanisms, remains unclear, and further studies are necessary to have a clear picture of the mechanisms involved. In our opinion, it is the nitrogen quality in food, and not the amount of caloric intake, that determines the balance of deposited/consumed rpWAT in our study.

4.1. Clinical Implications

Our data suggest that it may be useful to reconsider some aspects of metabolic roles of dietary nitrogen supply in animals, as well as in humans. NEAA should be considered hidden enemies introduced through proteins, which, when introduced in excess, shorten lifespan and probably directly modulate, inhibit or blunt the synthetic activities promoted by EAA. We believe that integrating the nitrogen supply provided by diets through the supplementation of EAA, in order to increase the EAA/NEAA ratio to at least >1, should be the pivotal intervention that may most efficiently improve the life expectancy of malnourished people of any age.

The usual paradigm of clinical nutrition assumes that whatever is lacking should be provided. However, this does not seem to be true for NEAA. A better alternative would be the provision of sufficient amounts of balanced formulations of EAA, because these would better promote and maintain those metabolic pathways responsible for the synthesis of the NEAA as needed, and also of their precursors and derivatives. Indeed, balanced formulations of EAA and the unbalancing of EAA/NEAA ratios >1, promote the gene expression and activity of mTOR, PGC-1-alpha, SIRT-1, eNOS and also promote mitochondriogenesis [11]. These factors are known to be involved with optimal metabolic performances in any physiological or pathological condition and at any age, and also are effective in vitro in inducing apoptosis in cancer cells [19]. An unresolved question is now if NEAA, on the contrary, inhibit some of the pathways epigenetically activated by EAA.

4.2. Study limitations

Our study has some limitations that need to be discussed. We used an EAA-100% formulation tailored to human needs, and thus presently used as a nutritional supplement for humans. Furthermore, the impossibility, in our experimental settings, to conduct precise bromatological analyses of the AAs content provided by the StD, so to control the possible variations that may exist among batches even when provided by the same producer, is of some concern and causes possible unexpected bias.

We also did not separately evaluate the contributions of individual AAs with respect to body changes. However, these probably had a mild influence on the overall results of the study. Therefore, investigating the effects of individual, or of a few, AAs, although interesting from a doctrinal point of view, would not reflect the complexity of nutritional needs and survival requirements linked to optimal animal nutrition and metabolism. This complexity is also demonstrated by testing with a known deficiency diet, such as that based only on casein protein and the peculiar amino acids ratios provided by casein.

5. Conclusions

We investigated the effects of different diets providing the same amount of carbohydrates, lipids, micronutrients and nitrogen, but containing various proteins or free EAA/NEAA ratios, on lifespan in mice. To our knowledge, this is the first report showing that diets providing nitrogen as free EAA are compatible with a prolonged lifespan in mice. The most relevant finding of our study was the inverse relationship between NEAA dietary content and lifespan. On the contrary, the diet with the highest amount of EAA increased lifespan and maintained low BW, while reducing systemic inflammation and preserving a balanced protein metabolism. On the contrary, the diet with a reduction of just less than 20% in EAA content compared to that usually provided by food proteins (about 45/49%) triggered the rapid catabolic processes characterized by rapid muscle mass loss, and led to precocious death of animals. We confirmed that casein, although among the reference proteins for rodents, is a protein that does not allow a lifespan comparable to that allowed by standard laboratory diets and providing adequate amounts of sulphur-containing AAs, which are insufficiently present in casein. However, in casein diets we could observe that a formulation of free AAs reproducing casein AAs content promoted the longest survival, in our opinion probably consequent to a more elevated absorption of methionine and cisteine.

It is commonly claimed that lifespan is affected by the amount of calories consumed [57]. Our data suggest that this is an oversimplified assumption. On the contrary, lifespan is conditioned by EAA and NEAA dietary content, since this ratio modulates phenotypic modifications in different organs, especially adipose and muscle tissues, and induces profound biological modifications. If we evaluate a diet in terms of the extension of lifespan, the total AAs content provided by any dietary protein should not be considered the optimal parameter. Indeed, our study suggests that an elevated intake of NEAA, provided by normal nutritional and food proteins, negatively affects health and correlates with lifespan, at least in mice. So, the concept of "optimal nutrition", being very hard to define anyway because it depends on so many variables (the aims of diet, sex, age, health, environment, species etc.), should be deeply revised on the basis of the present data. We think that the ratio among EAA and NEAA is the most likely factor responsible for the health-promoting effects of proteins in any diet, and eventually for prolonged or reduced survival, at least in rodents.

These data also led us to the question of why some AAs are provided exclusively with diet, whereas others can be synthesized by the organism itself. The origin and evolutionary significance of the relationships between EAA and NEAA is not known. We suggest as an hypothesis worth to be further explored, that the excessive introduction of NEAA may trigger certain natural selection mechanisms connected with the shortening of lifespan.

Author Contributions: Conceptualization, F.S.D., G.C. and C.R.; Methodology, G.C. and C.R.; Software, C.R. and G.C.; Formal Analysis, V.F., E.P., G.C.; Investigation, G.C. and C.R.; Data Curation, G.C., C.R. V.F.; Writing—Original Draft Preparation, G.C., C.R., V.F. and E.P.; Writing—Review, E.M., A.P., R.C. and F.S.D.; Writing—Editing. C.R., G.C., V.F.; Supervision, F.S.D.; Project Administration, F.S.D.; Funding Acquisition, F.S.D. and G.C.

Abbreviations

AAs, amino acids; BAT, brown adipose tissue; BW, body weight; BL, body length; EAA, essential amino acids; Hpg, haptoglobin; NEAA, non-essential amino acids; N, nitrogen; NLR, neutrophils-lymphocytes ratio; OW, organ weight; rpWAT, retroperitoneal white adipose tissue; StD, standard diet.

References

1. Pasini, E.; Corsetti, G.; Aquilani, R.; Romano, C.; Picca, A.; Calvani, R.; Dioguardi, F.S. Protein-amino acid metabolism disarrangements: The hidden enemy of chronic age-related conditions. *Nutrients* **2018**, *10*, 391. [CrossRef] [PubMed]
2. Guigoz, Y. The mini nutritional assessment review of the literature: What does it tell us? *J. Nutr. Health Aging* **2006**, *10*, 466–485. [PubMed]
3. Wu, G. Amino acids: Metabolism, functions, and nutrition. *Amino Acids* **2009**, *37*, 1–17. [CrossRef] [PubMed]
4. Hou, Y.; Yin, Y.; Wu, G. Dietary essentiality of "nutritionally non-essential amino acids" for animals and humans. *Exp. Biol. Med. (Maywood)* **2015**, *240*, 997–1007. [CrossRef] [PubMed]
5. Borman, A.; Wood, T.R.; Balck, H.C.; Anderson, E.G.; Oesterling, M.J.; Womack, M.; Rose, W.C. The role of arginine in growth with some observations on the effects of argininic acid. *J. Biol. Chem.* **1946**, *166*, 585–594. [PubMed]
6. Reeds, P.J. Dispensable and indispensable amino acids for humans. *J. Nutr.* **2000**, *130*, 1835S–1840S. [CrossRef] [PubMed]
7. Ren, W.; Yin, Y.; Liu, G.; Yu, X.; Li, Y.; Yang, G.; Li, T.; Wu, G. Effect of dietary arginine supplementation on reproductive performance of mice with porcine circovirus type 2 infection. *Amino Acids* **2012**, *42*, 2089–2094. [CrossRef]
8. Rose, W.C.; Oesterling, M.J.; Womack, M.J. Comparative growth on diets containing ten and 19 amino acids, with further observations upon the role of glutamic and aspartic acids. *Biol. Chem.* **1948**, *176*, 753–762.
9. Wu, G.; Wu, Z.; Dai, Z.; Yang, Y.; Wang, W.; Liu, C.; Wang, B.; Wang, J.; Yin, Y. Dietary requirements of "nutritionally non-essential amino acids" by animals and humans. *Amino Acids* **2013**, *44*, 1107–1113. [CrossRef]

10. Civitarese, A.E.; Carling, S.; Heilbronn, L.K.; Hulver, M.H.; Ukropcova, B.; Deutsch, W.A.; Smith, S.R.; Ravussin, E.; CALERIE Pennington Team. Calorie restriction increases muscle mitochondrial biogenesis in healthy humans. *PLoS Med.* **2007**, *4*, e76. [CrossRef]
11. D'Antona, G.; Ragni, M.; Cardile, A.; Tedesco, L.; Dossena, M.; Bruttini, F.; Caliaro, F.; Corsetti, G.; Bottinelli, R.; Carruba, M.O.; et al. Branched-chain amino acid supplementation promotes survival and supports cardiac and skeletal muscle mitochondrial biogenesis in middle-aged mice. *Cell Metab.* **2010**, *12*, 362–372. [CrossRef] [PubMed]
12. Corsetti, G.; Pasini, E.; D'Antona, G.; Nisoli, E.; Flati, V.; Assanelli, D.; Dioguardi, F.S.; Bianchi, R. Morphometric changes induced by amino acid supplementation in skeletal and cardiac muscles of old mice. *Am. J. Cardiol.* **2008**, *101*, S26–S34. [CrossRef] [PubMed]
13. Flati, V.; Pasini, E.; D'Antona, G.; Speca, S.; Toniato, E.; Martinotti, S. Intracellular mechanisms of metabolism regulation: The role of signaling via the mammalian target of rapamycin pathway and other routes. *Am. J. Cardiol.* **2008**, *101*, 16E–21E. [CrossRef] [PubMed]
14. Stacchiotti, A.; Corsetti, G.; Lavazza, A.; Rezzani, R. Microscopic features of mitochondria rejuvenation by amino acids. In *Current Microscopy Contributions to Advances in Science and Technology*; Méndez-Vilas, A., Ed.; Formatex Research Center: Badajoz, Spain, 2012; pp. 286–294.
15. Corsetti, G.; Stacchiotti, A.; Tedesco, L.; D'Antona, G.; Pasini, E.; Dioguardi, F.S.; Nisoli, E.; Rezzani, R. Essential amino acid supplementation decreases liver damage induced by chronic ethanol consumption in rats. *Int. J. Immunopathol. Pharmacol.* **2011**, *24*, 611–619. [CrossRef] [PubMed]
16. Tedesco, L.; Corsetti, G.; Ruocco, C.; Ragni, M.; Rossi, F.; Carruba, M.O.; Valerio, A.; Nisoli, E. A specific amino acid formula prevents alcoholic liver disease in rodents. *Am. J. Physiol. Gastrointest. Liver Physiol.* **2018**, *314*, G566–G582. [CrossRef] [PubMed]
17. Corsetti, G.; D'Antona, G.; Ruocco, C.; Stacchiotti, A.; Romano, C.; Tedesco, L.; Dioguardi, F.S.; Rezzani, R.; Nisoli, E. Dietary supplementation with essential amino acids boots the beneficial effects of rosuvastatin on mouse kidney. *Amino Acids* **2014**, *6*, 2189–2203. [CrossRef]
18. Corsetti, G.; Romano, C.; Pasini, E.; Marzetti, E.; Calvani, R.; Picca, A.; Flati, V.; Dioguardi, F.S. Diet enrichment with a specific essential free amino acid mixture improves healing of undressed wounds in aged rats. *Exp. Geront.* **2017**, *96*, 138–145. [CrossRef] [PubMed]
19. Bonfili, L.; Cecarini, V.; Cuccioloni, M.; Angeletti, M.; Flati, V.; Corsetti, G.; Pasini, E.; Dioguardi, F.S.; Eleuteri, A.M. Essential amino acid mixtures drive cancer cells to apoptosis through proteasome inhibition and autophagy activation. *FEBS J.* **2017**, *284*, 1726–1737. [CrossRef]
20. Dioguardi, F.S. Clinical use of amino acids as dietary supplement: Pros and cons. *J. Cachexia Sarcopenia Muscle* **2011**, *2*, 75–80. [CrossRef]
21. Wanders, D.; Forney, L.A.; Stone, K.P.; Burk, D.H.; Pierse, A.; Gettys, T.W. FGF21 mediates the thermogenic and insulin-sensitizing effects of dietary methionine restriction but not its effects on hepatic lipid metabolism. *Diabetes* **2017**, *66*, 858–867. [CrossRef]
22. Cummings, N.E.M.; Williams, E.M.; Kasza, I. Restoration of metabolic health by decreased consumption of branched-chain amino acids. *J. Physiol.* **2018**, *596*, 623–645. [CrossRef] [PubMed]
23. Wanders, D.; Stone, K.P.; Dille, K.; Simon, J.; Pierse, A.; Gettys, T.W. Metabolic responses to dietary leucine restriction involve remodeling of adipose tissue and enhanced hepatic insulin signaling. *Biofactors* **2015**, *41*, 391–402. [CrossRef] [PubMed]
24. Simpson, S.J.; Le Couteur, D.G.; Raubenheimer, D.; Solon-Biet, S.M.; Cooney, G.J.; Cogger, V.C.; Fontana, L. Dietary protein, aging and nutritional geometry. *Ageing Res. Rev.* **2017**, *39*, 78–86. [CrossRef] [PubMed]
25. Le Couteur, D.G.; Solon-Biet, S.; Wahl, D.; Cogger, V.C.; Willcox, B.J.; Willcox, D.C.; Raubenheimer, D.; Simpson, S.J. New Horizons: Dietary protein, ageing and the Okinawan ratio. *Age Ageing* **2016**, *45*, 443–447. [CrossRef] [PubMed]
26. Le Couteur, D.G.; Solon-Biet, S.; Cogger, V.C.; Mitchell, S.J.; Senior, A.; de Cabo, R.; Raubenheimer, D.; Simpson, S.J. The impact of low-protein high-carbohydrate diets on aging and lifespan. *Cell Mol. Life Sci.* **2016**, *73*, 1237–1252. [CrossRef]
27. Corsetti, G.; Pasini, E.; Romano, C.; Calvani, R.; Picca, A.; Marzetti, E.; Flati, V.; Dioguardi, F.S. Body weight loss and tissue wasting in late middle-aged mice on slightly imbalanced essential/non-essential amino acids diet. *Front. Med. (Lausanne)* **2018**, *17*, 136. [CrossRef] [PubMed]

28. Pasini, E.; Aquilani, R.; Dioguardi, F.S.; D'Antona, G.; Gheorghiade, M.; Taegtmeyer, H. Hypercatabolic syndrome: Molecular basis and effects of nutritional supplements with amino acids. *Am. J. Cardiol.* **2008**, *101*, 11E–15E. [CrossRef]
29. Reeves, P.G.; Forrest, H.; Nielsen, F.H.; Fahey, G.C., Jr. AIN-93 Purified diets for laboratory rodents: Final report of the american institute of nutrition ad hoc writing committee on the reformulation of the AIN-76A rodent diet. *J. Nutr.* **1993**, *123*, 1939–1951. [CrossRef] [PubMed]
30. Blouet, C.; Mariotti, F.; Azzout-Marniche, D.; Bos, C.; Mathé, V.; Tomé, D.; Huneau, J.F. The reduced energy intake of rats fed a high-protein low-carbohydrate diet explains the lower fat deposition, but macronutrient substitution accounts for the improved glycemic control. *J. Nutr.* **2006**, *136*, 1849–1854. [CrossRef] [PubMed]
31. French, T. Acute phase proteins. In *The Clinical Chemistry of Laboratory Animals*; Loeb, W.F., Quimby, F.W., Eds.; Pergamon Press: Oxford, UK, 1989; Volume 1, pp. 201–235.
32. Ouellet, G.; Malhotra, R.; Penne, E.L.; Usvya, L.; Levin, N.W.; Kotanko, P. Neutrophil-lymphocyte ratio as a novel predictor of survival in chronic hemodialysis patients. *Clin. Nephrol.* **2016**, *85*, 191–198. [CrossRef]
33. Prats-Puig, A.; Gispert-Saüch, M.; Díaz-Roldán, F.; Carreras-Badosa, G.; Osiniri, I.; Planella-Colomer, M.; Mayol, L.; de Zegher, F.; Ibánez, L.; Bassols, J.; et al. Neutrophil-to-lymphocyte ratio: An inflammation marker related to cardiovascular risk in children. *Thromb. Haemost.* **2015**, *114*. [CrossRef]
34. Evan's Awesome A/B Tools. Available online: http://www.evanmiller.org/ab-testing/survival-curves.html (accessed on 8 May 2019).
35. Volpi, E.; Kobayashi, H.; Sheffield-Moore, M.; Mittendorfer, B.; Wolfe, R.R. Essential amino acids are primarily responsible for the amino acid stimulation of muscle protein anabolism in healthy elderly adults. *Am. J. Clin. Nutr.* **2003**, *78*, 250–258. [CrossRef] [PubMed]
36. Mitrache, C.; Passweg, J.R.; Libura, J.; Petrikkos, L.; Seiler, W.O.; Gratwohl, A.; Stähelin, H.B.; Tichelli, A. Anemia: An indicator for malnutrition in the elderly. *Ann. Hematol.* **2001**, *80*, 295–298. [CrossRef] [PubMed]
37. Ou, S.M.; Chen, Y.T.; Hung, S.C.; Shih, C.J.; Lin, C.H.; Chiang, C.K.; Tarng, D.C. Taiwan Geriatric Kidney Disease (TGKD) Research Group: Association of estimated glomerular filtration rate with all-cause and cardiovascular mortality: The role of malnutrition-inflammation-cachexia syndrome. *J. Cachexia Sarcopenia Muscle* **2016**, *7*, 144–151. [CrossRef] [PubMed]
38. Shih, A.W.; McFarlane, A.; Verhovsek, M. Haptoglobin testing in hemolysis: Measurement and interpretation. *Am. J. Hematol.* **2014**, *89*, 443–447. [CrossRef] [PubMed]
39. Irwin, D.C.; Hyen Baek, J.; Hassell, K.; Nuss, R.; Eigenberger, P.; Lisk, C.; Loomis, Z.; Maltzahn, J.; Stenmark, K.R.; Nozik-Grayck, E.; et al. Hemoglobin-induced lung vascular oxidation, inflammation, and remodeling contribute to the progression of hypoxic pulmonary hypertension and is attenuated in rats with repeated-dose haptoglobin administration. *Free Radic. Biol. Med.* **2015**, *82*, 50–62. [CrossRef] [PubMed]
40. Romano, C.; Corsetti, G.; Pasini, E.; Flati, V.; Dioguardi, F.S. Dietary modifications of nitrogen intake decreases inflammation and promotes rejuvenation of spleen in aged mice. *J. Food Nutr. Res.* **2018**, *6*, 419–432. [CrossRef]
41. Potier, M.; Darcela, N.; Tome, D. Protein, amino acids and the control of food intake. *Curr. Opin. Clin. Nutr. Metab. Care* **2009**, *12*, 54–58. [CrossRef]
42. Dubos, R.; Schaedler, R.W.; Costello, R. Lasting biological effects of early environmental influences. 1. Conditioning of adult size by prenatal and postnatal nutrition. *J. Exp. Med.* **1968**, *127*, 783–799. [CrossRef]
43. Goettsch, M. Comparative protein requirement of the rat and mouse for growth, reproduction and lactation using casein diets. *J. Nutr.* **1960**, *70*, 307–312. [CrossRef]
44. Miner-Williams, W.; Deglaire, A.; Benamouzig, R.; Fuller, M.F.; Tomé, D.; Moughan, P.J. Endogenous proteins in terminal ileal digesta of adult subjects fed a casein-based diet. *Am. J. Clin. Nutr.* **2012**, *96*, 508–515. [CrossRef] [PubMed]
45. Jin, U.-H.; Lee, S.-O.; Sridharan, G.; Lee, K.; Davidson, L.A.; Jayaraman, A.; Chapkin, R.S.; Alaniz, R.; Safe, S. Microbiome-derived tryptophan metabolites and their aryl hydrocarbon receptor-dependent agonist and antagonist activities. *Mol. Pharmacol.* **2014**, *85*, 777–788. [CrossRef] [PubMed]
46. He, L.; Wu, L.; Xu, Z.; Li, T.; Yao, K.; Cui, Z.; Yin, Y.; Wu, G. Low-protein diets affect ileal amino acid digestibility and gene expression of digestive enzymes in growing and finishing pigs. *Amino Acids* **2015**, *48*, 21–30. [CrossRef] [PubMed]

47. Rondanelli, M.; Aquilani, R.; Verri, M.; Boschi, F.; Pasini, E.; Perna, S.; Faliva, A.; Condino, A.M. Plasma kinetics of essential amino acids following their ingestion as free formula or as dietary protein components. *Aging Clin. Exp. Res.* **2017**, *29*, 801–805. [CrossRef] [PubMed]
48. Jäger, R.; Kerksick, C.M.; Campbell, B.I.; Cribb, P.J.; Wells, S.D.; Skwiat, T.M.; Purpura, M.; Ziegenfuss, T.N.; Ferrando, A.A.; Arent, S.M.; et al. International Society of Sports Nutrition Position Stand: Protein and exercise. *J. Int. Soc. Sports Nutr.* **2017**, *14*, 20. [CrossRef] [PubMed]
49. Ables, G.P.; Johnson, J.E. Pleiotropic responses to methionine restriction. *Exp. Gerontol.* **2017**, *94*, 83–88. [CrossRef] [PubMed]
50. Levitt, D.G.; Levitt, M.D. Human serum albumin homeostasis: A new look at the roles of synthesis, catabolism, renal and gastrointestinal excretion, and the clinical value of serum albumin measurements. *Int. J. Gen. Med.* **2016**, *9*, 229–255. [CrossRef] [PubMed]
51. Gowda, S.; Desai, P.B.; Kulkarni, S.S.; Hull, V.V.; Math, A.A.; Vernekar, S.N. Markers of renal function tests. *N. Am. J. Med. Sci.* **2010**, *2*, 170–173.
52. Miller, R.A.; Chrisp, C.; Atchley, W. Differential longevity in mouse stocks selected for early life growth trajectory. *J. Gerontol. A Biol. Sci. Med. Sci.* **2000**, *55*, B455–B461. [CrossRef]
53. He, Q.; Morris, B.J.; Grove, J.S.; Petrovitch, H.; Ross, W.; Masaki, K.H.; Rodriguez, B.; Chen, R.; Donlon, T.A.; Willcox, D.C.; et al. Shorter men live longer: Association of height with longevity and FOXO3 genotype in american men of japanese ancestry. *PLoS ONE* **2014**, *9*, e94385. [CrossRef] [PubMed]
54. Aquilani, R.; Zuccarelli, G.C.; Condino, A.M.; Catani, M.; Rutili, C.; Del Vecchio, C.; Pisano, P.; Verri, M.; Iadarola, P.; Viglio, S.; et al. Despite inflammation, supplemented essential amino acids may improve circulating levels of albumin and hemoglobin in patients after hip fractures. *Nutrients* **2017**, *9*, 637. [CrossRef] [PubMed]
55. Boselli, M.; Aquilani, R.; Maestri, R.; Achilli, M.P.; Arrigoni, N.; Pasini, E.; Condino, A.M.; Boschi, F.; Dossena, M.; Buonocore, D.; et al. Inflammation and rehabilitation outcomes in patients with nontraumatic intracranial hemorrhage. *NeuroRehabilitation* **2018**, *42*, 449–456. [CrossRef] [PubMed]
56. Cheng, Y.; Meng, Q.; Wang, C.; Li, H.; Huang, Z.; Chen, S.; Xiao, F.; Guo, F. Leucine deprivation decreases fat mass by stimulation of lipolysis in white adipose tissue and upregulation of uncoupling protein 1 (UCP1) in brown adipose tissue. *Diabetes* **2010**, *59*, 17–25. [CrossRef] [PubMed]
57. Fontana, L.; Partridge, L.; Longo, V.D. Extending healthy life span–from yeast to humans. *Science* **2010**, *328*, 321–326. [CrossRef]

4

Germinated Pigmented Rice (*Oryza Sativa* L. cv. Superhongmi) Improves Glucose and Bone Metabolisms in Ovariectomized Rats

Soo Im Chung [1], Su Noh Ryu [2] and Mi Young Kang [1,*]

1 Department of Food Science and Nutrition, Brain Korea 21 Plus, Kyungpook National University, Daegu 41566, Korea; zizibe0312@nate.com
2 Department of Agricultural Science, Korea National Open University, Seoul 03087, Korea; ryusn@knou.ac.kr
* Correspondence: mykang@knu.ac.kr

Abstract: The effect of germinated Superhongmi, a reddish brown pigmented rice cultivar, on the glucose profile and bone turnover in the postmenopausal-like model of ovariectomized rats was determined. The ovariectomized Sprague-Dawley rats were randomly divided into three dietary groups (n = 10): normal control diet (NC) and normal diet supplemented with non-germinated Superhongmi (SH) or germinated Superhongmi (GSH) rice powder. After eight weeks, the SH and GSH groups showed significantly lower body weight, glucose and insulin concentrations, levels of bone resorption markers and higher glycogen and 17-β-estradiol contents than the NC group. The glucose metabolism improved through modulation of adipokine production and glucose-regulating enzyme activities. The GSH rats exhibited a greater hypoglycemic effect and lower bone resorption than SH rats. These results demonstrate that germinated Superhongmi rice may potentially be useful in the prevention and management of postmenopausal hyperglycemia and bone turnover imbalance.

Keywords: pigmented rice; germination; Superhongmi; bone metabolism; glucose

---

1. Introduction

Germination is considered as a simple, effective, and inexpensive method of improving the nutritional quality of rice [1]. The soaking of rice grains in water for a few days induces slight germination which causes an increase in nutrient bioavailability and absorption [2]. During germination, biochemical changes occur including the release of free and bound materials and the activation of dormant enzymes which break down large molecular substances, resulting in the generation of bioactive compounds and an increase in nutrients [3]. Germinated rice has been found to have higher amounts of bioactive compounds such as γ-oryzanol, γ-aminobutyric acid (GABA), tocopherols, and tocotrienols than non-germinated rice [4,5]. Moreover, it has been shown to possess strong antidiabetic, antihyperlipidemic, and antioxidative properties [1,6].

Pigmented rice cultivars with black, purple, red, or brown pericarp are known for their higher nutritional value and greater antioxidant potential than non-pigmented cultivars [7,8]. They contain high amounts of anthocyanins, phenolic compounds and bioactive components [9,10] and their consumption has been associated with a reduced risk of diabetes and cardiovascular disease [11]. Investigations on various pigmented cultivars revealed that ingestion of pigmented rice could improve the lipid and glucose profiles in mice, delay the starch and sugar absorption in rats, and suppress postprandial blood sugar elevation in human subjects [12,13].

Menopause, the permanent cessation of menstruation, promotes metabolic syndromes and increases the risk of diabetes, dyslipidemia, and obesity in women [14]. An elevation in the concentrations of glucose, insulin, cholesterol, and triglyceride has been observed in postmenopausal women relative to premenopausal ones [14–16]. Menopause is also believed to be associated with the pathogenesis of osteoporosis, a metabolic bone disorder characterized by enhanced bone fragility and increased fracture risk, in elderly women [17]. The rapid decrease of the ovarian hormone estrogen after menopause is regarded as the primary cause of these metabolic dysfunctions [14]. The surgical removal of ovaries, known as ovariectomy, mimics the estrogen-deficient condition in postmenopausal women. Hence, ovariectomized animal models are widely used in investigating the pathophysiological changes associated with menopause and in developing therapeutic strategies against menopause-induced metabolic disorders [18].

Superhongmi is a new pigmented rice cultivar with a reddish brown pericarp developed in Korea. Recent studies have shown that germinated Superhongmi rice has a strong antioxidant capacity and could improve the lipid metabolism in ovariectomized rats [19,20]. To further explore the therapeutic potential of Superhongmi rice against metabolic dysfunctions, particularly those caused by menopause, the present study investigated the effect of germinated Superhongmi rice on the glucose metabolism and bone turnover in the postmenopausal-like model of ovariectomized rats.

2. Materials and Methods

2.1. Rice Samples and Chemicals

Whole grains of Superhongmi rice were obtained from the department of Agricultural Science, Korea National Open University. They were grown from May to October 2014 in Dangjin, Chungcheongnam-do, South Korea. All chemicals and standards used in this study were of analytical grade and purchased from Merck KGaA (Darnstadt, Germany) and Sigma-Aldrich, Inc. (Steinhein, Germany).

2.2. Rice Germination

Dehusked whole rice grains were germinated following the method of Wu et al. [21] with slight modifications. The grains (50 g) were washed twice with distilled water to remove any dirt and placed evenly in a tray overlaid with cotton pads and cheesecloth. Distilled water (100 mL) was added and the whole tray was covered with a clean transparent plastic wrap with holes to allow for ventilation and incubated at 30 °C in an oven. The grains were regularly checked every 12 h to ensure there was no foul odor and fungal growth. After 72 h, the germinated rice grains, including the emerged radicles, were dried at 50 °C for 2 h, ground and pulverized (200–300 μm) using a grinding machine (HMF-3250S, Hanil Electronics, Seoul, South Korea), packed in hermetically sealed Ziploc plastic bags, and stored at −20 °C until further analysis. For the non-germinated samples, 50 g rice grains were washed, dried, ground (200–300 μm), and stored using the same method described above for the germinated grains. Both the germinated and non-germinated rice samples were analyzed for their bioactive compounds γ-oryzanol, GABA, phytic acid, tocols (tocopherols and tocotrienols), and policosanol, based on previously described methods [22–26] and for their proximate compositions using the methods of AOAC [27]. The results are shown in Table 1.

2.3. Animals and Diet

Thirty female ovariectomized Sprague-Dawley rats (10-week-old), weighing approximately 229 g each, were purchased from Central Laboratory Animal Inc. (Seoul, Korea). The animals were individually housed in a hanging stainless steel cage in a room (25 ± 2 °C, 50% relative humidity) with 12/12 h light-dark cycle and fed initially with a pelletized chow diet and distilled water ad libitum for 1 week. They were then randomly divided into three dietary groups (n = 10): normal control diet (NC) and NC diet supplemented with either 20% (w/w) non-germinated Superhongmi (SH) or germinated Superhongmi (GSH) rice powder. They were fed for 8 weeks and allowed free access to distilled water. The composition of the experimental diet (Table 2) was based on the AIN-93M diet [28]. At the end of the experimental period, the rats were anaesthetized with carbon dioxide by inhalation following a 12-h fast. The blood samples were drawn from the inferior vena cava into a heparin-coated tube and centrifuged at 1000× g for 15 min at 4 °C to obtain the plasma. The liver, heart, kidney, and white adipose tissues (perirenal and inguinal) were removed, rinsed with physiological saline, weighed, and stored at −70 °C until analysis. The current study protocol was approved by the Ethics Committee of Kyungpook National University for animal studies (approval No. 2015-0087).

Table 1. Bioactive components and proximate composition of Superhongmi rice powder.

Bioactive Compound	Non-Germinated	Germinated
γ-Oryzanol (mg/100 g rice)	33.21 ± 2.66	51.96 ± 1.99 [1,*]
GABA (mg/100 g rice)	98.54 ± 3.96	1102.02 ± 11.63 *
Phytic acid (mg/100 g rice)	2.01 ± 0.09	4.02 ± 0.14 *
Tocols (µg/100 g rice)	133.69 ± 8.62	256.79 ± 6.98 *
Policosanol (mg/100 g rice)	21.69 ± 1.02	26.51 ± 1.24 *
Proximate composition (% dry basis)		
Carbohydrates	76.58 ± 0.91 *	53.92 ± 0.98
Crude protein	7.11 ± 0.12 *	5.71 ± 0.41
Crude fat	2.31 ± 0.19	3.58 ± 0.17 *
Crude ash	1.34 ± 0.04 *	1.11 ± 0.02
Moisture	12.66 ± 0.32	35.68 ± 0.61 *

[1] Values are means ± standard error (n = 3); * indicates significant difference ($p < 0.05$) between germinated and non-germinated samples.

Table 2. Composition of experimental diets (%).

	NC [1]	SH	GSH
Casein	14.0	12.4	12.2
Sucrose	10.0	10.0	10.0
Dextrose	15.5	15.5	15.5
Corn starch	46.6	28.7	29.1
Cellulose	5.00	5.00	5.00
Soybean oil	4.00	3.50	3.24
Mineral mix	3.50	3.50	3.50
Vitamin mix	1.00	1.00	1.00
L-Cystine	0.18	0.18	0.18
Choline bitartrate	0.25	0.25	0.25
Non-germinated rice	-	20.0	-
Germinated rice	-	-	20.0
Total	100	100	100
Kcal	380	380	380

[1] NC, normal control diet (AIN-93M); SH, normal diet + non-germinated Superhongmi rice powder; GSH, normal diet + germinated Superhongmi rice powder.

2.4. Determination of Glucose Profile and Plasma Adipokine Levels

The levels of blood glucose and plasma insulin were determined using Accu-Chek Active Blood Glucose Test Strips (Roche Diagnostics, Berlin, Germany) and enzyme-linked immunosorbent assay (ELISA) kits (TMB Mouse Insulin ELISA kit, Shibayagi Co., Gunma, Japan), respectively. The hepatic glycogen level was determined using the anthrone-H_2SO_4 method with glucose as standard [29]. The homeostasis model assessment of insulin resistance (HOMA-IR) index was calculated using the equation described by Vogeser et al. [30]. The following plasma adipokines were analyzed using commercial assay kits: adiponectin (Shibayagi Co., Gunma, Japan), leptin (Cayman Chemical, Ann Arbor, MI, USA), resistin (B-Bridge International Inc., Santa Clara, CA, USA), and tumor necrosis factor (TNF)-α (Abcam, Cambridge, MA, USA).

2.5. *Determination of Hepatic Glucose-Regulating Enzymes Activities*

The liver tissue was homogenized in a buffer solution containing triethanolamine, EDTA, and dithiothreitol and centrifuged at 1000× *g* at 4 °C for 15 min [31]. The pellet was removed and the supernatant was centrifuged at 10,000× *g* at 4 °C for 15 min. The resulting precipitate served as the mitochondrial fraction and the supernatant was further centrifuged at 105,000× *g* at 4 °C for 1 h. The resulting precipitate and supernatant served as the microsome and cytosol fractions, respectively. The protein content was measured using the Bradford protein assay [32]. The phosphoenolpyruvate carboxykinase (PEPCK) activity was determined based on the method of Bentle and Lardy [33]. The absorbance of the assay mixture was measured at 340 nm. The glucokinase (GK) activity was measured following the method described by Davidson and Arion [34]. The reaction mixture was incubated at 37 °C for 10 min and the change in absorbance at 340 nm was recorded. The glucose-6-phosphatase (G6pase) activity was determined using the method of Alegre et al. [35]. The reaction mixture was incubated at 37 °C for 4 min and the change in absorbance at 340 nm was recorded. The enzyme activities were expressed as μmol/min/mg protein.

2.6. *Measurement of Bone Metabolism Biochemical Markers*

The levels of calcium and alkaline phosphatase (ALP) were measured using Ca and ALP assay kits (Cobas, Indianopolis, IN, USA), respectively. The levels of 17-β-estradiol, intact parathyroid hormone (PTH), osteocalcin, *N*-terminal telopeptide of type 1 collagen (NTx-1) and *C*-terminal telopeptide of type 1 collagen (CTx-1) were analyzed using commercial assay kits (MyBiosource Inc., San Diego, CA, USA).

2.7. *Statistical Analysis*

All data are presented as the mean ± standard error (SE). The data were evaluated by one-way ANOVA using a Statistical Package for Social Sciences software program version 19.0 (SPSS Inc., Chicago, IL, USA) and the differences between the means were assessed using Tukey's test. An independent *t*-test was used to assess the difference between the germinated and non-germinated rice samples. Statistical significance was considered at $p < 0.05$.

3. Results

3.1. *Body and Organ Weights*

The final body weight markedly decreased in both SH (389 g) and GSH (374 g) groups relative to that of the control group (403 g) (Table 3). The feed intake and feed efficiency ratio were lowest in the GSH group and highest in the NC group. The white adipose tissue weight was lowest in GSH rats (8.56 g), followed by the SH group (9.04 g), then the NC group (10.26 g). The weights of liver and heart were significantly lower in the SH and GSH groups compared to that of the NC group.

3.2. *Glucose Profile*

As shown in Table 4, the final blood glucose level was lowest in the GSH group (5.04 nmol/L), followed by the SH group (5.61 nmol/L), then the NC group (6.98 nmol/L). The plasma insulin level was also lowest in the GSH group (3.39 mU/L) and highest in the NC group (4.93 mU/L). Accordingly, the HOMA-IR index was highest in the NC group (1.49), followed by the SH group (0.97), then the GSH group (0.78). Both the SH and GSH groups showed significantly higher hepatic glycogen level (149–153 mg/g) than the NC group (94.7 mg/g).

Table 3. Body weight gain and weights of organs and adipose tissue in ovariectomized rats fed with germinated Superhongmi rice powder.

Parameter	NC	SH	GSH
Initial weight (g)	229.24 ± 1.25	228.32 ± 1.18	228.14 ± 0.79
Final weight (g)	402.65 ± 5.33 [c]	388.69 ± 4.92 [b]	374.25 ± 5.41 [a]
Weight gain (g)	174.68 ± 5.63 [c]	160.24 ± 4.72 [b]	148.32 ± 3.30 [a]
Feed intake (g/week)	181.58 ± 4.32 [c]	162.25 ± 3.20 [b]	149.44 ± 3.41 [a]
Feed efficiency ratio	0.16 ± 0.00 [c]	0.14 ± 0.00 [b]	0.12 ± 0.00 [a]
White adipose tissue weight (g)	10.26 ± 0.19 [c]	9.04 ± 0.19 [b]	8.56 ± 0.12 [a]
Organ weight (g)			
Liver	2.88 ± 0.01 [c]	2.57 ± 0.02 [b]	2.50 ± 0.01 [a]
Heart	0.26± 0.01 [b]	0.23 ± 0.01 [a]	0.22 ± 0.01 [a]
Kidney	0.40 ± 0.01	0.39 ± 0.02	0.39 ± 0.04

[a–c] Values are means ± SE (n = 10). Means in the same row not sharing a common superscript are significantly different at $p < 0.05$. NC, normal control diet (AIN-93M); SH, normal diet + non-germinated Superhongmi; GSH, normal diet + germinated Superhongmi rice.

Table 4. Glucose profile, adipokine level, and glucose-regulating enzyme activity in ovariectomized rats fed with germinated Superhongmi rice powder.

Parameter	NC	SH	GSH
Initial blood glucose (mmol/L)	4.98 ± 0.02	5.01 ± 0.02	5.08 ± 0.02
Final blood glucose (mmol/L)	6.98 ± 0.05 [c]	5.61 ± 0.03 [b]	5.04 ± 0.03 [a]
Plasma insulin (mU/L)	4.93 ± 0.03 [c]	3.91 ± 0.05 [b]	3.39 ± 0.01 [a]
Hepatic glycogen (mg/g liver)	94.68 ± 2.26 [a]	149.25 ± 2.78 [b]	152.88 ± 3.07 [b]
HOMA-IR index	1.49 ± 0.00 [c]	0.97 ± 0.02 [b]	0.78 ± 0.00 [a]
Plasma adipokine			
Adiponectin (ng/mL)	0.26 ± 0.03 [a]	0.48 ± 0.03 [b]	0.71 ± 0.06 [c]
Leptin (ng/mL)	3.76 ± 0.27	3.32 ± 0.33	3.36 ± 0.26
Resistin (ng/mL)	32.55 ± 0.12 [c]	22.88 ± 1.43 [b]	18.25 ± 1.05 [a]
TNF-α (μg/mL)	9.58 ± 0.81 [c]	7.25 ± 0.58 [b]	4.51 ± 0.12 [a]
Hepatic glucose-regulating enzymes (μmol/min/mg protein)			
PEPCK	3.74 ± 0.87 [c]	2.98 ± 0.52 [b]	1.18 ± 0.41 [a]
GK	1.62 ± 0.13 [a]	2.89 ± 0.19 [b]	2.98 ± 0.22 [b]
G6pase	76.95 ± 1.32 [c]	68.33 ± 1.47 [b]	47.58 ± 1.51 [a]
GK/G6pase ratio	0.02 ± 0.00 [a]	0.04 ± 0.00 [b]	0.06 ± 0.00 [c]

[a–c] Values are means ± SE (n = 10). Means in the same row not sharing a common superscript are significantly different at $p < 0.05$. NC, normal control diet (AIN-93M); SH, normal diet + non-germinated Superhongmi rice; GSH, normal diet + germinated Superhongmi rice; HOMA-IR, homeostasis model of insulin resistance = (fasting insulin × fasting glucose)/22.5; TNF, tumor necrosis factor; PEPCK, phosphoenolpyruvate carboxynase; GK, glucokinase; G6pase, glucose-6-phosphatase.

3.3. *Plasma Adipokine Level*

The adiponectin level was highest in the GSH group (0.71 ng/mL) and lowest in the NC group (0.26 ng/mL) (Table 4). On the other hand, the levels of resistin and TNF-α were lowest in the GSH group and highest in the NC group. No significant difference was found in the leptin level among the animal groups.

3.4. *Hepatic Glucose-Regulating Enzymes Activities*

The hepatic PEPCK and G6pase activities were lowest in GSH rats and highest in the NC group (Table 4). Both the SH and GSH rats exhibited significantly higher GK activity (2.89–2.98 μmol/min/mg protein) than the control ones (1.62 μmol/min/mg protein). The GK to G6pase ratio was highest in the GSH group (0.06), followed by the SH group (0.04), then the NC group (0.02).

3.5. Biochemical Markers of Bone Metabolism

The GSH group showed significantly higher levels of 17-β-estradiol (0.87 ng/mL) and lower levels of intact PTH (18.05 pg/mL), NTx-1 (121.44 nmol/L), and CTx-1 (13.29 nmol/L) than the NC and SH groups (Table 5). No significant difference was found in the calcium and osteocalcin contents among the groups. The ALP level, on the other hand, was below 0.50 μg/L in all groups.

Table 5. Biochemical markers of bone metabolism in ovariectomized rats fed with germinated Superhongmi rice powder.

	NC	SH	GSH
17-β-estradiol (ng/mL)	0.47 ± 0.03 ᵃ	0.52 ± 0.02 ᵃ	0.87 ± 0.05 ᵇ
Intact PTH (pg/mL)	22.58 ± 0.63 ᵇ	21.22 ± 1.02 ᵇ	18.05 ± 0.57 ᵃ
Calcium (mg/dL)	9.65 ± 0.53	10.68 ± 0.43	10.58 ± 0.58
Osteocalcin (ng/mL)	13.55 ± 1.23	13.16 ± 0.73	12.57 ± 0.54
Alkaline phosphatase (μg/L)	$<0.50 \pm 0.00$	$<0.50 \pm 0.00$	$<0.50 \pm 0.00$
NTx-1 (nmol/L)	181.58 ± 2.37 ᶜ	145.25 ± 1.23 ᵇ	121.44 ± 3.45 ᵃ
CTx-1 (nmol/mL)	23.71 ± 0.85 ᶜ	18.69 ± 0.65 ᵇ	13.29 ± 1.58 ᵃ

[a–c] Values are means ± SE ($n = 10$). Means in the same row not sharing a common superscript are significantly different at $p < 0.05$. NC, normal control diet (AIN-93M); SH, normal diet + non-germinated Superhongmi rice; GSH, normal diet + germinated Superhongmi rice; PTH, parathyroid hormone; NTx-1, *N*-terminal telopeptide of type 1 collagen; CTx-1, C-terminal telopeptide of type 1 collagen.

4. Discussion

Ovarian hormone deficiency resulting from menopause or ovariectomy increases the risk of diabetes, obesity, dyslipidemia, and osteoporosis [14,17,36]. The present study analyzed the effect of germinated Superhongmi rice, a reddish-brown pigmented cultivar, on the glucose and bone metabolisms in the postmenopausal-like model of ovariectomized rats. Results showed that diet supplementation of germinated and non-germinated Superhongmi rice powder significantly decreased the body weight gain, amount of body fat, blood glucose level, and plasma insulin concentrations and increased the hepatic glycogen level in ovariectomized rats. Both the SH and GSH animal groups also exhibited a markedly lower HOMA-IR index—an indicator of insulin resistance—than the control group, suggesting an increase in the insulin sensitivity in these animals. Studies in the past have also shown that pigmented rice could lower the body weight gain and improve the glucose metabolism in both laboratory animals and human subjects [12,13]. Between the two Superhongmi rice-fed groups, the GSH rats exhibited a greater body weight-lowering effect and hypoglycemic activity than the SH group. Germinated rice, especially pigmented cultivar, contains substantially higher amounts of bioactive compounds than non-germinated rice [4,5,19]. In the present study, γ-oryzanol, GABA, phytic acid, tocols, and policosanol were significantly higher in a germinated rice sample than that of the non-germinated one. γ-oryzanol, GABA, and phytic acid have hypolipidemic, hypoglycemic, and anti-obesity effects [4,7,37–39]. The tocols and policosanol possess antioxidative and antidiabetic property [4,40,41]. Hence, the strong hypoglycemic activity observed in GSH rats relative to the SH group is probably due to the increased amounts of bioactives in the germinated Superhongmi rice. This increase in the bioactive content is caused by the breaking down of the cell wall during germination, releasing the free and bound materials, and the activation of dormant enzymes associated with the synthesis of bioactive compounds [3].

The metabolism of glucose is influenced by adipokines and glucose-regulating enzymes. The ovariectomized rats fed with germinated Superhongmi rice powder showed the lowest resistin and TNF-α levels and highest adiponectin concentration. They also exhibited the lowest PEPCK and G6pase activities and highest GK activity and GK/G6pase ratio. The adipokines resistin and TNF-α regulate the lipid and glucose metabolisms and their elevated levels have been associated with the progression of obesity and diabetes [42–44]. The adiponectin, on the other hand, induces insulin-sensitizing effects and its enhanced expression has been shown to improve insulin sensitivity and glucose tolerance while its deficiency could induce insulin resistance [42]. An elevated level of adiponectin has also been reported to protect postmenopausal women against the development of diabetes [45]. The PEPCK, GK, and G6pase are major enzymes associated with glucose metabolism, wherein PEPCK and G6pase are involved in the regulation of gluconeogenesis and hepatic glucose output and an increase in their activities could result in an increased production of glucose [46,47]. The GK enzyme, on the other hand, is involved in glucose homeostasis and its enhanced activity has been associated with an increased glycogen level and reduced blood glucose content [48]. The GK/G6pase ratio, which reflects the balance between glucose uptake and output, was highest in GSH rats, indicating an enhanced glucose metabolism in these animals. Thus, the increase in adiponectin level and GK activity and the reduction in resistin and TNF-α concentrations and PEPCK and G6pase activities are possibly responsible for the improved glucose profile found in the rice-fed ovariectomized rats, particularly the GSH group.

Menopause and ovariectomy cause metabolic dysfunctions due to the rapid decrease of the estrogen hormone [14]. In the present study, the GSH rats showed significantly higher amount of 17-β-estradiol—the most potent form of estrogen—than the control group, suggesting that the germinated Superhongmi rice was able to inhibit the ovariectomy-induced reduction of estrogen level in these animals. Estrogen plays a central role in the regulation of bone metabolism, and administration of 17-β-estradiol has been reported to decrease the rate of bone turnover and prevent bone loss in postmenopausal women [49–51]. The ovariectomized rats fed with germinated Superhongmi rice also exhibited relatively low levels of intact PTH, NTx-1, and CTx-1, which are biochemical markers of bone resorption, indicating a reduced bone turnover in the GSH group. Increased bone resorption and imbalanced bone turnover are considered the main cause of the rapid rate of bone loss and enhanced risk of bone fracture in postmenopausal women [51,52]. Rice cultivars with colored pericarp, such as Superhongmi, are rich in antioxidant compounds such as anthocyanins, tocols, γ-oryzanol, and phytic acid [53] and germination could further increase the amount of these antioxidant compounds. Germinated Superhongmi rice has been previously reported to contain a substantial amount of antioxidant compounds and to have a strong antioxidant capacity [19]. Past investigations revealed that dietary antioxidants could prevent bone loss in postmenopausal women and ovariectomized animals and may be useful in the prevention and treatment of osteoporosis [54,55]. Since oxidative stress plays a central role in the pathogenesis of osteoporosis [56,57], the antioxidant compounds present in germinated Superhongmi rice may have been partly responsible for the improved bone metabolism observed in GSH rats.

5. Conclusions

The pigmented rice Superhongmi significantly reduced the body weight gain, glucose level, insulin concentration, and bone turnover in the postmenopausal-like model of ovariectomized rats through a mechanism involving the regulation of adipokine production and modulation of glucose-regulating enzyme activities. Germination for 72 h further enhanced the hypoglycemic effect and bone metabolism-improving action of this pigmented rice cultivar which may have been due to the increased amounts of various bioactive compounds such as GABA, γ-oryzanol, and tocols. Germinated Superhongmi rice may be beneficial as a functional food with therapeutic potential against menopause-induced hyperglycemia and bone turnover imbalance.

Acknowledgments: This research was supported by Basic Science Research Program through the National Research Foundation of Republic of Korea funded by the Ministry of Education (2014R1A1A2056797), and Next-Generation BioGreen21 Program (PJ011089).

Author Contributions: S.I.C. and M.Y.K. conceived and designed the experiments; S.N.R. offered rice samples, S.I.C. performed the experiments and analyzed the data; S.I.C. and M.Y.K. wrote the paper. All authors approved the final version of the manuscript.

References

1. Wu, F.; Yang, N.; Toure, A.; Jin, Z.; Xu, X. Germinated brown rice and its role in human health. *Crit. Rev. Food Sci. Nutr.* **2013**, *53*, 451–463. [CrossRef] [PubMed]
2. Patil, S.B.; Khan, M.K. Germinated brown rice as a value added rice product: A review. *J. Food Sci. Technol.* **2011**, *48*, 661–667. [CrossRef] [PubMed]
3. Moongngarm, A.; Saetung, N. Comparison of chemical compositions andbioactive compounds of germinated rough rice and brown rice. *Food Chem.* **2010**, *122*, 782–788. [CrossRef]
4. Cho, D.H.; Lim, S.T. Germinated brown rice and its bio-functional compounds. *Food Chem.* **2016**, *196*, 259–271. [CrossRef] [PubMed]
5. Ng, L.T.; Huang, S.H.; Chen, Y.T.; Su, C.H. Changes of tocopherols, tocotrienols, γ-oryzanol, and γ-aminobutyric acid levels in the germinated brown rice of pigmented and nonpigmented cultivars. *J. Agric. Food Chem.* **2013**, *61*, 12604–12611. [CrossRef] [PubMed]
6. Mohd, E.N.; Abdul, K.K.K.; Amom, Z.; Azlan, A. Antioxidant activity of white rice, brown rice and germinated brown rice (in vivo and in vitro) and the effects on lipid peroxidation and liver enzymes in hyperlipidaemic rabbits. *Food Chem.* **2013**, *141*, 1306–1312. [CrossRef] [PubMed]
7. Kang, M.Y.; Rico, C.W.; Bae, H.J.; Lee, S.C. Antioxidant capacity of newly developed pigmented rice cultivars in Korea. *Cereal Chem.* **2013**, *90*, 497–501. [CrossRef]
8. Min, B.; McClung, A.M.; Chen, M.H. Phytochemicals and antioxidant capacities in rice brans of different color. *J. Food Sci.* **2011**, *76*, C117–C126. [CrossRef] [PubMed]
9. Deng, G.F.; Xu, X.R.; Zhang, Y.; Li, D.; Gan, R.Y.; Li, H.B. Phenolic compounds and bioactivities of pigmented rice. *Crit. Rev. Food Sci. Nutr.* **2013**, *53*, 296–306. [CrossRef] [PubMed]
10. Frank, T.; Reichardt, B.; Shu, Q.; Engel, K.H. Metabolite profiling of colored rice (*Oryza sativa* L.) grains. *J. Cereal Sci.* **2012**, *55*, 112–119. [CrossRef]
11. Ling, W.H.; Cheng, Q.X.; Ma, J.; Wang, T. Red and black rice decrease atherosclerotic plaque formation and increase antioxidant status in rabbits. *J. Nutr.* **2001**, *131*, 1421–1426. [PubMed]
12. Bae, H.J.; Rico, C.W.; Ryu, S.N.; Kang, M.Y. Hypolipidemic, hypoglycemic and antioxidantive effects of a new pigmented rice cultivar "Superjami" in high fat-fed mice. *J. Korean Soc. Appl. Biol. Chem.* **2014**, *57*, 685–691. [CrossRef]
13. Shimoda, H.; Aitani, M.; Tanaka, J.; Hitoe, S. Purple rice extract exhibits preventive activities on experimental diabetes models and human subjects. *J. Rice Res.* **2015**, *3*, 137. [CrossRef]
14. Carr, M.C. The emergence of the metabolic syndrome with menopause. *J. Clin. Endocrinol. Metab.* **2003**, *88*, 2404–2411. [CrossRef] [PubMed]
15. Akahoshi, M.; Soda, M.; Nakashima, E.; Shimaoka, K.; Seto, S.; Yano, K. Effects of menopause on trends of serum cholesterol, blood pressure, and body mass index. *Circulation* **1996**, *94*, 61–66. [CrossRef] [PubMed]
16. Otsuki, M.; Kasayama, S.; Morita, S.; Asanuma, N.; Saito, H.; Mukai, M.; Koga, M. Menopause, but not age, is an independent risk factor for fasting plasma glucose levels in nondiabetic women. *Menopause* **2007**, *14*, 404–407. [CrossRef] [PubMed]
17. Ji, M.X.; Yu, Q. Primary osteoporosis in postmenopausal women. *Chronic Dis. Transl. Med.* **2015**, *1*, 9–13. [CrossRef]
18. Brinton, R.D. Minireview: Translational animal models of human menopause: Challenges and emerging opportunities. *Endocrinology* **2012**, *153*, 3571–3578. [CrossRef] [PubMed]
19. Chung, S.I.; Lo, L.M.P.; Kang, M.Y. Effect of germination on the antioxidant capacity of pigmented rice (*Oryza sativa* L. cv. Superjami and Superhongmi). *Food Sci. Technol. Res.* **2016**, *22*, 387–394. [CrossRef]
20. Lo, L.M.P.; Kang, M.Y.; Yi, S.J.; Chung, S.I. Dietary supplementation of germinated pigmented rice (*Oryza sativa* L.) lowers dyslipidemia risk in ovariectomized Sprague-Dawley rats. *Food Nutr. Res.* **2016**, *60*. [CrossRef] [PubMed]
21. Wu, F.; Chen, H.; Yang, N.; Wang, J.; Duan, X.; Jin, Z.; Xu, X. Effect on germination time on physicochemical properties of brown rice flour and starch from different rice cultivars. *J. Cereal Sci.* **2013**, *58*, 263–271. [CrossRef]
22. Chakuton, K.; Puangpronpitag, D.; Nakornriab, M. Phytochemical Content and Antioxidant Activity of Colored and Non-colored Thai Rice Cultivars. *Asian J. Plant Sci.* **2012**, *11*, 285–293.

23. Islam, M.A.; Becerra, J.X. Analysis of chemical components involved in germination process of rice variety Jhapra. *J. Sci. Res.* **2012**, *4*, 251–262. [CrossRef]
24. Jeng, T.L.; Shih, Y.J.; Ho, P.T.; Lai, C.C.; Lin, Y.W. γ -Oryzanol, tocol and mineral compositions in different grain fractions of giant embryo rice mutants. *J. Sci. Food Agric.* **2012**, *92*, 1468–1474. [CrossRef] [PubMed]
25. Kim, N.H.; Kwak, J.; Baik, J.Y.; Yoon, M.R.; Lee, J.S.; Yoon, S.W.; Kim, I.H. Changes in lipid substances in rice during grain development. *Phytochemistry* **2015**, *116*, 170–179. [CrossRef] [PubMed]
26. Konwachara, T.; Ahromrit, A. Effect of cooking on functional properties of germinated black glutinous rice (KKU-URL012). *Songklanakarin J. Sci. Technol.* **2014**, *36*, 283–290.
27. Association of Official Analytical Chemists Inc. *AOAC Official Methods of Analysis*; Association of Official Analytical Chemists Inc.: Arlington, VA, USA, 2003.
28. American Institute of Nutrition. Report of ad hoc committee on standards for nutritional studies. *J. Nutr.* **1977**, *107*, 1340–1347.
29. Seifter, S.; Dayton, S.; Navic, B.; Muntwyler, E. The estimation of glycogen with the anthrone reagent. *Arch. Biochem.* **1950**, *25*, 191–200. [PubMed]
30. Vogeser, M.; Konig, D.; Frey, I.; Predel, H.G.; Parhofer, K.G.; Berg, A. Fasting serum insulin and the homeostasis model of insulin resistance (HOMA-IR) in the monitoring of lifestyle interventions in obese persons. *Clin. Biochem.* **2007**, *40*, 964–968. [CrossRef] [PubMed]
31. Hulcher, F.H.; Oleson, W.H. Simplified spectrophotometric assay for microsomal 3-hydroxy-3-methylglutaryl CoA reductase by measurement of coenzyme A. *J. Lipid Res.* **1973**, *14*, 625–631. [PubMed]
32. Bradford, M.M. A rapid sensitive method for the quantitation of microgram quantities of protein utilizing the principle of protein-dye binding. *Anal. Biochem.* **1976**, *72*, 248–254. [CrossRef]
33. Bentle, L.A.; Lardy, H.A. Interaction of anions and divalent metal ions with phosphoenolpyruvate carboxykinase. *J. Biol. Chem.* **1976**, *251*, 2916–2921. [PubMed]
34. Davidson, A.L.; Arion, W.J. Factors underlying significant underestimations of glucokinase activity in crude liver extracts: Physiological implications of higher cellular activity. *Arch. Biochem. Biophys.* **1987**, *253*, 156–167. [CrossRef]
35. Alegre, M.; Ciudad, C.J.; Fillat, C.; Guinovart, J.J. Determination of glucose-6-phosphatase activity using the glucose dehydrogenase-coupled reaction. *Anal. Biochem.* **1988**, *173*, 185–189. [CrossRef]
36. Seidlova-Wuttke, D.; Nguyen, B.T.; Wuttke, W. Long-term effects of ovariectomy on osteoporosis and obesity in estrogen-receptor-β-deleted mice. *Comp. Med.* **2012**, *62*, 8–13. [PubMed]
37. Kim, S.M.; Rico, C.W.; Lee, S.C.; Kang, M.Y. Modulatory effect of rice bran and phytic acid on glucose metabolism in high fat-fed C57BL/6N mice. *J. Clin. Biochem. Nutr.* **2010**, *47*, 12–17. [CrossRef] [PubMed]
38. Son, M.J.; Rico, C.W.; Nam, S.H.; Kang, M.Y. Influence of oryzanol and ferulic acid on the lipid metabolism and antioxidative status in high fat-fed mice. *J. Clin. Biochem. Nutr.* **2010**, *46*, 150–156. [CrossRef] [PubMed]
39. Son, M.J.; Rico, C.W.; Nam, S.H.; Kang, M.Y. Effect of oryzanol and ferulic acid on the glucose metabolism of mice fed with high fat diet. *J. Food Sci.* **2011**, *76*, H7–H10. [CrossRef] [PubMed]
40. Chauhan, K.; Chauhan, B. Policosanol: Natural wax component with potent health benefits. *Int. J. Med. Pharm. Sci.* **2015**, *5*, 15–24.
41. Lee, J.Y.; Choi, H.Y.; Kang, Y.R.; Chang, H.B.; Chun, H.S.; Lee, M.S.; Kwon, Y.I. Effects of long-term supplementation of policosanol on blood cholesterol/glucose levels and 3-hydroxy-3methylglutaryl coenzyme a reductase activity in a rat model fed high cholesterol diets. *Food Sci. Biotechnol.* **2016**, *25*, 899–904. [CrossRef]
42. Jung, U.J.; Choi, M.S. Obesity and its metabolic complications: The role of adipokines and the relationship between obesity, inflammation, insulin resistance, dyslipidemia and nonalcoholic fatty lover disease. *Int. J. Mol. Sci.* **2014**, *15*, 6184–6223. [CrossRef] [PubMed]
43. Silha, J.V.; Weiler, H.A.; Murphy, L.J. Plasma adipokines and body composition in response to modest dietary manipulations in the mouse. *Obesity* **2006**, *14*, 1320–1329. [CrossRef] [PubMed]
44. Steppan, C.M.; Bailey, S.T.; Bhat, S.; Brown, E.J.; Banerjee, R.R.; Wright, C.M.; Patel, H.R.; Ahima, R.S.; Lazar, M.A. The hormone resistin links obesity to diabetes. *Nature* **2001**, *409*, 307–312. [CrossRef] [PubMed]
45. Darabi, H.; Raeisi, A.; Kalantarhormozi, M.R.; Ostovar, A.; Assadi, M.; Asadipooya, K.; Vahdat, K.; Dobaradaran, S.; Nabipour, I. Adiponectin as protective factor against progression toward type 2 diabetes mellitus in postmenopausal women. *Medicine* **2015**, *94*, e1347. [CrossRef] [PubMed]

46. She, P.; Shiota, M.; Shelton, K.D.; Chalkley, R.; Postic, C.; Magnuson, M.A. Phosphoenolpyruvate carboxykinase is necessary for the integration of hepatic energy metabolism. *Mol. Cell. Biol.* **2000**, *20*, 6508–6517. [CrossRef] [PubMed]
47. Schaftingen, E.V.; Gerin, I. The glucose-6-phosphatase system. *Biochem. J.* **2002**, *362*, 513–532. [CrossRef] [PubMed]
48. Coope, G.J.; Atkinson, A.M.; Allott, C.; McKerrecher, D.; Johnstone, C.; Pike, K.G. Predictive blood glucose lowering efficacy by glucokinase activators in high fat fed female zucker rats. *Br. J. Pharmacol.* **2003**, *149*, 328–335. [CrossRef] [PubMed]
49. Curran, M.P.; Wagstaff, A.J. Spotlight on estradiol and norgestimate as hormone therapy in postmenopausal women. *Treat. Endocrinol.* **2002**, *1*, 127–129. [CrossRef] [PubMed]
50. Ettinger, B. Use of low-dosage 17 beta-estradiol for the prevention of osteoporosis. *Clin. Ther.* **1993**, *15*, 950–962. [PubMed]
51. Vaananen, H.K.; Harkonen, P.L. Estrogen and bone metabolism. *Maturitas* **1996**, *23*, S65–S69. [CrossRef]
52. Seibel, M.J. Biochemical markers of bone turnover part II: Clinical applications in the management of osteoporosis. *Clin. Biochem. Rev.* **2006**, *27*, 123–138. [PubMed]
53. Goufo, P.; Trindade, H. Rice antioxidants: Phenolic acids, flavonoids, anthocyanins, proanthocyanidins, tocopherols, tocotrienols, γ-oryzanol, and phytic acid. *Food Sci. Nutr.* **2014**, *2*, 75–104. [CrossRef] [PubMed]
54. Franca, N.A.G.; Camargo, M.B.; Lazaretti-Castro, M.; Martini, L.A. Antioxidant intake and bone status in a cross-sectional study of Brazilian women with osteoporosis. *Nutr. Health* **2013**, *22*, 133–142. [CrossRef] [PubMed]
55. Muhammad, N.; Luke, D.A.; Shuid, A.N.; Mohamed, N.; Soelaiman, I.N. Tocotrienol supplementation in postmenopausal osteoporosis: Evidence from a laboratory study. *Clinics* **2013**, *68*, 1338–1343. [CrossRef]
56. Altindag, O.; Erel, O.; Soran, N.; Celik, H.; Selek, S. Total oxidative/anti-oxidative status and relation to bone mineral density in osteoporosis. *Rheumatol. Int.* **2008**, *28*, 317–321. [CrossRef] [PubMed]
57. Sendur, O.F.; Turan, Y.; Tastaban, E.; Serter, M. Antioxidant status in patients with osteoporosis: A controlled study. *Jt. Bone Spine* **2009**, *76*, 514–518. [CrossRef] [PubMed]

5

Bone-Protective Effects of Dried Plum in Postmenopausal Women: Efficacy and Possible Mechanisms

Bahram H. Arjmandi [1,2,*], Sarah A. Johnson [3], Shirin Pourafshar [1,2], Negin Navaei [1,2,4], Kelli S. George [1,2], Shirin Hooshmand [5], Sheau C. Chai [6] and Neda S. Akhavan [1,2]

1 Department of Nutrition, Food and Exercise Sciences, College of Human Sciences, Florida State University, Tallahassee, FL 32306, USA; sp12r@my.fsu.edu (S.P.); negin.navaei@life.edu (N.N.); ksg15c@my.fsu.edu (K.S.G.); nsa08@my.fsu.edu (N.S.A.)
2 Center for Advancing Exercise and Nutrition Research on Aging (CAENRA), College of Human Sciences, Florida State University, Tallahassee, FL 32306, USA
3 Department of Food Science and Human Nutrition, College of Health and Human Sciences, Colorado State University, Fort Collins, CO 80523, USA; Sarah.Johnson@colostate.edu
4 Department of Nutrition, College of Graduate and Undergraduate Studies, Life University, Marietta, GA 30060, USA
5 School of Exercise and Nutritional Sciences, College of Health & Human Services, San Diego State University, San Diego, CA 92182, USA; shooshmand@mail.sdsu.edu
6 Department of Behavioral Health and Nutrition, College of Health Sciences, University of Delaware, Newark, DE 19716, USA; scchai@udel.edu
* Correspondence: barjmandi@fsu.edu

Abstract: Osteoporosis is an age-related chronic disease characterized by a loss of bone mass and quality, and is associated with an increased risk of fragility fractures. Postmenopausal women are at the greatest risk of developing osteoporosis due to the cessation in ovarian hormone production, which causes accelerated bone loss. As the demographic shifts to a more aged population, a growing number of postmenopausal women will be afflicted with osteoporosis. Certain lifestyle factors, including nutrition and exercise, are known to reduce the risk of developing osteoporosis and therefore play an important role in bone health. In terms of nutrition, accumulating evidence suggests that dried plum (*Prunus domestica* L.) is potentially an efficacious intervention for preventing and reversing bone mass and structural loss in an ovariectomized rat model of osteoporosis, as well as in osteopenic postmenopausal women. Here, we provide evidence supporting the efficacy of dried plum in preventing and reversing bone loss associated with ovarian hormone deficiency in rodent models and in humans. We end with the results of a recent follow-up study demonstrating that postmenopausal women who previously consumed 100 g dried plum per day during our one-year clinical trial conducted five years earlier retained bone mineral density to a greater extent than those receiving a comparative control. Additionally, we highlight the possible mechanisms of action by which bioactive compounds in dried plum exert bone-protective effects. Overall, the findings of our studies and others strongly suggest that dried plum in its whole form is a promising and efficacious functional food therapy for preventing bone loss in postmenopausal women, with the potential for long-lasting bone-protective effects.

Keywords: bioactive compounds; functional foods; menopause; nutrition; polyphenols; (poly)phenols; prune; osteopenia; osteoporosis

1. Introduction

The postmenopausal period typically occupies one-third of a woman's life [1], and it is estimated that by the year 2020, more than 46 million women in the United States (U.S.) will be postmenopausal [2]. Menopause is associated with the development of numerous chronic diseases [3], due to an abrupt cessation of ovarian hormone production, namely estrogen. Osteoporosis is a chronic and debilitating age-related skeletal disease characterized by the loss of bone mass and a deterioration of the microstructural properties of bone, resulting in an increased propensity for fragility fractures [4]. Osteoporosis is responsible for more than 1.5 million fractures per year in the U.S., with most occurring in postmenopausal women [5]. Osteoporosis and its related bone fractures are a major public health concern as they are associated with increased morbidity and mortality, a poor quality of life, and a large economic burden [6,7]. Approximately 44 million men and women over the age of 50 have osteoporosis or low bone mass in the U.S. [3]. Diminished estrogen levels associated with menopause result in an initial phase of rapid bone loss, followed by a period of a slower deterioration of the skeleton [8]. This rapid phase of bone loss occurs within the first five to 10 years following the cessation of menses or the surgical removal of the ovaries [9]. As the demographic shifts to a more aged population, the prevalence and incidence of osteoporosis are likely to continue to increase, with affected individuals being at a greater risk of falls, fragility fractures, and therefore morbidity and mortality [3]. As such, therapeutic strategies that can delay, slow down, or prevent bone loss in aging individuals, and particularly in postmenopausal women, are critically needed.

Hormone replacement therapy is a logical therapeutic strategy for postmenopausal women since age-related chronic disease development typically begins after the cessation of ovarian hormone production. However, evidence from the Women's Health Initiative indicates that the risks associated with hormone replacement therapy outweigh its benefits, making the exploration of alternative therapies necessary [10]. Although the Food and Drug Administration has approved several anti-resorptive pharmacological agents such as bisphosphonates and denosumab, as well as the bone-forming pharmacological agent teriparatide, these drugs are associated with adverse side effects, are costly, and often have low compliance [11]. Therefore, it is imperative that safe and cost-effective therapeutic strategies, aside from medications, that can delay, slow down, or prevent bone loss in postmenopausal women be identified, investigated for efficacy, and disseminated for public use.

It is well-known that certain lifestyle factors, including diet and nutrition, play an important role in bone health. In fact, research has demonstrated that certain foods (i.e., functional foods) and their bioactive compounds, including nutrient and non-nutrient compounds, have bone-protective effects [12]. Of the functional foods investigated for their bone-protective properties, the most efficacious have typically been in the form of fruits and vegetables. The findings from our studies [13–15] and others [16,17] suggest that dried plum (*Prunus domestica* L.) is the most effective in preventing and reversing bone loss among the fruits and vegetables investigated. This has also been demonstrated by Mühlbauer et al. [18,19], who examined the effects of 60 fruits and vegetables on bone. Their findings indicated that onion and dried plum had the most potent bone-protective effects. Though the consumption of fruits and vegetables for general health and well-being is encouraged, in terms of bone health, not all fruits and vegetables offer the same benefits. For instance, while certain fruits such as dried plum and to some extent blueberries exert bone-protective effects [20], in our observations [14], the same may not be true for other fruits such as raisins and dates. We are using a conditional term for the effectiveness of blueberry on bone, because our findings [20], as well as those of Zhang et al. [21,22], are preliminary at this point and await confirmation in human studies. The reasons for these discrepancies in the efficacy among fruits and vegetables remain unknown.

Due to the bioactive compound content and composition of dried plum, as well as promising preclinical and clinical research findings, dried plum has been and continues to be investigated as a potential functional food with respect to bone health. Numerous studies in cells, rodent models of postmenopausal osteoporosis, and postmenopausal women have demonstrated its efficacy and have identified possible mechanisms of action. Studies have aimed to identify specific bioactive compounds in dried plum responsible for its bone-protective properties. The present review provides an overview of dried plum, including its nutritional and bioactive compound composition, and provides evidence from preclinical and clinical studies supporting the efficacy of dried plum in preventing and reversing bone loss in postmenopausal women, as well as evidence to support possible mechanisms of action, and bioactive compounds in dried plum responsible for its efficacy. Additionally, gaps in the research and promising new areas of investigation are discussed.

A literature search was performed using the PubMed database and Google Scholar. The following keywords, alone and in combination, were used: bone, dried plum, menopause, osteopenia, osteoporosis, ovariectomy, ovariectomized, plum, postmenopausal, and prune. Preclinical studies using rodent models of postmenopausal osteoporosis and clinical trials with postmenopausal women were included in this review.

2. Dried Plum: A Promising Functional Food for Bone Health

The U.S., primarily California, is a major producer of dried plum, with approximately 99% of the U.S. and 40% of the world supply grown in California. Dried plum was previously referred to as prunes until a formal name change was requested and approved by the Food and Drug Administration in 2001 [23]. It is most commonly known for its effects on gastrointestinal motility and research has been and continues to be conducted with respect to gastrointestinal health to support these observations. In addition, dried plum has been investigated for its antimicrobial, cancer-preventive, cardiometabolic, neurological, and bone-protective effects [24,25].

To date, the most notable research has been in the area of bone metabolism and health. The unique ability of dried plum to promote bone health is likely related to its bioactive compound composition. Dried plum is rich in nutrient bioactive compounds including dietary fiber, vitamin K, boron, copper, magnesium, manganese, among others, many of which are known to positively influence bone [23–25]. It is also rich in non-nutrient bioactive compounds including (poly)phenols such as chlorogenic acids (e.g., chlorogenic acid, neochlorogenic acid, cryptochlorogenic acid) and proanthocyanidins [24,25]. Dried plum has been ranked as having one of the highest oxygen radical absorbance capacities among the commonly consumed fruits and vegetables. It has been suggested that this is likely to be primarily due to its (poly)phenolic compound composition and content, as dried plum is low in ascorbic acid, carotenoids, and vitamin E [23]. In addition, previous research has demonstrated that phenolic compounds, including those found in dried plum, exert bone-protective effects and profoundly affect bone metabolism [25]. For instance, rutin, a flavonoid commonly found in plums and various berries, has been reported to inhibit ovariectomy-induced bone loss in a rat model of osteoporosis [26]. Nonetheless, the question still remains as to which bioactive component(s) of dried plum are responsible for its bone-protective effects. The answer may simply be that the whole fruit is more efficacious than its isolated components due to the additive and/or synergistic effects of these components within the food matrix.

3. Dried Plum and Bone Health: Rodent Models of Postmenopausal Osteoporosis

Previous studies investigating the role of dried plum on bone health in rodent models of postmenopausal osteoporosis are summarized in Table 1. Our laboratory [27] was the first to report the bone-protective effects of dried plum both in general, and specifically in an established rat model of postmenopausal osteoporosis [28]. We showed that ovariectomy led to significant declines in the bone mineral density (BMD) of the 4th lumbar vertebrae and femurs, as well as a decrease in the tibial trabecular bone area compared to sham-operated (Sham) rats. However, ovariectomized (Ovx) rats that received 25% of the diet as dried plum for 45 days did not lose bone, while those receiving 5% of the diet as dried plum lost bone similarly to Ovx rats not receiving dried plum (Figure 1). Despite this, we also found that dried plum dose-dependently increased circulating insulin-like growth factor-I (IGF-I) levels, while having no effect on tartrate-resistant acid phosphatase-5b (TRAP-5b) levels. At that time, TRAP-5b was considered to be a biomarker of bone resorption. Therefore, these results suggested that dried plum prevented bone loss, in part, by increasing the rate of bone formation, but not through inhibiting bone resorption.

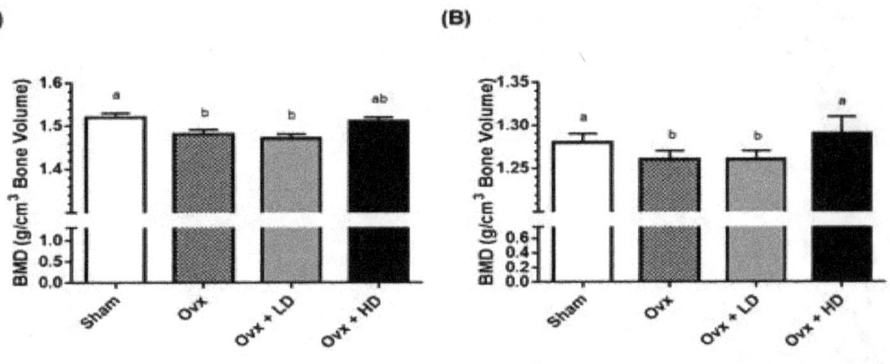

Figure 1. (**A**) Effects of ovariectomy and dried plum on bone density of right femur; (**B**) Effects of ovariectomy and dried plum on bone density of 4th lumbar spine. Bars represent mean ± standard error of the mean. Bars that do not share the same letters are significantly ($p < 0.05$) different from each other. BMD, bone mineral density; HD, high dose (25%) dried plum; LD, low dose (5%) dried plum; Ovx, ovariectomized; Sham, sham-operated.

We next asked the question: could the addition of dried plum to the diet restore bone mass after bone loss has occurred? Toward this end, our laboratory [27] used an Ovx rat model of postmenopausal osteoporosis to evaluate the ability of dried plum at different doses to reverse bone loss. In this study, 90-day-old female Sprague-Dawley rats were divided into six groups: Sham control, Ovx control, Ovx + 17β-estradiol (E_2), Ovx + 5% of the diet as dried plum, Ovx + 15% of the diet as dried plum, and Ovx + 25% of the diet as dried plum for 60 days. Interestingly, the consumption of all doses of dried plum (5%, 15%, and 25%) effectively restored femoral and tibial BMD to the same extent as E_2, while only the group receiving 25% dried plum showed the restoration of 4th lumbar BMD (Figure 2). At the time in which this study was conducted, the loss of bone volume accompanied by the loss of trabecular connectivity was generally believed to be an irreversible process [29]. To our knowledge, our study was the first to demonstrate that an agent of any kind could reverse the loss of trabecular microstructures including the bone volume/total volume, connectivity density, trabecular number, trabecular separation, and structure model index (Figure 3).

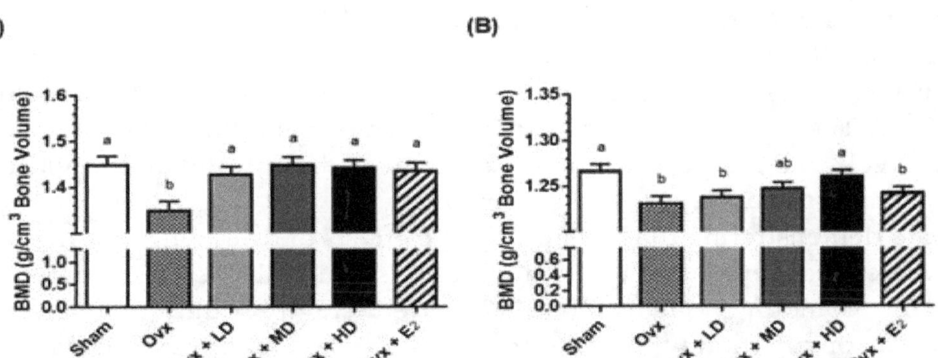

Figure 2. (**A**) Effects of ovariectomy, dried plum, and estrogen on bone density of right femur; (**B**) Effects ovariectomy, dried plum, and estrogen on bone density of 4th lumbar spine. Bars represent mean ± standard error of the mean. Bars that do not share the same letters are significantly ($p < 0.05$) different from each other. BMD, bone mineral density; E_2, 17β-estradiol, LD, low dose (5%) dried plum; high dose (25%) dried plum; MD, medium dose (15%) dried plum; Ovx, ovariectomized; Sham, sham-operated.

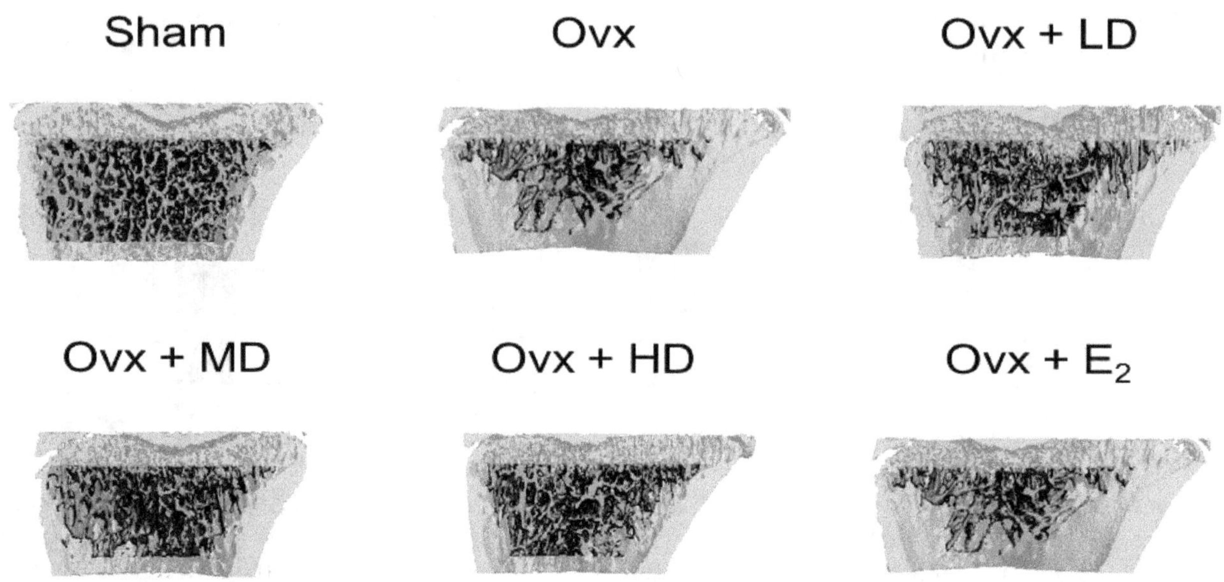

Figure 3. Representative images of proximal tibia demonstrating the effect of ovariectomy, dried plum, and estrogen on trabecular bone structure. E_2, 17β-estradiol; LD, high dose (25%) dried plum; low dose (5%) dried plum; MD, medium dose (15%) dried plum, Ovx, ovariectomized; Sham, sham-operated.

We next sought to evaluate the efficacy of several potentially bone-protective functional foods and bioactive compounds (i.e., dried plum, figs, dates, raisins, blueberries, dried plum (poly)phenols, fructooligosaccharides (FOS), and β-hydroxy-β-methylbutyrate, alone and in combination, on the bone mass and quality in Ovx rats after bone loss had already occurred [14]. Our findings revealed that the group receiving 5% FOS + 7.5% dried plum in their diet had the greatest reversal of BMD loss in the right femur and 4th lumbar spine, 4th lumbar spine calcium loss, and trabecular separation. Interestingly, none of the treatments altered the serum or urinary markers of bone turnover. The findings of this study suggest that the addition of prebiotic FOS to dried plum improves its efficacy in restoring bone mass and quality after bone loss has occurred. Although the mechanisms remain unknown, FOS has been demonstrated to increase the absorption of minerals, including calcium and magnesium, in the colon [30]. Additionally, considering that FOS is a prebiotic, it is likely that the combination of FOS and dried plum worked through gut microbiota-related mechanisms including an increase in mineral absorption. Importantly, the dose of dried plum (i.e., 7.5% of the diet) that was efficacious in combination with FOS was lower than what was previously found to be effective. This suggests that the addition of FOS to dried plum may improve the efficacy of dried plum and should be further investigated. These findings will be particularly important if they can be translated to humans, as it could be a novel strategy for reducing the amount of dried plum an individual would need to consume on a daily basis to achieve the same outcomes.

In addition to demonstrating the bone-protective effects of dried plum alone and in combination with FOS, we have also demonstrated in numerous studies that soy is a potentially efficacious functional food for promoting bone health [31–35]. We therefore sought to determine the efficacy of a soy-based diet in combination with 7.5% dried plum, 5% FOS, or 7.5% dried plum + 5% FOS on reversing bone loss in a rat model of postmenopausal osteoporosis. We found that the combination of a soy-based diet with dried plum, FOS, or both, significantly improved the whole body BMD and femoral BMD, while the combination of all components (i.e., soy, dried plum, and FOS) had the most pronounced effect on lumbar BMD [15]. All interventions were noted to improve the biomechanical properties of bone, as demonstrated by the increased ultimate load. The serum biomarker results suggest that these improvements may have been due, in part, to their ability to enhance bone formation and reduce bone resorption, as shown by increases in blood alkaline phosphatase (ALP) and decreased urinary deoxypyridinoline (Dpd).

Other investigators have also demonstrated the bone-protective effects of dried plum in rodent models postmenopausal osteoporosis. Rendina et al. [16] showed that feeding 25% of the diet as dried plum for four weeks to female Ovx C57BL/6J mice prevented the loss of BMD and bone mineral content (BMC) of the spine, and trabecular microarchitectural properties of the vertebrae and proximal tibiae, resulting in greater bone strength and stiffness in the vertebrae. Additionally, feeding dried plum in the diet at 15% and 25% doses restored myeloid and lymphoid levels to that of the sham-operated mice and suppressed ex vivo concanavalin A stimulated lymphocyte tumor necrosis factor-α production in splenocytes.

In another study, Rendina et al. [36] reported the results of a study comparing the bone-protective effects of dried plum with other fruits (i.e., dried apple, apricot, grape, and mango) in Ovx C57BL/6 mice over an eight-week period. They demonstrated that dried plum had superior anabolic effects on the trabecular bone microarchitectural properties of the vertebrae, was able to prevent tibial bone loss, and restored the trabecular biomechanical properties of the spine when compared with the other fruits. In addition, dried plum was more efficacious than the other fruits in enhancing plasma glutathione peroxidase activity, downregulating osteoclast differentiation, upregulating osteoblast activity, and suppressing Ovx-induced apoptosis.

Smith et al. [37] reported the findings of a study out of the same laboratory in which they compared the effects of six weeks of dried plum supplementation to treatment with parathyroid hormone (PTH). Treatment with dried plum at doses of 15% and 25% in the diet restored the whole body and femoral BMD to that of the Sham group and improved the trabecular bone volume and cortical thickness. Systemic blood biomarkers of bone metabolism (i.e., *N*-terminal procollagen type 1 and Dpd) were reduced, indicating a reduction in bone turnover. Dynamic bone histomorphometric analysis of the tibial metaphysis revealed that dried plum restored the Ovx-induced increase in the cancellous bone formation rate and mineralizing surface to that of the Sham group. Dried plum also upregulated the gene expression of *bone morphogenetic protein 2*, a regulator of osteogenesis, and *IGF-I* while downregulating the *nuclear factor T cell activator 1*, a transcription factor involved in the regulation of osteoclast differentiation. Compared with that of the effects of PTH on bone, dried plum reduced the rate of bone turnover, rather than increasing the rate of bone formation.

In summary, our data and others strongly suggest that dried plum is an efficacious functional food for preventing and reversing the loss of bone mass and structural properties in a rat model of postmenopausal osteoporosis. We have also shown that dried plum dose-dependently increases systemic and local indices of bone formation, e.g., serum and mRNA levels of ALP. These findings suggest that dried plum prevents and reverses bone loss, primarily through enhanced bone formation.

Table 1. Preclinical studies investigating the role of dried plum on bone health in rodent models of postmenopausal osteoporosis.

Reference	Model	Number	Groups	Duration	Primary Outcomes	Primary Findings
Arjmandi et al., 2001 [27]	Sham and Ovx female 90-day old Sprague-Dawley rats	48	(1) Sham control, (2) Ovx control, (3) Ovx + 5% dried plum, or (4) Ovx + 25% dried plum	45 days	BMD and % mineral content of right femur and 4th lumbar vertebrae; trabecular total area and bone area; cortical total area, bone area, marrow space, endosteal perimeter, and periosteal perimeter; serum ALP, TRAP, and IGF-1	Compared to Ovx control: 4th lumbar vertebrae and femur BMD and trabecular bone area were significantly ↑ in the 25% dried plum group
Deyhim et al., 2005 [38]	Sham and Ovx female 90-day old Sprague-Dawley rats	80	(1) Sham control, (2) Ovx control, (3) Ovx + 17β-estradiol, (4) Ovx + 5% dried plum, (5) Ovx + 15% dried plum, (6) Ovx + 25% dried plum	60 days	BMD of femur, left tibiae, and 4th lumbar; biomechanical properties (length, cortical area, unit yield force, and unit ultimate force); trabecular microarchitectural properties (BV/TV), Tb N, Tb S, Tb Th, ConnDens, SMI); serum IGF-1, ALP, and TRAP; urinary Dpd	Compared to Ovx control: Femur and tibia BMD were ↑ in all dried plum groups, 4th lumbar BMD tended to be significantly and was significantly ↑ in the 15% and 25% dried plum groups, respectively; unit yield force tended to be significantly ↑ in all dried plum groups; Tb S was significantly ↑ in all dried plum groups while Tb N and Tb Th were significantly ↑ in 15% and 25% dried plum groups and BV/TV and ConnDens were significantly ↑ in 25% dried plum group; urinary Dpd tended to be significantly ↓ in all dried plum groups
Arjmandi et al., 2010 [14]	Sham and Ovx female 90-day old Sprague-Dawley rats	180	(1) Sham control, (2) Ovx control, (3) Ovx + 2% FOS, (4) Ovx + 5% FOS + 7.5% dried plum, (5) Ovx + 2% FOS + 5% dried plum, (6) Ovx + 2% FOS + dried plum polyphenols, (7) Ovx + 2% FOS + dried plum juice, (8) Ovx + 2% FOS + dried plum puree, or (9) Ovx + 2% FOS + dried plum pulp/skins	60 days	BMD and BMC of whole body, right femur, and 4th lumbar vertebrae; bone histomorphometric parameters (BV/TV, Tb N, Tb S, Tb Th, ConnDens, and SMI); 4th lumbar calcium content; serum osteocalcin and IGF-1; serum and urinary calcium, magnesium, and phosphorus; urinary Dpd	Compared to Ovx control: 4th lumbar vertebrae and femur BMD were significantly ↑ in 5% FOS + 7.5% dried plum group with tendency to significantly ↓ loss of lumbar vertebrae calcium, and significantly ↓ trabecular separation
Johnson et al., 2011 [15]	Sham and Ovx female 90-day old Sprague-Dawley rats	72	(1) Sham control, (2) Ovx control, (3) Ovx + soy, (4) Ovx + soy + dried plum, Ovx + soy + FOS, or (5) Ovx + soy + dried plum + FOS	60 days	BMD and BMC of the whole body, right femur, and 4th lumbar vertebrae; femoral strength; bone histomorphometric parameters (BV/TV, Tb N, Tb S, Tb Th, and MS/BS); serum total ALP; urinary creatinine and Dpd	Compared to Ovx control: Whole body and 4th lumbar BMD tended to be significantly ↑ in Ovx + soy + dried plum group and was significantly increased in Ovx + soy + dried plum + FOS group, and right femur BMD was significantly ↑; Tb Th tended to be significantly ↑ and Tb Sp, and MS/BS tended to be significantly ↓ in Ovx + soy + dried plum + FOS group; serum ALP and urinary Dpd tended to be significantly ↓ in Ovx + soy + dried plum group and urinary Dpd was significantly ↓ in Ovx + soy + dried plum + FOS group
Rendina et al., 2012 [16]	Sham and Ovx female 90-day old C57BL/6J mice	59	(1) Sham control, (2) Ovx control, (3) Ovx + 5% dried plum, (4) Ovx + 15% dried plum, (5) Ovx + 25% dried plum	4 weeks	BMA, BMC, and BMD of the 4th to 5th lumbar vertebrae; bone microarchitecture parameters of tibia and 4th lumbar vertebrae (BV/TV, Tb N, Tb S, Tb Th, ConnDens, and SMI); biomechanical properties of trabecular bone (total force, stiffness, size-independent stiffness, and Von Mises stresses); plasma PINP and IGF-1; Runx2, osteocalcin, and NFATc1 bone gene expression	Compared to Ovx control: BMC and BMD were significantly ↑ in 25% dried plum group; BV/TV and vertebra Tb N were significantly ↑ in 15% and 25% dried plum groups, tibia Tb N was increased in 25% dried plum group, tibia Tb S was significantly ↓ in 15% and 25% dried plum groups while vertebra Tb S was significantly decreased in 25% dried plum group; vertebra ConnDens and SMI were significantly ↑ and ↓, respectively, in 15% and 25% dried plum groups while vertebra apparent mean/density tended to be ↑ in 15% dried plum group and was significantly ↑ in 25% dried plum group; tibia ConnDens and SMI, were significantly ↑ and ↓, respectively, in 15% and 25% dried plum groups while apparent mean density was increased in 25% dried plum group; vertebra total force, stiffness, and size-independent stiffness were significantly ↑ and Von Mises stresses was significantly ↓ in 15% and 25% dried plum groups; PINP, NFATc1, and Runx2 were significantly ↓ in all dried plum groups while IGF-1 was significantly ↑ in 15% dried plum group and osteocalcin was significantly decreased in 15% and 25% dried plum groups

Table 1. *Cont.*

Reference	Model	Number	Groups	Duration	Primary Outcomes	Primary Findings
Rendina et al., 2013 [36]	Sham and Ovx female 90-day old C57BL/6J mice	68	(1) Sham control, (2) Ovx control, (3) Ovx + 25% dried plum, (4) Ovx + 25% dried apple, (5) Ovx + 25% dried apricot, (6) Ovx + 25% dried grape, (7) Ovx + 25% dried mango	8 weeks	BMA, BMC, and BMD of the whole body and 4th and 5th lumbar vertebrae; bone microarchitecture parameters of tibia and 4th lumbar vertebrae (BV/TV, Tb N, Tb S, Tb Th, ConnDens, SMI, and trabecular density); biomechanical properties of trabecular bone (total force, stiffness, size-independent stiffness); plasma GPx; bone marrow gene expression of NFATc1, Col1a1, ALP, osteocalcin, Bak1; flushed femur expression of Bak1, Casp3, Casp9	25% dried plum compared to Ovx control: Whole body and vertebra BMA, BMD, and BMC were significantly ↑, vertebra and tibia BV/TV were significantly ↑; vertebra Tb N, Tb Th, Tb Sp, ConnDens and trabecular density were significantly ↑ and SMI was significantly ↓; proximal tibia Tb N and trabecular density were significantly ↑; vertebra total force, stiffness, and size independent stiffness and tibia size independent stiffness were significantly ↑; plasma GPx was significantly ↑; NFATc1 was significantly ↓ and Col1a1 tended to be ↑, bone marrow Bak1 was significantly ↑, and Casp9 was significantly ↓
Smith et al., 2014 [37]	Sham and Ovx female 6-month old Sprague-Dawley rats	84	(1) Sham control, (2) Ovx control, (3) Ovx + 5% dried plum, (4) Ovx + 15% dried plum, (5) Ovx + 25% dried plum, (6) Ovx + PTH	6 weeks	BMA, BMC, and BMD of the whole body, femur, and 4th and 5th lumbar vertebrae; bone microarchitecture parameters of tibia and 4th lumbar vertebrae (BV/TV, Tb N, Tb S, Tb Th, ConnDens, and SMI); dynamic bone histomorphometry (proximal tibia metaphysis BFR, MS/BS, and MAR; tibial cancellous MS/bone area, and BFR/BV; tibial cortical bone periosteal BFR, periosteal MS, periosteal MAR, endocortical BFR, endocortical MS, and endocortical MAR), plasma PINP; urinary Dpd; bone gene expression of NFATc1, Col1a1, ALP, osteocalcin, Runx2, BMP 2 and 4, IFG-1, RANKL, OPG	Compared to Ovx control: Whole body and femur BMD was significantly ↑ in all dried plum groups; vertebral BMD was significantly ↑ in 15% and 25% dried plum groups and tended to be significantly increased in 5% dried plum group; vertebral BV/TV and Tb N significantly ↑ and Tb S and ConnDens significantly ↓ in all dried plum groups, whereas Tb Th and SMI ↑ and ↑, respectively, in 15% and 25% dried plum groups; proximal tibia metaphysis Tb Sp ↓ in 15% and 25% dried plum groups; tibial mid-diaphysis cortical thickness ↑ in all dried plum groups while cortical area tended to be significantly ↑ in 5% dried plum group; plasma PINP was significantly ↓ in all dried plum groups; urinary Dpd tended to be significantly decreased and was significantly decreased in 5% and 15% dried plum groups, respectively; proximal tibial metaphysis BFR tended to be significantly ↓ in 5% dried plum group and was significantly ↓ in 15% and 25% dried plum groups, MS/BS was significantly ↓ in 15% and 25% dried plum groups, and MAR was significantly ↓ in 15% dried plum group and tended to be significantly ↓ in 5% and 25% dried plum groups; tibial cancellous MS/bone area and BFR/BV were significantly ↓ in all dried plum groups; tibial endocortical MAR was significantly ↓ in the 5% dried plum group and tended to be significantly reduced in the 15% and 25% dried plum groups; relative abundance of NFATc1 was significantly ↓ and BMP4 was significantly ↑ in all dried plum groups, while Col1a1 tended to be significantly reduced in all dried plum groups and IGF-1 was significantly ↑ in 25% dried plum group and tended to be significantly ↑ in 15% dried plum group
Pawlowski et al., 2014 [39]	Ovx female 3-month old Sprague-Dawley rats	44	(1) Control, (2) grape seed extract-high, (3) grape seed extract-low, (4) blueberry-high, (5) blueberry-low, (6) dried plum-high, (7) dried plum-low, (8) grape-high, (9) grape-low, (10) resveratrol-high, (11) resveratrol-low, (12) soy isoflavone-glycosylated, (13) soy isoflavone-genistein aglycone	10 days	Urine calcium (^{45}Ca and total calcium); serum BALP; urinary NTx	Bone calcium retention was significantly ↑ in dried plum-high group compared to baseline

Table 1. *Cont.*

Reference	Model	Number	Groups	Duration	Primary Outcomes	Primary Findings
Léotoing et al., 2016 [40]	Ovx female 5-month old Wistar rats	84	(1) Sham control, (2) Ovx control, (3) high chlorogenic acid dried plum, (4) low chlorogenic acid dried plum, (5) high chlorogenic acid dried plum juice, (6) low chlorogenic acid dried plum juice, (7) low chlorogenic acid dried plum + fiber	90 days	Total femoral BMD, metaphyseal BMD, and diaphyseal BMD; total BMC; blood osteocalcin, CPII, CTX-II, and CRI; urinary Dpd and calcium; BRI	Compared to Ovx control: Total femoral BMD and metaphyseal BMD were significantly ↑ in low chlorogenic acid dried plum + fiber and low chlorogenic acid dried plum juice group and tended to be significantly ↑ in all other dried plum groups; diaphyseal BMD was significantly ↑ in high chlorogenic acid dried plum, low chlorogenic acid dried plum + fiber and the low chlorogenic acid dried plum juice groups; total BMC was significantly ↑ in all low chlorogenic acid dried plum groups and tended to be significantly ↑ in high chlorogenic acid dried plum groups; blood osteocalcin was significantly ↓ in high chlorogenic acid dried plum, low chlorogenic acid dried plum + fiber, and low chlorogenic acid dried plum juice groups and tended to be significantly ↓ in the other dried plum groups; urinary Dpd was significantly ↓ in low chlorogenic acid dried plum + fiber and low chlorogenic acid dried plum juice groups and tended to be significantly ↓ in the other dried plum groups; BRI tended to be ↓ in all high chlorogenic acid dried plum groups and tended to be ↑ in all low chlorogenic acid dried plum groups; all groups had significantly ↑ calciurea; CPII and CRI were significantly ↑ in high chlorogenic acid dried plum group

BALP, bone alkaline phosphatase; BMA, bone mineral area; BMC, bone mineral content; BMD, bone mineral density; BFR, bone formation rate; BMP, bone morphogenetic proteins; BRI, bone remodeling index; BSAP, bone-specific alkaline phosphatase; BV/TV, bone volume to total volume ratio; ^{45}Ca, calcium-45; Col1a1, type 1 collagen; ConnDens, connectivity density; CPII, C-propeptide of type II collagen; CRI, cartilage remodeling index; CTX-II, C-terminal telopeptides of type II collagen; Dpd, deoxypyridinoline; HP, helical peptide; IGF-1, insulin-like growth factor-1, IGFBP-3, insulin-like growth factor binding protein-3; IL-6, interleukin-6; MAR, mineral apposition rate; MS, mineralizing surface; MS/BS, mineral surface as percent of bone surface; NFATc1, nuclear factor of activated T cells; NTx, cross-linked N-telopeptides of type 1 collagen; OPG, osteoprotegerin; PINP, N-terminal propeptide of type 1 procollagen; PTH, parathyroid hormone; RANKL, receptor activator of nuclear factor kappa-B ligand; Runx2, runt-related protein 2; Tb N, trabecular number; Tb Sp, trabecular separation; Tb Th, trabecular thickness; TRAP, tartrate-resistant acid phosphatase; TNF-α, tumor necrosis factor-alpha; Ovx, ovariectomized; Sham, sham-operated; SMI, structural model index.

4. Dried Plum and Bone Health: Clinical Trials in Postmenopausal Women

Previously conducted clinical trials investigating the role of dried plum on bone health in postmenopausal women are summarized in Table 2. To our knowledge, our laboratory was the first to evaluate the bone-protective properties of dried plum in humans. Initially, we reported the findings of a three-month clinical trial evaluating the efficacy of dried plum versus dried apple (comparative control) on the biomarkers of bone formation in postmenopausal women [41]. Here, we showed that the consumption of 100 g/day dried plum significantly increased the serum markers of bone formation, namely total ALP, bone-specific ALP (BALP), and IGF-1 by 12, 6, and 17%, respectively. The increase in BALP is important as studies have shown that clinically relevant doses of bone-forming agents such as sodium fluoride, growth hormone, and PTH take several months to moderately increase the serum levels of BALP [42]. Interestingly, the serum and urinary biomarkers of bone resorption were not affected by either intervention. These observations further support our hypothesis that dried plum prevents and reverses bone loss through enhanced bone formation.

To evaluate whether a longer treatment period would lead to an improvement in bone mass, we conducted a one-year clinical trial comparing the effects of the daily consumption of 100 g dried plum to 75 g dried apple (comparative control) on BMD and the biomarkers of bone turnover in 100 osteopenic postmenopausal women. We found that dried plum consumption significantly improved the BMD of the ulna and lumbar spine compared with the dried apple control (Figure 4) [13]. Additionally, dried plum consumption led to significantly decreased serum TRAP-5b and BALP levels. Osteocalcin and C-reactive protein levels were significantly lower in the dried plum group than in the apple group. Although the findings of our initial three-month clinical trial indicated that BALP levels increased following dried plum consumption, this was not observed in our one-year clinical trial. We cannot offer a definitive reason for this discrepancy. However, variation is inherent in bone biomarkers due to intra- and inter-individual variability, analytical reasons, and sample stability. For these reasons, BMD remains the gold-standard for evaluating bone health [43].

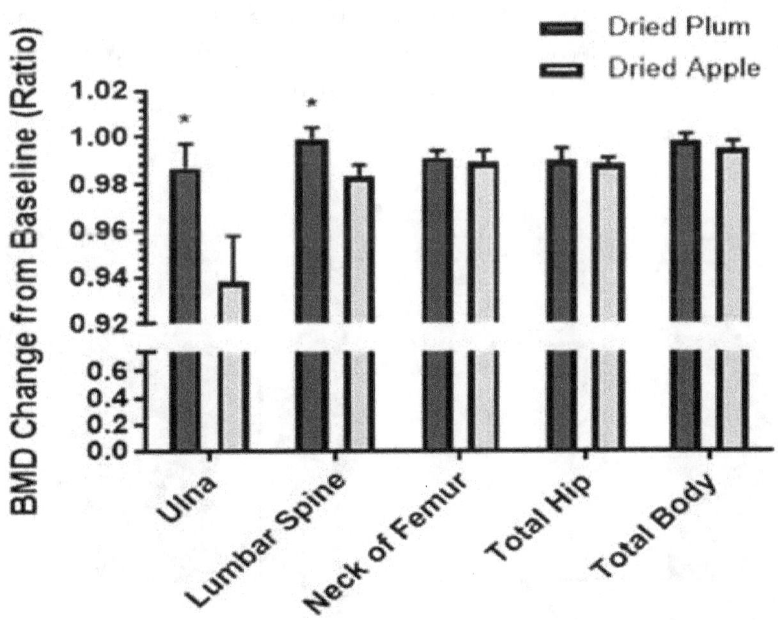

Figure 4. Change from baseline (ratio) in bone mineral density (BMD) from baseline to one-year following daily consumption of 100 g dried plum or 75 g dried apple. Bars represent mean ± standard error of the mean. * Denotes significant ($p < 0.05$) difference between groups.

We later investigated the potential mechanisms of action by which dried plum exerted these effects. We showed that compared to the baseline, dried plum increased receptor activator of nuclear factor kappa-B ligand levels by +1.99% versus +18.33% in the control group, increased the osteoprotegerin levels by +4.87% versus −2.15% in the control group, and decreased serum sclerostin levels by −1.12% in the dried plum group versus +3.78% in the control group [44]. While these percent changes did not reach statistical significance, they are clearly promising preliminary findings. Collectively, these findings suggest that dried plum prevents bone loss in postmenopausal women through the suppression of bone turnover.

Next, we [45] reported the findings of a six-month clinical trial evaluating the effects of resistance training with and without dried plum at a dose of 90 g in postmenopausal breast cancer survivors. While both groups were found to increase upper and lower body strength, no improvements were observed in the body composition or BMD. Interestingly, both groups displayed improvements in the blood biomarkers of bone turnover, with no added effect of dried plum observed.

Our successive six-month clinical trial evaluated the efficacy of two doses of dried plum (50 g versus 100 g) in preventing bone loss in older postmenopausal women [46]. Our findings confirmed dried plums' ability to prevent the loss of total body BMD and indicated that a lower dose of dried plum (i.e., 50 g) may be as effective as 100 g of dried plum. This study also demonstrated a reduction in serum TRAP-5b in both dried plum groups.

Most recently, we evaluated whether or not individuals who received the dried plum intervention in our previous one-year clinical trial conducted five years prior were able to retain BMD to a greater extent than those who received the dried apple intervention. Of the 100 women who completed the initial clinical trial, 20 came back for a follow-up visit. All participants, irrespective of group assignment, reported that they did not regularly consume dried plums. We found that individuals that received the dried plum intervention (n = 8) in our previous one-year clinical trial retained BMD of the ulna and lumbar spine to a greater extent than those who received the dried apple intervention (n = 12) (unpublished data, Figure 5). Although these findings are preliminary, they suggest that women in the dried plum group retained bone density in the lumbar spine and ulna to a greater extent than those in the dried apple group over the course of five years, even in the absence of regular dried plum consumption. These findings should be interpreted with caution as the influence of other factors including diet, physical activity, and medications have not been evaluated. Nonetheless, these findings are promising and further research is needed to evaluate the extent to which bone density is retained following the cessation of an intervention with dried plum.

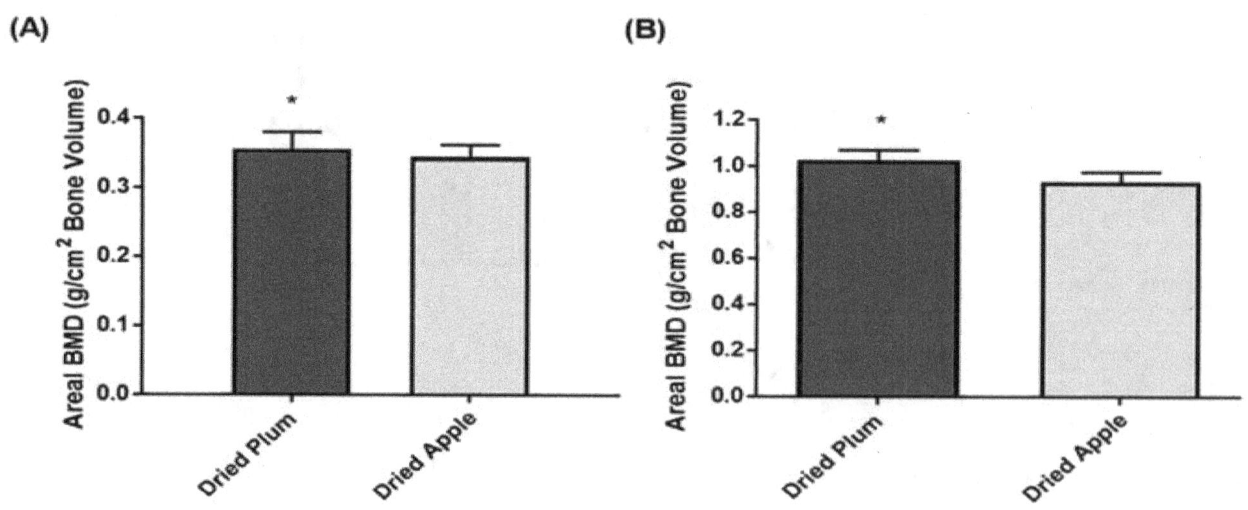

Figure 5. Bone mineral density (BMD) of the (**A**) ulna and (**B**) lumbar spine five years following one-year intervention study with daily consumption of 100 g dried plum or 75 g dried apple. Bars represent mean ± standard error of the mean. * Values were significantly ($p < 0.05$) different between groups.

Table 2. Clinical trials investigating the role of dried plum on bone health in postmenopausal women.

Reference	Design	Population	Number	Intervention	Duration	Primary Outcomes	Primary Findings
Arjmandi et al., 2002 [41]	RCT	Postmenopausal women	58	100 g/day dried plum or 75 g/day dried apple (comparative control)	3 months	Serum IGF-1, IGFBP-3, AP, TRAP, BSAP, calcium, phosphorus, and magnesium, urinary Dpd, HP, and creatinine	↑ IGF-1, AP, and BSAP compared to baseline in dried plum group
Hooshmand et al., 2011 [13]	RCT	Postmenopausal women with osteopenia	160	100 g/day dried plum or 75 g/day dried apple (comparative control)	12 months	Whole body, lumbar spine, hip, and forearm BMD; serum BALP, osteocalcin, TRAP-5b, and CRP	↑ ulna and lumbar spine BMD in dried plum group compared to dried apple ($p < 0.05$), ↓ BALP in dried plum group compared to baseline
Hooshmand et al., 2014 [44]	RCT	Postmenopausal women with osteopenia	160	100 g/day dried plum or 75 g/day dried apple (comparative control)	12 months	Serum Dpd, RANKL, OPG, and sclerostin	Non-significant ↑ in RANKL, RANKL/OPG ratio, and sclerostin, and ↓ in OPG compared to baseline in dried apple group, non-significant ↑ in OPG and RANKL and ↓ in sclerostin in dried plum group compared to baseline
Simonavice et al., 2014 [45]	Non-randomized intervention trial	Postmenopausal breast cancer survivors	23	Resistance exercise with/without 90 g/day dried plum	6 months	Whole body, lumbar spine, femur, and forearm BMD; serum BAP, TRAP-5b, and CRP	No significant effects
Hooshmand et al., 2016 [46]	RCT	Older postmenopausal women	48	0, 50, or 100 g/day dried plum	6 months	Whole body, lumbar spine, hip, and forearm BMD; serum hs-CRP, IGF-1, BAP, TRAP-5b, BAP/TRAP-5b ratio, sclerostin, 25-OH vitamin D, RANKL, OPG, calcium, and phosphorus	↑ whole body BMD in both dried plum groups compared to control, ↓ TRAP-5b at 3 and 6 months in dried plum groups compared to control, ↑ BAP/TRAP-5b ratio at 6 months in both dried plum groups compared to baseline

BMD, bone mineral density; BSAP, bone-specific alkaline phosphatase; CRP, C-reactive protein; Dpd, deoxypyridinoline; HP, helical peptide; hs-CRP, high-sensitivity CRP; IGF-1, insulin-like growth factor-1, IGFBP-3, insulin-like growth factor binding protein-3; OPG, osteoprotegerin; RANKL, receptor activator of nuclear factor kappa-B ligand; RCT, randomized controlled trial; TRAP, tartrate-resistant acid phosphatase.

5. Bioactive Compounds and Possible Mechanisms of Action

Dried plum is known to contain several bioactive compounds including dietary fiber, vitamins (e.g., vitamin K), minerals (e.g., boron, copper), and (poly)phenolic compounds such as chlorogenic acids (i.e., chlorogenic acid, neochlorogenic acid, and cryptochlorogenic acid) and proanthocyanidins [24,25]. The exact nutrients and/or components contributing to the bone-protective effects of dried plum are unknown. However, many of these compounds are known to exert bone-protective effects and therefore likely work additively and/or synergistically.

Among the compounds found in dried plum is boron, which is a trace element critical for bone health as a deficiency or excess in consumption of boron can be harmful to bone. Dried plum contains a higher amount of boron than most fruits. In fact, the content of boron in 47.7 g dried plum (~5 dried plums) is about 1.1 mg [23]. The average daily intake of boron is about 1–2 mg/day, depending on sex and age, among other factors [47]. Boron has been shown to stimulate bone growth and bone metabolism [48], and play an important role in preserving BMD, bone microarchitecture, and bone strength [49–51]. A study by Chapin et al. [52] showed that rats fed diets containing 20 or more mg boron/100 g diet had a significantly improved vertebral strength. These authors also demonstrated that rats fed a boric acid diet of 200 ppm or more for nine weeks not only had a significant increase in the boron content of their bone, but retained their bone boron content three-fold greater than the controls 32 weeks after exposure to the diet ended. This suggests that boron has the ability to accumulate in bone, and though the half-life of boron in bone is uncertain, it may be similar to that of calcium, where the half-life is significantly longer than in tissue. This action of boron may play a role in the maintenance of bone density over long periods of time, even without regular consumption.

Another mineral abundant in dried plum important for bone health is potassium [53,54]. One hundred grams of dried plum contains 732 mg. Tucker et al. [55] investigated both the cross-sectional and longitudinal relationships between potassium and BMD using a Framingham Heart Study database and concluded that potassium contributes to the maintenance of BMD in men and women. Additionally, higher intakes of potassium have been shown to reduce bone resorption, particularly in the face of high protein intake [56].

Dried plum is also a good source of copper. A 47.7 g serving of dried plum provides 0.13 mg, which is 31.2% of the dietary reference intake. Copper is a cofactor for lysyl oxidase, which is involved in the cross-linking of collagen and elastin [24,57]. In an in vivo study by Yee et al. [57], Ovx Sprague-Dawley rats placed on a copper deficient diet had more severe osteopenia than the copper adequate diet. Copper may in part contribute to the beneficial properties of dried plum on bone, giving an additive effect.

Dried plum is rich in vitamin K and a 47.7 g serving of dried plum provides 348 mg vitamin K, or 15.6% of the dietary reference intake [53]. Vitamin K is important for bone health as it promotes a calcium balance [58]. Additionally, it is a cofactor for the γ-carboxylation of osteocalcin, a bone matrix protein secreted by osteoblasts that promotes normal bone mineralization by regulating the growth of hydroxyapatite crystals [58]. A study by Braam et al. [59] demonstrated that supplementation with vitamin K at the level of 1 mg daily for three years attenuated the loss of BMD in the lumbar spine.

Among the (poly)phenols found in dried plum, chlorogenic acids (e.g., neochlorogenic acid, cryptochlorigenic acid, and chlorogenic acid) are the most abundant. In fact, 100 g of dried plum is estimated to contain between 108 and 153 mg chlorogenic acids. Previous research has demonstrated that chlorogenic acids are bone-protective. For instance, Zhou et al. [60] demonstrated that supplementing Ovx rats with chlorogenic acid led to improved BMD and microarchitecture, and an increased proliferation of osteoblast precursors and osteoblast differentiation, as well as increases in bone formation biomarkers. Despite this, Léotoing et al. [40] demonstrated that the bone-protective effects of dried plum is not dependent on the content of chlorogenic acids. As the authors pointed out, it is important to consider that dried plum contains other (poly)phenols such as quercetin, rutin, proanthocyanidins, among others, as well as dietary fiber in the form of soluble and insoluble fiber including pectin, fructans, hemicelluloses, and cellulose [23,40], which may be responsible for the effects of dried plum on bone. (Poly)phenols and their metabolites are known to not only act as antioxidants themselves [53,61,62], but to also activate endogenous antioxidant and inhibit inflammatory signaling pathways [63,64]. Considering that bone loss has been linked to oxygen-derived free radicals in the bone microenvironment, an imbalance in antioxidant defenses, and oxidative stress [65,66], as well as a pro-inflammatory state [67], it is possible that other dried plum (poly)phenols and their metabolites work through this mechanism. In fact, we and others have demonstrated the antioxidant and anti-inflammatory properties of dried plum [68,69]. Dried plum has a high oxygen radical absorbance capacity (ORAC) compared with many commonly consumed fruits and vegetables [70]. More recently, Kayano et al. [61], have isolated several ortho-diphenolic and mono hydroxyl phenolic compounds with ORAC values as high as 4.68 units of Trolox equivalent per mg of dried plum. Therefore, the beneficial effects of dried plum on bone may be partly mediated through its antioxidant properties.

Importantly, dried plum is rich in soluble and insoluble fibers, including pectin, fructans, hemicelluloses, and cellulose [23,40], which are known to increase mineral absorption (e.g., calcium) [71]. For instance, fibers are fermented by colonic bacteria, resulting in the production of short-chain fatty acids (SCFA). SCFAs enhance calcium absorption through reductions in the pH of the intestinal lumen and increasing the solubility of calcium, thereby facilitating passive diffusion through exchanges of luminal calcium with cellular hydrogen, and increasing the permeability of gut epithelial cells and paracellular transport [40,71,72]. Dietary fiber, including prebiotic dietary fibers, as well as (poly)phenolic compounds, have been shown to alter the microbial composition in the gut [71,73,74]. As such, it is possible that chronic dried plum consumption induces changes in the gut microbiome, thereby increasing SCFA production. It is also possible that these changes in the gut microbiome promote bone health through other mechanisms including those involving the immune system. However, this has yet to be investigated and is therefore speculative.

Lastly, previous research has shown that dried plum rich in chlorogenic acid increases bone calcium retention in an Ovx rodent model of postmenopausal osteoporosis [39]. Although changes in biomarkers of bone turnover were not noted, the observation that bone calcium retention was greater is consistent with the notion that dried plum reduces bone turnover. This is an interesting finding that warrants further investigation.

6. Conclusions

The bone-protective effects of dried plum in postmenopausal women have been supported by several animal studies and confirmed in randomized controlled trials. The exact mechanisms by which dried plum exerts these effects remains unknown. Additionally, it is unclear as to which bioactive compound(s) in dried plum is/are responsible for its bone-protective properties. Considering that many of the bioactive compounds present in dried plum have been shown to modulate bone metabolism, it is likely that there are additive and/or synergistic effects among these compounds. In addition to preventing bone loss in postmenopausal women, our recent findings suggest that the bone-protective effects of dried plum may be long-lasting, thereby contributing to the maintenance of bone density after regular consumption has ceased.

The findings of our previously conducted clinical trials indicate that dried plum is most efficacious in preventing bone loss in the ulna and lumbar spine. Although the reason for this is not currently known, both vertebra and ulna contain more trabecular bone than other sites (e.g., femur). In fact, vertebra and ulna contain more than 60% and up to 50% trabecular bone, respectively. Bone turnover is known to be greater in trabecular bone than cortical bone [75,76]. The body of literature suggests that dried plum slows the rate of bone turnover. As such, it is likely that dried plum has a more pronounced effect of reducing bone loss at these sites through reductions in trabecular bone turnover.

An important point to consider with any nutritional intervention, including functional foods, is caloric intake. The addition of dried plum to the diet contributes approximately 120 kcal and 240 kcal for 50 g and 100 g doses, respectively [23]. In our previous clinical trials, study participants were advised to maintain their usual diet and physical activity patterns throughout the duration of the study. We did not observe significant changes in nutritional intake, including calories, nor in body weight. Considering that self-reported dietary intake and physical activity are known to have limitations, including measurement error, it is therefore unknown as to whether our study participants made alterations in their diets or physical activity to maintain their body weight. Dried plum is high in dietary fiber which alters the transit time and may increase satiety, thereby reducing the overall caloric intake. Logically, one would assume that the addition of dried plum to the diet would displace other calories. However, this is speculative and needs future confirmation.

Future research should aim not only to better understand the mechanisms by which dried plum consumption contributes to bone health, including the involvement of the gut microbiome, but also to elucidate the long-term maintenance of such effects, including their role in fracture prevention. With respect to feasibility, we have observed good study participant treatment compliance and retention with long-term dried plum consumption at doses of 50 g (six months) and 100 g (one year). Study participants were generally willing to commit to the regular consumption of dried plum in order to improve their bone health and avoid taking osteoporosis medications. Our study participants were educated on ways to incorporate dried plum into their diets (e.g., in their meals) in an effort to promote compliance. Nonetheless, there are challenges with any long-term dietary intervention. For this reason, it is important that future studies aim to establish the lowest dose of dried plum or alternative dosing methods (e.g., intermittent dosing regimens) that provide the same efficacy as 100 g/day. Additionally, the combination of other foods and/or bioactive compounds that show promise for bone health, such as FOS, with dried plum should be further investigated, as this may enhance its efficacy. Finally, many of the previously conducted clinical trials evaluating the bone-protective effects of dried plum had small sample sizes, which may have contributed to null findings. Therefore, future large-scale clinical trials are needed to further establish the bone-protective effects of dried plum in postmenopausal women.

Acknowledgments: This work was funded in part by the California Dried Plum Board and the United States Department of Agriculture.

References

1. Barrett-Connor, E. Epidemiology and the Menopause: A Global Overview. *Int. J. Fertil. Menopausal. Stud.* **1993**, *38* (Suppl. 1), 6–14. [PubMed]
2. American Congress of Obstetricians and Gynecologists. 2011 Women's Health Stats and Facts. Available online: https://www.acog.org/-/media/NewsRoom/MediaKit.pdf (accessed on 14 April 2017).
3. Facts and Statistics. International Osteoporosis Foundation. Available online: https://www.iofbonehealth.org/facts-statistics (accessed on 14 April 2017).
4. Raisz, L.G. Pathogenesis of Osteoporosis: Concepts, Conflicts, and Prospects. *J. Clin. Investig.* **2005**, *115*, 3318–3325. [CrossRef] [PubMed]
5. Kamienski, M.; Tate, D.; Vega, M. The Silent Thief: Diagnosis and Management of Osteoporosis. *Orthop. Nurs.* **2011**, *30*, 162–171. [CrossRef] [PubMed]
6. Burge, R.; Dawson-Hughes, B.; Solomon, D.H.; Wong, J.B.; King, A.; Tosteson, A. Incidence and Economic Burden of Osteoporosis-Related Fractures in the United States, 2005–2025. *J. Bone Miner. Res.* **2007**, *22*, 465–475. [CrossRef] [PubMed]
7. Looker, A.C.; Borrud, L.G.; Dawson-Hughes, B.; Shepherd, J.A.; Wright, N.C. Osteoporosis or Low Bone Mass at the Femur Neck or Lumbar Spine in Older Adults: United States, 2005–2008. *NCHS Data Brief* **2012**, *93*, 1–8.
8. Demontiero, O.; Vidal, C.; Duque, G. Aging and Bone Loss: New Insights for the Clinician. *Ther. Adv. Musculoskelet. Dis.* **2012**, *4*, 61–76. [CrossRef] [PubMed]

9. Almeida, M.; Laurent, M.R.; Dubois, V.; Claessens, F.; O'Brien, C.A.; Bouillon, R.; Vanderschueren, D.; Manolagas, S.C. Estrogens and Androgens in Skeletal Physiology and Pathophysiology. *Physiol. Rev.* **2017**, *97*, 135–187. [CrossRef] [PubMed]
10. Rossouw, J.E.; Anderson, G.L.; Prentice, R.L.; LaCroix, A.Z.; Kooperberg, C.; Stefanick, M.L.; Jackson, R.D.; Beresford, S.A.; Howard, B.V.; Johnson, K.C.; et al. Risks and Benefits of Estrogen Plus Progestin in Healthy Postmenopausal Women: Principal Results from the Women's Health Initiative Randomized Controlled Trial. *JAMA* **2002**, *288*, 321–333. [CrossRef] [PubMed]
11. Kayser, J.; Ettinger, B.; Pressman, A. Postmenopausal Hormonal Support: Discontinuation of Raloxifene Versus Estrogen. *Menopause* **2001**, *8*, 328–332. [CrossRef] [PubMed]
12. Cashman, K.D. Diet, Nutrition, and Bone Health. *J. Nutr.* **2007**, *137*, 2507S–2512S. [PubMed]
13. Hooshmand, S.; Chai, S.C.; Saadat, R.L.; Payton, M.E.; Brummel-Smith, K.; Arjmandi, B.H. Comparative Effects of Dried Plum and Dried Apple on Bone in Postmenopausal Women. *Br. J. Nutr.* **2011**, *106*, 923–930. [CrossRef] [PubMed]
14. Arjmandi, B.H.; Johnson, C.D.; Campbell, S.C.; Hooshmand, S.; Chai, S.C.; Akhter, M.P. Combining Fructooligosaccharide and Dried Plum Has the Greatest Effect on Restoring Bone Mineral Density among Select Functional Foods and Bioactive Compounds. *J. Med. Food* **2010**, *13*, 312–319. [CrossRef] [PubMed]
15. Johnson, C.D.; Lucas, E.A.; Hooshmand, S.; Campbell, S.; Akhter, M.P.; Arjmandi, B.H. Addition of Fructooligosaccharides and Dried Plum to Soy-Based Diets Reverses Bone Loss in the Ovariectomized Rat. *Evid. Based Complement. Alternat. Med.* **2011**, *2011*, 836267. [CrossRef] [PubMed]
16. Rendina, E.; Lim, Y.F.; Marlow, D.; Wang, Y.; Clarke, S.L.; Kuvibidila, S.; Lucas, E.A.; Smith, B.J. Dietary Supplementation with Dried Plum Prevents Ovariectomy-Induced Bone Loss While Modulating the Immune Response in C57bl/6j Mice. *J. Nutr. Biochem.* **2012**, *23*, 60–68. [CrossRef] [PubMed]
17. Halloran, B.P.; Wronski, T.J.; VonHerzen, D.C.; Chu, V.; Xia, X.; Pingel, J.E.; Williams, A.A.; Smith, B.J. Dietary Dried Plum Increases Bone Mass in Adult and Aged Male Mice. *J. Nutr.* **2010**, *140*, 1781–1787. [CrossRef] [PubMed]
18. Mühlbauer, R.C.; Lozano, A.; Reinli, A. Onion and a Mixture of Vegetables, Salads, and Herbs Affect Bone Resorption in the Rat by a Mechanism Independent of Their Base Excess. *J. Bone Miner. Res.* **2002**, *17*, 1230–1236. [CrossRef] [PubMed]
19. Mühlbauer, R.C.; Lozano, A.; Reinli, A.; Wetli, H. Various Selected Vegetables, Fruits, Mushrooms and Red Wine Residue Inhibit Bone Resorption in Rats. *J. Nutr.* **2003**, *133*, 3592–3597. [PubMed]
20. Devareddy, L.; Hooshmand, S.; Collins, J.K.; Lucas, E.A.; Chai, S.C.; Arjmandi, B.H. Blueberry Prevents Bone Loss in Ovariectomized Rat Model of Postmenopausal Osteoporosis. *J. Nutr. Biochem.* **2008**, *19*, 694–699. [CrossRef] [PubMed]
21. Zhang, J.; Lazarenko, O.P.; Blackburn, M.L.; Shankar, K.; Badger, T.M.; Ronis, M.J.; Chen, J.R. Feeding Blueberry Diets in Early Life Prevent Senescence of Osteoblasts and Bone Loss in Ovariectomized Adult Female Rats. *PLoS ONE* **2011**, *6*, e24486. [CrossRef] [PubMed]
22. Zhang, J.; Lazarenko, O.P.; Blackburn, M.L.; Badger, T.M.; Ronis, M.J.; Chen, J.R. Blueberry Consumption Prevents Loss of Collagen in Bone Matrix and Inhibits Senescence Pathways in Osteoblastic Cells. *Age (Dordr)* **2013**, *35*, 807–820. [CrossRef] [PubMed]
23. Bowen, P.E. Role of Commodity Boards in Advancing the Understanding of the Health Benefits of Whole Foods: California Dried Plums. *Nutr. Today* **2017**, *52*, 19–25. [CrossRef] [PubMed]
24. Stacewicz-Sapuntzakis, M. Dried Plums and Their Products: Composition and Health Effects—An Updated Review. *Crit. Rev. Food Sci. Nutr.* **2013**, *53*, 1277–1302. [CrossRef] [PubMed]
25. Hooshmand, S.; Arjmandi, B.H. Viewpoint: Dried Plum, an Emerging Functional Food That May Effectively Improve Bone Health. *Ageing Res. Rev.* **2009**, *8*, 122–127. [CrossRef] [PubMed]
26. Horcajada-Molteni, M.N.; Crespy, V.; Coxam, V.; Davicco, M.J.; Rémésy, C.; Barlet, J.P. Rutin Inhibits Ovariectomy-Induced Osteopenia in Rats. *J. Bone Miner. Res.* **2000**, *15*, 2251–2258. [CrossRef] [PubMed]
27. Arjmandi, B.H.; Lucas, E.A.; Juma, S.; Soliman, A.; Stoecker, B.J.; Khalil, D.A.; Smith, B.J.; Wang, C. Prune Prevents Ovariectomy-Induced Bone Loss in Rats. *J. Am. Nutraceutical Assoc.* **2001**, *4*, 50–56.
28. Kalu, D.N. The Ovariectomized Rat Model of Postmenopausal Bone Loss. *Bone Miner.* **1991**, *15*, 175–191. [CrossRef]

29. Lane, N.E.; Haupt, D.; Kimmel, D.B.; Modin, G.; Kinney, J.H. Early Estrogen Replacement Therapy Reverses the Rapid Loss of Trabecular Bone Volume and Prevents Further Deterioration of Connectivity in the Rat. *J. Bone Miner. Res.* **1999**, *14*, 206–214. [CrossRef] [PubMed]
30. Tokunaga, T. Novel Physiological Function of Fructooligosaccharides. *Biofactors* **2004**, *21*, 89–94. [CrossRef] [PubMed]
31. Devareddy, L.; Khalil, D.A.; Korlagunta, K.; Hooshmand, S.; Bellmer, D.D.; Arjmandi, B.H. The Effects of Fructo-Oligosaccharides in Combination with Soy Protein on Bone in Osteopenic Ovariectomized Rats. *Menopause* **2006**, *13*, 692–699. [CrossRef] [PubMed]
32. Devareddy, L.; Khalil, D.A.; Smith, B.J.; Lucas, E.A.; Soung, D.Y.; Marlow, D.D.; Arjmandi, B.H. Soy Moderately Improves Microstructural Properties without Affecting Bone Mass in an Ovariectomized Rat Model of Osteoporosis. *Bone* **2006**, *38*, 686–693. [CrossRef] [PubMed]
33. Arjmandi, B.H.; Lucas, E.A.; Khalil, D.A.; Devareddy, L.; Smith, B.J.; McDonald, J.; Arquitt, A.B.; Payton, M.E.; Mason, C. One Year Soy Protein Supplementation Has Positive Effects on Bone Formation Markers but Not Bone Density in Postmenopausal Women. *Nutr. J.* **2005**, *4*, 8. [CrossRef] [PubMed]
34. Arjmandi, B.H.; Khalil, D.A.; Smith, B.J.; Lucas, E.A.; Juma, S.; Payton, M.E.; Wild, R.A. Soy Protein Has a Greater Effect on Bone in Postmenopausal Women Not on Hormone Replacement Therapy, as Evidenced by Reducing Bone Resorption and Urinary Calcium Excretion. *J. Clin. Endocrinol. Metab.* **2003**, *88*, 1048–1054. [CrossRef] [PubMed]
35. Arjmandi, B.H.; Birnbaum, R.; Goyal, N.V.; Getlinger, M.J.; Juma, S.; Alekel, L.; Hasler, C.M.; Drum, M.L.; Hollis, B.W.; Kukreja, S.C. Bone-Sparing Effect of Soy Protein in Ovarian Hormone-Deficient Rats Is Related to Its Isoflavone Content. *Am. J. Clin. Nutr.* **1998**, *68*, 1364S–1368S. [PubMed]
36. Rendina, E.; Hembree, K.D.; Davis, M.R.; Marlow, D.; Clarke, S.L.; Halloran, B.P.; Lucas, E.A.; Smith, B.J. Dried Plum's Unique Capacity to Reverse Bone Loss and Alter Bone Metabolism in Postmenopausal Osteoporosis Model. *PLoS ONE* **2013**, *8*, e60569. [CrossRef] [PubMed]
37. Smith, B.J.; Bu, S.Y.; Wang, Y.; Rendina, E.; Lim, Y.F.; Marlow, D.; Clarke, S.L.; Cullen, D.M.; Lucas, E.A. A Comparative Study of the Bone Metabolic Response to Dried Plum Supplementation and Pth Treatment in Adult, Osteopenic Ovariectomized Rat. *Bone* **2014**, *58*, 151–159. [CrossRef] [PubMed]
38. Deyhim, F.; Stoecker, B.J.; Brusewitz, G.H.; Devareddy, L.; Arjmandi, B.H. Dried Plum Reverses Bone Loss in an Osteopenic Rat Model of Osteoporosis. *Menopause* **2005**, *12*, 755–762. [CrossRef] [PubMed]
39. Pawlowski, J.W.; Martin, B.R.; McCabe, G.P.; Ferruzzi, M.G.; Weaver, C.M. Plum and Soy Aglycon Extracts Superior at Increasing Bone Calcium Retention in Ovariectomized Sprague Dawley Rats. *J. Agric. Food Chem.* **2014**, *62*, 6108–6117. [CrossRef] [PubMed]
40. Leotoing, L.; Wauquier, F.; Davicco, M.J.; Lebecque, P.; Gaudout, D.; Rey, S.; Vitrac, X.; Massenat, L.; Rashidi, S.; Wittrant, Y.; et al. The Phenolic Acids of Agen Prunes (Dried Plums) or Agen Prune Juice Concentrates Do Not Account for the Protective Action on Bone in a Rat Model of Postmenopausal Osteoporosis. *Nutr. Res.* **2016**, *36*, 161–173. [CrossRef] [PubMed]
41. Arjmandi, B.H.; Khalil, D.A.; Lucas, E.A.; Georgis, A.; Stoecker, B.J.; Hardin, C.; Payton, M.E.; Wild, R.A. Dried Plums Improve Indices of Bone Formation in Postmenopausal Women. *J. Womens Health Gend. Based Med.* **2002**, *11*, 61–68. [CrossRef] [PubMed]
42. Hodsman, A.B.; Fraher, L.J.; Watson, P.H.; Ostbye, T.; Stitt, L.W.; Adachi, J.D.; Taves, D.H.; Drost, D. A Randomized Controlled Trial to Compare the Efficacy of Cyclical Parathyroid Hormone Versus Cyclical Parathyroid Hormone and Sequential Calcitonin to Improve Bone Mass in Postmenopausal Women with Osteoporosis. *J. Clin. Endocrinol. Metab.* **1997**, *82*, 620–628. [CrossRef] [PubMed]
43. Wheater, G.; Elshahaly, M.; Tuck, S.P.; Datta, H.K.; van Laar, J.M. The Clinical Utility of Bone Marker Measurements in Osteoporosis. *J. Transl. Med.* **2013**, *11*, 201. [CrossRef] [PubMed]
44. Hooshmand, S.; Brisco, J.R.; Arjmandi, B.H. The Effect of Dried Plum on Serum Levels of Receptor Activator of Nf-Kappab Ligand, Osteoprotegerin and Sclerostin in Osteopenic Postmenopausal Women: A Randomised Controlled Trial. *Br. J. Nutr.* **2014**, *112*, 55–60. [CrossRef] [PubMed]
45. Simonavice, E.; Liu, P.Y.; Ilich, J.Z.; Kim, J.S.; Arjmandi, B.; Panton, L.B. The Effects of a 6-Month Resistance Training and Dried Plum Consumption Intervention on Strength, Body Composition, Blood Markers of Bone Turnover, and Inflammation in Breast Cancer Survivors. *Appl. Physiol. Nutr. Metab.* **2014**, *39*, 730–739. [CrossRef] [PubMed]

46. Hooshmand, S.; Kern, M.; Metti, D.; Shamloufard, P.; Chai, S.C.; Johnson, S.A.; Payton, M.E.; Arjmandi, B.H. The Effect of Two Doses of Dried Plum on Bone Density and Bone Biomarkers in Osteopenic Postmenopausal Women: A Randomized, Controlled Trial. *Osteoporos. Int.* **2016**, *27*, 2271–2279. [CrossRef] [PubMed]
47. Trumbo, P.; Yates, A.A.; Schlicker, S.; Poos, M. Dietary Reference Intakes: Vitamin A, Vitamin K, Arsenic, Boron, Chromium, Copper, Iodine, Iron, Manganese, Molybdenum, Nickel, Silicon, Vanadium, and Zinc. *J. Am. Diet. Assoc.* **2001**, *101*, 294–301. [CrossRef]
48. Nielsen, F.H.; Hunt, C.D.; Mullen, L.M.; Hunt, J.R. Effect of Dietary Boron on Mineral, Estrogen, and Testosterone Metabolism in Postmenopausal Women. *FASEB J.* **1987**, *1*, 394–397. [CrossRef]
49. Nielsen, F.H. Biochemical and Physiologic Consequences of Boron Deprivation in Humans. *Environ. Health Perspect.* **1994**, *102* (Suppl. 7), 59–63. [CrossRef] [PubMed]
50. Nielsen, F.H. Is Boron Nutritionally Relevant? *Nutr. Rev.* **2008**, *66*, 183–191. [CrossRef] [PubMed]
51. Zofkova, I.; Davis, M.; Blahos, J. Trace Elements Have Beneficial, as Well as Detrimental Effects on Bone Homeostasis. In *Physiol. Res.*; 2017. Available online: https://www.ncbi.nlm.nih.gov/pubmed/28248532 (accessed on 14 April 2017).
52. Chapin, R.E.; Ku, W.W.; Kenney, M.A.; McCoy, H. The Effects of Dietary Boric Acid on Bone Strength in Rats. *Biol. Trace Elem. Res.* **1998**, *66*, 395–399. [CrossRef] [PubMed]
53. Dismore, M.L.; Haytowitz, D.B.; Gebhardt, S.E.; Peterson, J.W.; Booth, S.L. Vitamin K Content of Nuts and Fruits in the US Diet. *J. Am. Diet. Assoc.* **2003**, *103*, 1650–1652. [CrossRef] [PubMed]
54. Stacewicz-Sapuntzakis, M.; Bowen, P.E.; Hussain, E.A.; Damayanti-Wood, B.I.; Farnsworth, N.R. Chemical Composition and Potential Health Effects of Prunes: A Functional Food? *Crit. Rev. Food Sci. Nutr.* **2001**, *41*, 251–286. [CrossRef] [PubMed]
55. Tucker, K.L.; Hannan, M.T.; Chen, H.; Cupples, L.A.; Wilson, P.W.; Kiel, D.P. Potassium, Magnesium, and Fruit and Vegetable Intakes Are Associated with Greater Bone Mineral Density in Elderly Men and Women. *Am. J. Clin. Nutr.* **1999**, *69*, 727–736. [PubMed]
56. Zwart, S.R.; Hargens, A.R.; Smith, S.M. The Ratio of Animal Protein Intake to Potassium Intake Is a Predictor of Bone Resorption in Space Flight Analogues and in Ambulatory Subjects. *Am. J. Clin. Nutr.* **2004**, *80*, 1058–1065. [PubMed]
57. Yee, C.D.; Kubena, K.S.; Walker, M.; Champney, T.H.; Sampson, H.W. The Relationship of Nutritional Copper to the Development of Postmenopausal Osteoporosis in Rats. *Biol. Trace Elem. Res.* **1995**, *48*, 1–11. [CrossRef] [PubMed]
58. Iwamoto, J.; Takeda, T.; Sato, Y. Effects of Vitamin K2 on Osteoporosis. *Curr. Pharm. Des.* **2004**, *10*, 2557–2576. [CrossRef] [PubMed]
59. Braam, L.A.; Knapen, M.H.; Geusens, P.; Brouns, F.; Hamulyák, K.; Gerichhausen, M.J.; Vermeer, C. Vitamin K1 Supplementation Retards Bone Loss in Postmenopausal Women between 50 and 60 Years of Age. *Calcif. Tissue Int.* **2003**, *73*, 21–26. [CrossRef] [PubMed]
60. Zhou, R.P.; Lin, S.J.; Wan, W.B.; Zuo, H.L.; Yao, F.F.; Ruan, H.B.; Xu, J.; Song, W.; Zhou, Y.C.; Wen, S.Y.; et al. Chlorogenic Acid Prevents Osteoporosis by Shp2/Pi3k/Akt Pathway in Ovariectomized Rats. *PLoS ONE* **2016**, *11*, e0166751. [CrossRef] [PubMed]
61. Kayano, S.; Kikuzaki, H.; Fukutsuka, N.; Mitani, T.; Nakatani, N. Antioxidant Activity of Prune (*Prunus domestica* L.) Constituents and a New Synergist. *J. Agric. Food Chem.* **2002**, *50*, 3708–3712. [CrossRef] [PubMed]
62. Nakatani, N.; Kayano, S.; Kikuzaki, H.; Sumino, K.; Katagiri, K.; Mitani, T. Identification, Quantitative Determination, and Antioxidative Activities of Chlorogenic Acid Isomers in Prune (*Prunus domestica* L.). *J. Agric. Food Chem.* **2000**, *48*, 5512–5516. [CrossRef] [PubMed]
63. Rahman, I.; Biswas, S.K.; Kirkham, P.A. Regulation of Inflammation and Redox Signaling by Dietary Polyphenols. *Biochem. Pharmacol.* **2006**, *72*, 1439–1452. [CrossRef] [PubMed]
64. Stevenson, D.E.; Hurst, R.D. Polyphenolic Phytochemicals—Just Antioxidants or Much More? *Cell Mol. Life Sci.* **2007**, *64*, 2900–2916. [CrossRef] [PubMed]
65. Garrett, I.R.; Boyce, B.F.; Oreffo, R.O.; Bonewald, L.; Poser, J.; Mundy, G.R. Oxygen-Derived Free Radicals Stimulate Osteoclastic Bone Resorption in Rodent Bone in Vitro and in Vivo. *J. Clin. Investig.* **1990**, *85*, 632–639. [CrossRef] [PubMed]
66. Callaway, D.A.; Jiang, J.X. Reactive Oxygen Species and Oxidative Stress in Osteoclastogenesis, Skeletal Aging and Bone Diseases. *J. Bone Miner. Metab.* **2015**, *33*, 359–370. [CrossRef] [PubMed]

67. Mundy, G.R. Osteoporosis and Inflammation. *Nutr. Rev.* **2007**, *65*, S147–S151. [CrossRef] [PubMed]
68. Igwe, E.O.; Charlton, K.E. A Systematic Review on the Health Effects of Plums (Prunus Domestica and Prunus Salicina). *Phytother. Res.* **2016**, *30*, 701–731. [CrossRef] [PubMed]
69. Hooshmand, S.; Kumar, A.; Zhang, J.Y.; Johnson, S.A.; Chai, S.C.; Arjmandi, B.H. Evidence for Anti-Inflammatory and Antioxidative Properties of Dried Plum Polyphenols in Macrophage Raw 264.7 Cells. *Food Funct.* **2015**, *6*, 1719–1725. [CrossRef] [PubMed]
70. McBride, J. Can Foods Forestall Aging? *Agric. Res.* **1999**, *47*, 14–17.
71. McCabe, L.; Britton, R.A.; Parameswaran, N. Prebiotic and Probiotic Regulation of Bone Health: Role of the Intestine and Its Microbiome. *Curr. Osteoporos. Rep.* **2015**, *13*, 363–371. [CrossRef] [PubMed]
72. Steves, C.J.; Bird, S.; Williams, F.M.; Spector, T.D. The Microbiome and Musculoskeletal Conditions of Aging: A Review of Evidence for Impact and Potential Therapeutics. *J. Bone Miner. Res.* **2016**, *31*, 261–269. [CrossRef] [PubMed]
73. Duda-Chodak, A.; Tarko, T.; Satora, P.; Sroka, P. Interaction of Dietary Compounds, Especially Polyphenols, with the Intestinal Microbiota: A Review. *Eur. J. Nutr.* **2015**, *54*, 325–341. [CrossRef] [PubMed]
74. Tuohy, K.M.; Conterno, L.; Gasperotti, M.; Viola, R. Up-Regulating the Human Intestinal Microbiome Using Whole Plant Foods, Polyphenols, and/or Fiber. *J. Agric. Food Chem.* **2012**, *60*, 8776–8782. [CrossRef] [PubMed]
75. Clarke, B. Normal Bone Anatomy and Physiology. *Clin. J. Am. Soc. Nephrol.* **2008**, *3* (Suppl. 3), S131–S139. [CrossRef] [PubMed]
76. Lespessailles, E.; Hambli, R.; Ferrari, S. Osteoporosis Drug Effects on Cortical and Trabecular Bone Microstructure: A Review of Hr-Pqct Analyses. *Bonekey Rep.* **2016**, *5*, 836. [CrossRef] [PubMed]

6

The Role of AOPP in Age-Related Bone Loss and the Potential Benefits of Berry Anthocyanins

Melissa M. Melough , Xin Sun and Ock K. Chun *

Department of Nutritional Sciences, University of Connecticut, Storrs, CT 06269, USA; melissa.melough@uconn.edu (M.M.M.); xin.sun@uconn.edu (X.S.)

* Correspondence: ock.chun@uconn.edu

Abstract: Age-related bone loss is a major factor in osteoporosis and osteoporotic fractures among the elderly. Because bone homeostasis involves a balance between bone formation and resorption, multiple mechanisms may induce age-dependent changes in bone. Oxidative stress is one such factor that contributes to the pathology of aging-associated osteoporosis (AAO). Advanced oxidation protein products (AOPP) are a biomarker of oxidant-mediated protein damage, and can also act to increase the production of reactive oxygen species (ROS), thereby perpetuating oxidative damage. AOPP is a relatively novel marker of oxidative stress, and its role in bone aging has not been fully elucidated. Furthermore, it has been theorized that dietary antioxidants may decrease AOPP levels, thereby reducing AAO risk, but a limited number of studies have been specifically targeted at addressing this hypothesis. Therefore, the objective of this review is to examine the findings of existing research on the role of AOPP in age-related bone loss, and the potential use of dietary antioxidants to mitigate the effects of AAOP on age-related bone loss. Cross-sectional studies have delivered mixed results, showing that AOPP levels are inconsistently associated with bone loss and aging. However, in vitro studies have documented multiple mechanisms by which AOPP may lead to bone loss, including upregulation of the JNK/p38 MAPK signaling pathways as well as increasing expression of sclerostin and of receptor activator of NFκB ligand (RANKL). Studies also indicate that antioxidants—especially berry anthocyanins—may be an effective dietary agent to prevent aging-associated bone deterioration by inhibiting the formation of AOPP and ROS. However, the understanding of these pathways in AAO has largely been based on in vitro studies, and should be examined in further animal and human studies in order to inform recommendations regarding dietary anthocyanin use for the prevention of AAO.

Keywords: AOPP; bone; aging; osteoporosis; antioxidants; berry anthocyanins

---

1. Introduction

Age-related bone loss is a primary contributor to osteoporosis and osteoporotic fractures in the elderly. Osteoporosis is considered a major public health threat for an estimated 44 million Americans, or 55% of the population aged 50 years and older [2]. Numerous studies employing various methods have dealt with the pathophysiology of postmenopausal osteoporosis [3], but aging-associated osteoporosis (AAO) has not been as well studied [4]. AAO is thought to be a type of low-turnover osteoporosis resulting from aging-associated calcium deficiency and an imbalance between bone resorption and formation [5].

Oxidative stress plays a central role in human aging and accelerates the aging process [6,7]. Bone density is maintained by two phases of bone remodeling: bone resorption by osteoclasts and bone formation by osteoblasts [8]. Emerging evidence indicates that the increased production of reactive oxygen species (ROS) in bone cells may activate bone resorption, resulting in a gradual decline in bone mass and density with aging [7]. Studies have shown that oxidative stress results in reduced bone formation, increased osteoblast and osteocyte apoptosis, and decreased bone mineral density (BMD) in aged mice [9]. Reduced BMD is one of the defining characteristics of osteoporosis, and correlates with bone strength and fracture risk [2]. Induced oxidative stress in young mice and rats has also been shown to reduce osteoblastogenesis and to increase osteoclast number and activity [10,11]. Loss of sex steroids potentiates the effects of aging by weakening defense mechanisms against oxidative stress [10]. Previous studies have clearly demonstrated that the bone turnover pattern remains relatively steady in advanced aging [12]. Based on this pattern, there is a reduction in bone formation as a result of a decreased recruitment of osteoblasts and an elevation of bone resorption that might result from enhanced activity of osteoclasts, which is the primary underlying mechanism of AAO [12].

Advanced oxidation protein products (AOPP) arise from the reaction between plasma proteins and chlorinated oxidants (e.g., hypochlorous acid, HOCl) by the H_2O_2-myeloperoxidase (MPO) system, and are di-tyrosine-containing cross-linking protein products considered to be novel markers of oxidant-mediated protein damage [13–15]. AOPP are mainly carried by albumin in the circulation, and oxidized albumin is rapidly cleared mainly through the uptake by the liver and spleen [16]. Like advanced glycation end products (AGEs), AOPP signal via the receptor for AGE (RAGE) in endothelial cells and induce endothelial dysfunction [17]. Increased plasma levels of AOPP have been found in many diseases, such as diabetes, uremia, obesity, coronary artery disease, and inflammatory bowel diseases. Evidence indicates that AOPP increase with age, and that AOPP can trigger cytosolic superoxide generation via the activation of nicotinamide adenine dinucleotide phosphate (NADPH) oxidase (NOX), which is a major source of ROS [18] (Figure 1). Therefore, AOPP may serve not only as markers of oxidant-mediated protein damage, but also as potential inducers of oxidative stress [15].

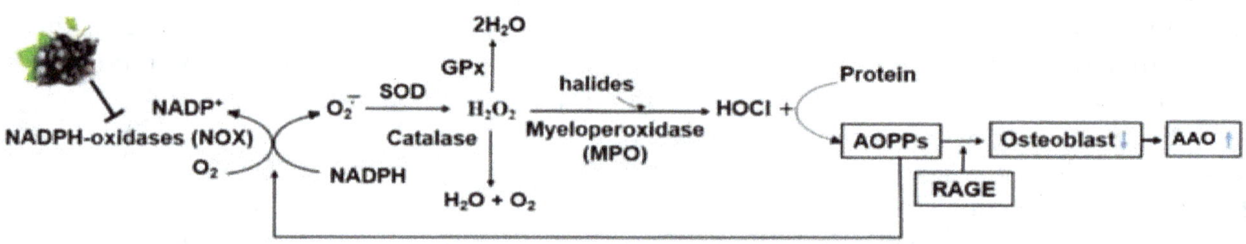

Figure 1. Potential mechanism of anthocyanins in lowering aging-associated osteoporosis (AAO) risk through inhibiting nicotinamide adenine dinucleotide phosphate (NADPH) oxidase (NOX)-mediated advanced oxidation protein products (AOPP) formation. GPx: glutathione peroxidase; RAGE: receptor for advanced glycation end products; SOD: superoxide dismutase.

Due to the public health relevance of AAO and the emerging evidence demonstrating the role of oxidative stress in bone aging, it is of great importance to characterize the ways in which AOPP may affect bone health and homeostasis. It has also been hypothesized that due to their antioxidant capacity, anthocyanins found in plants such as berries may prevent or reduce bone resorption and deterioration. Therefore, the purpose of this review is to examine the current state of knowledge regarding the role of AOPP in age-related bone loss and to assess the potential for the use of berry anthocyanins to reduce the formation of AOPP and improve bone-related outcomes in aging.

Articles included in this review were identified using PubMed and Web of Science. To examine the role of AOPP in bone loss, databases were searched for "AOPP bone loss". Other keywords added to this search were osteoporosis, osteoblasts, and osteoclasts. To find studies investigating the effects of anthocyanins on bone loss, databases were searched for "berry anthocyanin bone loss", and the following terms were added to expand the search: AOPP, antioxidant, osteoporosis. All articles for this review were published by May 2017. Publications identified by these methods were then limited to those describing cross-sectional analyses of AOPP and bone health in humans and animals, in vitro studies of cells treated with AOPP, and clinical trials or observational studies seeking to examine the effects of dietary antioxidants on AOPP and bone outcomes.

2. Aging-Associated Osteoporosis

Osteoporosis is a skeletal disease characterized by the deterioration of bone mass and microarchitecture, leading to increased fragility and predisposition to bone fractures [2]. While postmenopausal osteoporosis is related to estrogen deficiency and affects trabecular bone, aging-associated osteoporosis (AAO) primarily affects cortical bone and has many contributing factors including genetics, nutrition, physical activity, and physiological changes to bone [5]. Because bone loss appears to begin near age 40 and accelerates after age 60, age-related bone loss affects a growing number of men and women as the global population of older individuals increases [19].

One well-established physiological effect of bone aging is decreased bone mineral content, which is associated with increased brittleness and decreased fracture resistance [20]. Aging is also associated with morphological changes to bone such as thinning of the cortical walls and the overall slimming of the bones, as well as changes to proteins in bone, including collagen [20]. Increased bone resorption in aging may also contribute to reduced bone mineral density (BMD), and can be exacerbated by reductions in bone formation related to reduced osteoblastogenesis and increased adipogenesis in the bone marrow, which affects matrix formation and mineralization [21]. The etiology of osteoporosis is multifactorial and influenced by both genetic and environmental factors. Of particular interest to this review is the effect of oxidative stress.

3. AOPP as a Marker of Oxidative Stress in Bone

Studies indicate that oxidative stress may enhance bone resorption and disturb the coupling of bone resorption to bone formation, contributing to AAO [19,22]. Oxidative stress increases with age, as ROS production rises and the activities of antioxidant enzymes such as superoxide dismutase (SOD) and glutathione peroxidase simultaneously decrease [19,23]. The oxidative stress resulting from this imbalance can stimulate apoptosis of osteoblasts and osteocytes [24,25], and may reduce osteoblastogenesis [26] while also increasing the formation and activation of osteoclasts [10].

AOPP is a novel marker of oxidative stress that may be particularly important in the context of bones, both as a biological driver and a biomarker of bone degradation. Several cross-sectional studies have examined the relationship between bone status and AOPP in both humans and animals (Table 1). Zhang et al. demonstrated that among male Wistar rats, AOPP levels in both plasma and femurs increased with age, while SOD activity decreased [19]. AOPP was also associated with decreases in BMD, bone volume, trabecular thickness, and the rate of bone formation. Similarly, a 2015 study showed that plasma AOPP was associated with reduced BMD and increased markers of bone turnover among postmenopausal women [27]. Importantly, this study did not adjust for potential cofounding factors such as age, body mass index, diet, or smoking. Recent studies by a group in Italy linked lipid hydroperoxides—one marker of oxidative stress—to reduced BMD in postmenopausal women, but did not find significant relationships between AOPP and BMD [28]. Differences between these studies could reflect differences in study populations as well as the progression of bone disease or oxidative damage. The currently available cross-sectional study data provide weak evidence to support the link between AOPP and bone health. Given these mixed findings and important limitations to each study, alternative study designs that illuminate potential mechanisms of AOPP in bone are essential for understanding the relationship between AOPP and osteoporosis.

Table 1. Cross-sectional studies of AOPP and bone status in humans and animals.

Study	Population	Observations	Limitations
Zhang (2011) [19]	Young, adult, and old (n = 26 each) male Wistar rats	AOPP in plasma and femur increased with aging and were negatively associated with femur BMD	Sample size; potentially limited translatability to humans
Wu (2015) [27]	60 postmenopausal women with osteoporosis, 60 without osteoporosis	AOPP was associated with reduced BMD and increased bone turnover markers	Sample size; no adjustment for factors such as BMI, diet, or smoking; BMD assessed only at lumbar spine
Cervellati (2013) [28]	98 pre- and 93 post-menopausal women	No significant association between AOPP and bone status	Potential for residual confounding; AOPP assessed only in serum
Cervellati (2014) [22]	167 postmenopausal women	No significant association between AOPP and bone status	Potential for residual confounding; AOPP assessed only in serum

AOPP: advanced oxidation protein products; BMD: bone mineral density; BMI: body mass index.

Few interventional trials in animals have investigated the actions of AOPP on bone. One study showed that AOPP administration accelerated bone deterioration in aged male rats and that the AOPP-induced changes in bone turnover markers, trabecular BMD, and microstructural parameters could be completely prevented by the oral administration of the NOX inhibitor apocynin, suggesting that AOPP induced bone deterioration via the activation of NAPDH oxidase [4]. Another study showed that administration of the radical scavenger antioxidant melatonin reduced AOPP levels and other markers of oxidative stress in streptozotocin-induced diabetic male rats, leading to beneficial effects on bone healing in a short-term study [29]. Although not specific to osteoporosis, this suggests that AOPP may inhibit bone formation.

4. Mechanisms of Action of AOPP in Bone

Several in vitro studies that have challenged cells with AOPP have helped to clarify the mechanisms by which AOPP may impact bone (Table 2). A recent study using an osteocyte-like cell line (MLO-Y4) demonstrated that when cultured with AOPP-modified mouse serum albumin (AOPP-MSA), AOPP increased ROS generation and activated the c-Jun N-terminal kinase (JNK) and p38 mitogen-activated protein kinase (p38 MAPK) signaling pathways in a ROS-dependent manner, leading to apoptosis of these cells [30]. Upregulation of the JNK/p38 MAPK signaling pathways by AOPP also increased the expression of the protein sclerostin [30], which inhibits osteoblast function and bone formation by antagonizing the Wnt signaling pathway [31]. Through the JNK/p38 MAPK pathway, AOPP also upregulated the expression of receptor activator of NFκB ligand (RANKL) [30], which can upregulate osteoclastogenesis upon binding to its receptor [32].

A study using rat mesenchymal stem cells (MSC, which give rise to osteoblasts and osteocytes) demonstrated that exposure to AOPP-modified bovine serum albumin (AOPP-BSA) inhibited MSC proliferation, reduced alkaline phosphatase (ALP) activity, decreased collagen I mRNA levels, and inhibited bone nodule formation [33]. AOPP also increased ROS generation and upregulated the expression of RAGE [33]. In rat osteoblast-like cells, AOPP-modified rat serum albumin (AOPP-RSA) induced many of the same effects and provided evidence that AOPP may inhibit the proliferation of osteoblast-like cells through the ROS-dependent NFκB pathway [34].

Table 2. In vitro studies of the effect of AOPP on bone cells.

Study	Cell Type	Treatments	Outcome
Yu (2016) [30]	Osteocytic MLO-Y4 cells	Cultured with AOPP-MSA (25, 50, 100, or 200 μg/mL for 24 h or 200 μg/mL for 3, 6, 12, or 24 h)	AOPP triggered apoptosis and upregulated expression of sclerostin and RANKL in a JNK/p38 MAPK-dependent manner
Sun (2013) [33]	Rat MSC	Cultured with AOPP-BSA (50, 100, 200, or 400 μg/mL for 3 days or 200 μg/mL for 24, 48, or 72 h)	AOPP inhibited proliferation, reduced ALP activity and ALP and collagen I mRNA, increased ROS generation, upregulated RAGE expression
Zhong (2009) [34]	Rat osteoblast-like cells	Cultured with AOPP-RSA (50, 100, or 200 μg/mL for 24 h or 100 μg/mL for 24, 48, or 72 h)	AOPP inhibited proliferation, reduced ALP activity, downregulated expression of osteocalcin, induced ROS generation and NFκB phosphorylation

AOPP: advanced oxidation protein products; MLO-Y4: murine osteocyte-like cell line Y4; AOPP-MSA: AOPP-modified mouse serum albumin; RANKL: receptor activator of NFκB (nuclear factor κB) ligand; JNK: c-Jun N-terminal kinase; p38 MAPK: p38 mitogen-activated protein kinase; MSC: mesenchymal stem cells; AOPP-BSA: AOPP-modified bovine serum albumin; ALP: alkaline phosphatase; ROS: reactive oxygen species; RAGE: receptor for advanced glycation end products; AOPP-RSA: AOPP-modified rat serum albumin.

Taken together, these in vitro studies indicate that AOPP may act through the NFκB, JNK, and p38 MAPK signaling pathways to inhibit bone formation while promoting resorption. Previous reports have shown that the binding of RANKL to RANK causes recruitment of TNF receptor-associated factor 6 (TRAF6), which in turn activates NFκB, JNK, and MAPK, which induce nuclear factor of activated T cells (NFAT)c1, a key transcription factor for osteoclastogenesis [35,36]. Therefore, AOPP may disturb the balance between bone formation and resorption by upregulating osteoclastogenesis through these pathways.

Furthermore, it has also been documented that AGE-RAGE interaction induces the generation of ROS through the NOX pathway, resulting in the apoptosis of osteoblasts/MSC [37] and in the inhibition of the proliferation and differentiation of osteoblasts/MSC [38]. RAGE overexpression by lentiviral transfection has been shown to inhibit osteoblast proliferation through the suppression of the Wnt, phosphoinositide 3-kinase (PI3K), and extracellular signal-related kinase (ERK) pathways [38]. It has also been reported that RAGE plays a critical role in osteoclast maturation and activation [39], and RAGE expression in osteoclasts is age-dependent [40]. Studies using RAGE knockout mice have also shown that bone mass and bone biomechanical strength are increased with a decreased number of osteoclasts compared with wild-type mice [41]. Therefore, based on observations from the current literature, AOPP may inhibit osteoblastic activity and differentiation through the AOPP-RAGE-ROS pathway via the activation of NOX, which may be an important mechanism involved in the development of AAO.

5. Antioxidant Intake and Bone Health: Potential Benefits of Berry Anthocyanins

Because of the potential role of AOPP in aging-associated bone turnover, it is plausible that increased consumption of dietary antioxidants could reduce the formation of AOPP by inhibiting the NOX pathway, thereby lowering AAO risk. Two studies that support this hypothesis showed that murine osteoblastic MC3T3-E1 cells cultured with 2-deoxy-D-ribose (dRib) to induce oxidative damage could be rescued from dRib toxicity by the addition of the flavonoid antioxidants hesperetin [41] and myricetin [42], and that these antioxidant treatments markedly reduced AOPP along with other markers of oxidation. Melatonin is a well-studied antioxidant [43], and has also been shown to protect against H_2O_2-induced apoptosis of MSC [44]. The positive effects of dietary antioxidants on BMD and bone status have also been demonstrated in multiple cross-sectional investigations [45–47]. However, due to the inherent limitations of cross-sectional studies, this hypothesis should be further investigated using cohort studies or interventional trials.

Recently, considerable attention has been directed to the potential favorable effects of berries in enhancing bone health due to the antioxidant properties of anthocyanins in berries. Several studies indicate that blackcurrant anthocyanins exhibit a range of health benefits, including antioxidant [48,49] and anti-inflammatory effects [50,51], which could potentially improve bone remodeling. Several studies have utilized ovariectomized (OVX) animals to mimic the estrogen deficiency of menopause, and have found that supplementation with blueberry or blackcurrant attenuated the OVX-induced bone loss (Table 3) [52–54].

Table 3. Animal studies of the impact of berry antioxidants on ovariectomy-induced bone loss.

Study	Population	Treatments	Duration	Outcome
Li (2014) [52]	Female Sprague Dawley rats (total $n = 30$)	Randomized to sham operation, OVX control, and OVX blueberry treatment (10% w/w freeze-dried blueberry powder)	12 weeks	Blueberry inhibited bone resorption, bone loss, and the reduction of bone strength of OVX rats
Zheng (2016) [53]	Female C57BL/6J mice (total $n = 54$)	Randomized to sham operation or OVX, then further divided into control diet or diet containing 1% blackcurrant extract	4, 8, or 12 weeks	Blackcurrant attenuated OVX-induced bone loss as measured by BMD and trabecular volume; blackcurrant reduced bone resorption activity
Devareddy (2008) [54]	Female Sprague Dawley rats ($n = 30$)	Randomized to sham operation, OVX control, and OVX blueberry treatment (5% w/w dried blueberry powder)	100 days	Blueberry prevented OVX-induced loss of whole-body BMD; blueberry treatment group had lower serum osteocalcin

OVX: ovariectomized; BMD: bone mineral density.

However, evidence of bone-protective effects of berries outside of an estrogen-deficient model is still limited. In recent in vitro experiments using murine bone marrow macrophages, anthocyanins from blackcurrant, blackberry, and blueberry suppressed NOX (NOX1 and NOX2) mRNA expression by over 60% [51]. This reduction consequently downregulated nuclear factor (erythroid-derived 2)-like 2 (Nrf2) mRNA expression, suggesting that the NOX pathway was the major source of ROS production and that berry anthocyanins effectively inhibited the NOX pathway, thus reducing ROS production (Figure 1). In cultured RAW 264.7 macrophages, anthocyanins from blackcurrant, blueberry, and blackberry significantly inhibited lipopolysaccharide-induced inflammation as indicated by lower mRNA levels of TNFα and interleukin-1β, and lowered nuclear p65 levels, indicating decreased NFκB activity [51]. TNFα plays a central role in inflammation-mediated bone loss by augmenting osteoblastic RANKL-induced osteoclastogenesis and directly stimulates osteoclast formation [55,56]. These results indicate that berry anthocyanins may be an effective dietary agent in preventing aging-associated bone deterioration directly by inhibiting NOX-mediated AOPP formation and indirectly by reducing bone resorption through lowering ROS formation.

6. Conclusions

Oxidative stress contributes to the universal phenomenon of bone aging, and is a key factor in the development of AAO. AOPP is a biomarker of oxidative damage to protein and has been associated with lower BMD in both humans and animals in some observational studies. While not all observational studies confirmed the role of AOPP in AAO, the association between AOPP and bone loss is supported by several mechanistic studies elucidating the signaling pathways by which AOPP may reduce bone formation and/or increase bone resorption. Relatively little work has specifically examined how dietary antioxidants may impede bone aging through the reduction of AOPP. Studies that have addressed this hypothesis indicate that antioxidant consumption may be an effective method of inhibiting AOPP formation and lowering ROS formation in bone. Importantly, these findings are largely based on in vitro studies and should be expanded in future research examining how long-term consumption of dietary antioxidants reduces AOPP formation and mitigates aging-associated bone loss in older adulthood. This type of research may serve as a basis for future human clinical studies, which may ultimately lead to the development of dietary recommendations and strategies for the prevention of AAO.

Acknowledgments: This study was supported by the USDA National Institute of Food and Agriculture (NIFA) Seed Grant (Award Number 2016-67018-24492) to Ock K. Chun.

References

1. Yamagishi, S. Role of Advanced Glycation End Products (AGEs) in Osteoporosis in Diabetes. *Curr. Drug Targets* **2011**, *12*, 2096–2102. [CrossRef] [PubMed]
2. Alejandro, P.; Constantinescu, F. A Review of Osteoporosis in the Older Adult. *Clin. Geriatr. Med.* **2017**, *33*, 27–40. [CrossRef] [PubMed]
3. Raisz, L.G. Science in medicine Pathogenesis of osteoporosis: Concepts, conflicts, and prospects. *J. Clin. Investig.* **2005**, *115*, 3318–3325. [CrossRef] [PubMed]
4. Zeng, J.H.; Zhong, Z.M.; Li, X.D.; Wu, Q.; Zheng, S.; Zhou, J.; Ye, W.B.; Xie, F.; Wu, X.H.; Huang, Z.P.; et al. Advanced oxidation protein products accelerate bone deterioration in aged rats. *Exp. Gerontol.* **2014**, *50*, 64–71. [CrossRef] [PubMed]
5. Duque, G.; Troen, B.R. Understanding the mechanisms of senile osteoporosis: New facts for a major geriatric syndrome. *J. Am. Geriatr. Soc.* **2008**, *56*, 935–941. [CrossRef] [PubMed]
6. Wei, Y.H.; Lee, H.C. Oxidative Stress, Mitochondrial DNA Mutation, and Impairment of Antioxidant Enzymes in Aging. *Exp. Biol. Med.* **2002**, *227*, 671–682. [CrossRef]
7. Wauquier, F.; Leotoing, L.; Coxam, V.; Guicheux, J.; Wittrant, Y. Oxidative stress in bone remodelling and disease. *Trends Mol. Med.* **2009**, *15*, 468–477. [CrossRef] [PubMed]
8. Parfitt, A.M.; Chir, B. Bone remodeling and bone loss: Understanding the pathophysiology of osteoporosis. *Clin. Obstet. Gynecol.* **1987**, *30*, 789–811. [CrossRef] [PubMed]
9. Atashi, F.; Modarressi, A.; Pepper, M.S. The role of reactive oxygen species in mesenchymal stem cell adipogenic and osteogenic differentiation: A review. *Stem Cells Dev.* **2015**, *24*, 1150–1163. [CrossRef] [PubMed]
10. Garrett, I.R.; Boyce, B.F.; Oreffo, R.O.C.; Bonewald, L.; Poser, J.; Mundy, G.R. Oxygen-derived free radicals stimulate osteoclastic bone resorption in rodent bone in vitro and in vivo. *J. Clin. Investig.* **1990**, *85*, 632–639. [CrossRef] [PubMed]
11. Suzuki, T.; Katsumata, S.; Matsuxaki, H.; Suzuki, K. Dietary zinc deficiency induces oxidative stress and promotes tumor necrosis factor-α- and interleukin-1β-induced RANKL expressio in rat bone. *J. Clin. Biochem. Nutr.* **2016**, *58*, 122–129. [CrossRef] [PubMed]
12. Almeida, M.; Han, L.; Martin-Millan, M.; Plotkin, L.I.; Stewart, S.A.; Roberson, P.K.; Kousteni, S.; O'Brien, C.A.; Bellido, T.; Parfitt, A.M.; et al. Skeletal Involution by Age-associated Oxidative Stress and Its Acceleration by Loss of Sex Steroids. *J. Biol. Chem.* **2007**, *282*, 27285–27297. [CrossRef] [PubMed]
13. Hazen, S.L.; Hsu, F.F.; Heinecke, J.W. p-Hydroxyphenylacetaldehyde Is the Major Product of L-Tyrosine Oxidation by Activated Human Phagocytes. *J. Biol. Chem.* **1996**, *271*, 1861–1867. [CrossRef] [PubMed]
14. Heinecke, J.W.; Li, W.; Daehnke, H.L.; Goldstein, J.A. Dityrosine, a Specific Marker of Oxidation. *J. Biol. Chem.* **1993**, *268*, 4069–4077. [PubMed]
15. Witko-Sarsat, V.; Friedlander, M.; Capeillère-Blandin, C.; Nguyen-Khoa, T.; Nguyen, A.T.; Zingraff, J.; Jungers, P.; Descamps-Latscha, B. Advanced oxidation protein products as a novel marker of oxidative stress in uremia. *Kidney Int.* **1996**, *49*, 1304–1313. [CrossRef] [PubMed]
16. Iwao, Y.; Anraku, M.; Hiraike, M.; Kawai, K.; Nakajou, K.; Kai, T.; Suenaga, A.; Otagiri, M. The structural and pharmacokinetic properties of oxidized human serum albumin, advanced oxidation protein products (AOPP). *Drug Metab. Pharmacokinet.* **2006**, *21*, 140–146. [CrossRef] [PubMed]

17. Guo, Z.J.; Niu, H.X.; Hou, F.F.; Zhang, L.; Fu, N.; Nagai, R.; Lu, X.; Chen, B.H.; Shan, Y.X.; Tian, J.W.; et al. Advanced oxidation protein products activate vascular endothelial cells via a RAGE-mediated signaling pathway. *Antioxid. Redox Signal.* **2008**, *10*, 1699–1712. [CrossRef] [PubMed]
18. Sherman, S.S.; Tobin, J.D.; Hollis, B.W.; Gundberg, C.M.; Roy, T.A.; Plato, C.C. Biochemical parameters associated with low bone density in healthy men and women. *J Bone Min Res.* **1992**, *7*, 1123–1130. [CrossRef] [PubMed]
19. Zhang, Y.B.; Zhong, Z.M.; Hou, G.; Jiang, H.; Chen, J.T. Involvement of oxidative stress in age-related bone loss. *J. Surg. Res.* **2011**, *169*, e37–e42. [CrossRef] [PubMed]
20. Boskey, A.L.; Coleman, R. Aging and Bone. *J. Dent. Res.* **2010**, *89*, 1333–1348. [CrossRef] [PubMed]
21. Demontiero, O.; Vidal, C.; Duque, G. Aging and bone loss: New insights for the clinician. *Ther. Adv. Musculoskelet. Dis.* **2012**, *4*, 61–76. [CrossRef] [PubMed]
22. Cervellati, C.; Bonaccorsi, G.; Cremonini, E.; Romani, A.; Fila, E.; Castaldini, M.C.; Ferrazzini, S.; Fifanti, M.; Massari, L. Oxidative stress and bone resorption interplay as a possible trigger for postmenopausal osteoporosis. *Biomed. Res. Int.* **2014**, *2014*, 1–8. [CrossRef] [PubMed]
23. Sánchez-Rodríguez, M.A.; Ruiz-Ramos, M.; Correa-Muñoz, E.; Mendoza-Núñez, V.M. Oxidative stress as a risk factor for osteoporosis in elderly Mexicans as characterized by antioxidant enzymes. *BMC Musculoskelet. Disord.* **2007**, *8*, 1–7. [CrossRef] [PubMed]
24. Östman, B.; Michaëlsson, K.; Helmersson, J.; Gedeborg, R.; Melhus, H. Oxidative stress and bone mineral density in elderly men: Antioxidant activity of alpha-tocopherol. *Free Radic. Biol. Med.* **2009**, *47*, 668–673. [CrossRef] [PubMed]
25. Huang, C.; Lv, B.; Wang, Y. ProteinpPhosphatase 2A mediates oxidative stress induced apoptosis in osteoblasts. *Mediat. Inflamm.* **2015**, *2015*, 1–8. [CrossRef]
26. Almeida, M.; Han, L.; Martin-Millan, M.; O'Brien, C.A.; Manolagas, S.C. Oxidative stress antagonizes Wnt signaling in osteoblast precursors by diverting β-catenin from T cell factor- to forkhead box O-mediated transcription. *J. Biol. Chem.* **2007**, *282*, 27298–27305. [CrossRef] [PubMed]
27. Wu, Q.; Zhong, Z.M.; Pan, Y.; Zeng, J.H.; Zheng, S.; Zhu, S.Y.; Chen, J.T. Advanced Oxidation Protein Products as a Novel Marker of Oxidative Stress in Postmenopausal Osteoporosis. *Med. Sci. Monit.* **2015**, *21*, 2428–2432. [CrossRef] [PubMed]
28. Cervellati, C.; Bonaccorsi, G.; Cremonini, E.; Bergamini, C.M.; Patella, A.; Castaldini, C.; Ferrazzini, S.; Capatti, A.; Picarelli, V.; Pansini, F.S.; et al. Bone mass density selectively correlates with serum markers of oxidative damage in post-menopausal women. *Clin. Chem. Lab. Med.* **2013**, *51*, 333–338. [CrossRef] [PubMed]
29. Yildirimturk, S.; Batu, S.; Alatli, C.; Olgac, V.; Firat, D.; Sirin, Y. The effects of supplemental melatonin administration on the healing of bone defects in streptozotocin-induced diabetic rats. *J. Appl. Oral Sci.* **2016**, *24*, 239–249. [CrossRef] [PubMed]
30. Yu, C.; Huang, D.; Wang, K.; Lin, B.; Liu, Y.; Liu, S.; Wu, W.; Zhang, H. Advanced oxidation protein products induce apoptosis, and upregulate sclerostin and RANKL expression, in osteocytic MLO-Y4 cells via JNK/p38 MAPK activation. *Mol. Med. Rep.* **2016**, *15*, 543–550. [CrossRef] [PubMed]
31. Baron, R.; Kneissel, M. WNT signaling in bone homeostasis and disease: From human mutations to treatments. *Nat. Med.* **2013**, *19*, 179–192. [CrossRef] [PubMed]
32. Boyce, B.F.; Xing, L. Biology of RANK, RANKL, and osteoprotegerin. *Arthritis Res. Ther.* **2007**, *9*, S1. [CrossRef] [PubMed]
33. Sun, N.; Yang, L.; Li, Y.; Zhang, H.; Chen, H.; Liu, D.; Li, Q.; Cai, D. Effect of advanced oxidation protein products on the proliferation and osteogenic differentiation of rat mesenchymal stem cells. *Int. J. Mol. Med.* **2013**, *32*, 485–491. [CrossRef] [PubMed]
34. Zhong, Z.M.; Bai, L.; Chen, J.T. Advanced oxidation protein products inhibit proliferation and differentiation of rat osteoblast-like cells via NF-κB pathway. *Cell. Physiol. Biochem.* **2009**, *24*, 105–114. [CrossRef] [PubMed]
35. Naito, A.; Azuma, S.; Tanaka, S.; Miyazaki, T.; Takaki, S.; Takatsu, K.; Nakao, K.; Nakamura, K.; Katsuki, M.; Yamamoto, T.; et al. Severe osteopetrosis, defective interleukin-1 signalling and lymph node organogenesis in TRAF6-deficient mice. *Genes Cells* **1999**, *4*, 353–362. [CrossRef] [PubMed]
36. Takayanagi, H. The role of NFAT in osteoclast formation. *Ann. N. Y. Acad. Sci.* **2007**, *1116*, 227–237. [CrossRef] [PubMed]

37. Wautier, M.; Chappey, O.; Corda, S.; Stern, D.M.; Schmidt, A.M.; Wautier, J. Activation of NADPH oxidase by AGE links oxidant stress to altered gene expression via RAGE. *Am. J. Physiol. Endocrinol. Metab.* **2001**, *280*, E685–E694. [PubMed]
38. Li, G.; Xu, J.; Li, Z. Receptor for advanced glycation end products inhibits proliferation in osteoblast through suppression of Wnt, PI3K and ERK signaling. *Biochem. Biophys. Res. Commun.* **2012**, *423*, 684–689. [CrossRef] [PubMed]
39. Zhou, Z.; Immel, D.; Xi, C.X.; Bierhaus, A.; Feng, X.; Mei, L.; Nawroth, P.; Stern, D.M.; Xiong, W.C. Regulation of osteoclast function and bone mass by RAGE. *J. Exp. Med.* **2006**, *203*, 1067–1080. [CrossRef] [PubMed]
40. Cui, S.; Xiong, F.; Hong, Y.; Jung, J.U.; Li, X.S.; Liu, J.Z.; Yan, R.; Mei, L.; Feng, X.; Xiong, W.C. APPswe/AB regulation of osteoclast activation and RAGE expression in an age-dependent manner. *J. Bone Miner. Res.* **2011**, *26*, 1084–1098. [CrossRef] [PubMed]
41. Choi, E.M.; Kim, Y.H. Hesperetin attenuates the highly reducing sugar-triggered inhibition of osteoblast differentiation. *Cell Biol. Toxicol.* **2008**, *24*, 225–231. [CrossRef] [PubMed]
42. Lee, K.H.; Choi, E.M. Myricetin, a naturally occurring flavonoid, prevents 2-deoxy-d-ribose induced dysfunction and oxidative damage in osteoblastic MC3T3-E1 cells. *Eur. J. Pharmacol.* **2008**, *591*, 1–6. [CrossRef] [PubMed]
43. Reiter, R.J.; Tan, D.X.; Mayo, J.C.; Sainz, R.M.; Leon, J.; Czarnocki, Z. Melatonin as an antioxidant: Biochemical mechanisms and pathophysiological implications in humans. *Acta Biochim. Pol.* **2003**, *50*, 1129–1146. [PubMed]
44. Wang, F.W.; Wang, Z.; Zhang, Y.M.; Du, Z.X.; Zhang, X.L.; Liu, Q.; Guo, Y.J.; Li, X.G.; Hao, A.J. Protective effect of melatonin on bone marrow mesenchymal stem cells against hydrogen peroxide-induced apoptosis in vitro. *J. Cell. Biochem.* **2013**, *114*, 2346–2355. [CrossRef] [PubMed]
45. Rivas, A.; Romero, A.; Mariscal-Arcas, M.; Monteagudo, C.; López, G.; Lorenzo, L.; Ocaña-Peinado, F.M.; Olea-Serrano, F. Association between dietary antioxidant quality score (DAQs) and bone mineral density in Spanish women. *Nutr. Hosp.* **2012**, *27*, 1886–1893. [CrossRef] [PubMed]
46. Zhang, J.; Munger, R.G.; West, N.A.; Cutler, D.R.; Wengreen, H.J.; Corcoran, C.D. Antioxidant intake and risk of osteoporotic hip fracture in Utah: An effect modified by smoking status. *Am. J. Epidemiol.* **2006**, *163*, 9–17. [CrossRef] [PubMed]
47. De Franca, N.A.; Camargo, M.B.; Lazaretti-Castro, M.; Martini, L.A. Antioxidant intake and bone status in a cross-sectional study of Brazilian women with osteoporosis. *Nutr. Health* **2013**, *22*, 133–142. [CrossRef] [PubMed]
48. Shen, C.L.; von Bergen, V.; Chyu, M.C.; Jenkins, M.R.; Mo, H.; Chen, C.H.; Kwun, I.S. Fruits and dietary phytochemicals in bone protection. *Nutr. Res.* **2012**, *32*, 897–910. [CrossRef] [PubMed]
49. McGhie, T.K.; Walton, M.C.; Barnett, L.E.; Vather, R.; Martin, H.; Au, J.; Alspach, P.A.; Booth, C.L.; Kruger, M.C. Boysenberry and blackcurrant drinks increased the plasma antioxidant capacity in an elderly population but had little effect on other markers of oxidative stress. *J. Sci. Food Agric.* **2007**, *87*, 2519–2527. [CrossRef]
50. Kumazawa, Y.; Kawaguchi, K.; Takimoto, H. Immunomodulating Effects of Flavonoids on Acute and Chronic Inflammatory Responses Caused by Tumor Necrosis Factor α. *Curr. Pharm. Des.* **2006**, *12*, 4271–4279. [CrossRef] [PubMed]
51. Lee, S.G.; Kim, B.; Yang, Y.; Pham, T.X.; Park, Y.K.; Manatou, J.; Koo, S.I.; Chun, O.K.; Lee, J.Y. Berry anthocyanins suppress the expression and secretion of proinflammatory mediators in macrophages by inhibiting nuclear translocation of NF-κB independent of NRF2-mediated mechanism. *J. Nutr. Biochem.* **2014**, *25*, 404–411. [CrossRef] [PubMed]
52. Li, T.; Wu, S.M.; Xu, Z.Y.; Ou-Yang, S. Rabbiteye blueberry prevents osteoporosis in ovariectomized rats. *J. Orthop. Surg. Res.* **2014**, *9*, 56–62. [CrossRef] [PubMed]
53. Zheng, X.; Mun, S.; Lee, S.G.; Vance, T.M.; Hubert, P.; Koo, S.I.; Lee, S.K.; Chun, O.K. Anthocyanin-Rich Blackcurrant Extract Attenuates Ovariectomy-Induced Bone Loss in Mice. *J. Med. Food* **2016**, *19*, 390–397. [CrossRef] [PubMed]
54. Devareddy, L.; Hooshmand, S.; Collins, J.K.; Lucas, E.A.; Chai, S.C.; Arjmandi, B.H. Blueberry prevents bone loss in ovariectomized rat model of postmenopausal osteoporosis. *J. Nutr. Biochem.* **2008**, *19*, 694–699. [CrossRef] [PubMed]

55. Komine, M.; Kukita, A.; Kukita, T.; Ogata, Y.; Hotokebuchi, T.; Kohashi, O. Tumor necrosis factor-alpha cooperates with receptor activator of nuclear factor kappaB ligand in generation of osteoclasts in stromal cell-depleted rat bone marrow cell culture. *Bone* **2001**, *28*, 474–483. [CrossRef]
56. Fox, S.W.; Evans, K.E.; Lovibond, A.C. Transforming growth factor-β enables NFATc1 expression during osteoclastogenesis. *Biochem. Biophys. Res. Commun.* **2008**, *366*, 123–128. [CrossRef] [PubMed]

7

Identification of a Circulating Amino Acid Signature in Frail Older Persons with Type 2 Diabetes Mellitus: Results from the Metabofrail Study

Riccardo Calvani [1,2], Leocadio Rodriguez-Mañas [3], Anna Picca [1,2], Federico Marini [4], Alessandra Biancolillo [5], Olga Laosa [6], Laura Pedraza [6], Jacopo Gervasoni [1,2], Aniello Primiano [1,2], Giorgia Conta [4], Isabelle Bourdel-Marchasson [7], Sophie C. Regueme [7], Roberto Bernabei [1,2], Emanuele Marzetti [1,2,*], Alan J. Sinclair [8], Giovanni Gambassi [1,2] and on behalf of the European MID-Frail Consortium

1 Università Cattolica del Sacro Cuore, 00168 Rome, Italy; riccardo.calvani@gmail.com (R.C.); anna.picca1@gmail.com (A.P.); jacopo.gervasoni@policlinicogemelli.it (J.G.); anielloprim@gmail.com (A.P.); Roberto.Bernabei@unicatt.it (R.B.); giovanni.gambassi@unicatt.it (G.G.)

2 Fondazione Policlinico Universitario "Agostino Gemelli" IRCCS, 00168 Rome, Italy

3 Servicio de Geriatría, Hospital Universitario de Getafe, 28905 Madrid, Spain; leocadio.rodriguez@salud.madrid.org

4 Department of Chemistry, Sapienza Università di Roma, 00185 Rome, Italy; federico.marini@uniroma1.it (F.M.); giorgia.conta@uniroma1.it (G.C.)

5 Department of Physical and Chemical Sciences, Università degli Studi dell'Aquila, 67100 L'Aquila, Italy; alessandra.biancolillo@univaq.it

6 Foundation for Biomedical Research, Hospital Universitario de Getafe, 28905 Madrid, Spain; olga.laosa@salud.madrid.org (O.L.); laura.pedraza@salud.madrid.org (L.P.)

7 Centre Hospitalier Universitaire de Bordeaux, 33000 Bordeaux, France; isabelle.bourdel-marchasson@chu-bordeaux.fr (I.B.-M.); sophie.regueme@chu-bordeaux.fr (S.C.R.)

8 Foundation for Diabetes Research in Older People, Diabetes Frail Ltd., Luton LU1 3UA, UK; sinclair.5@btinternet.com

* Correspondence: emanuele.marzetti@policlinicogemelli.it

Abstract: Diabetes and frailty are highly prevalent conditions that impact the health status of older adults. Perturbations in protein/amino acid metabolism are associated with both functional impairment and type 2 diabetes mellitus (T2DM). In the present study, we compared the concentrations of a panel of circulating 37 amino acids and derivatives between frail/pre-frail older adults with T2DM and robust non-diabetic controls. Sixty-six functionally impaired older persons aged 70+ with T2DM and 30 age and sex-matched controls were included in the analysis. We applied a partial least squares-discriminant analysis (PLS-DA)-based analytical strategy to characterize the metabotype of study participants. The optimal complexity of the PLS-DA model was found to be two latent variables. The proportion of correct classification was 94.1 ± 1.9% for frail/pre-frail persons with T2DM and 100% for control participants. Functionally impaired older persons with T2DM showed higher levels of 3-methyl histidine, alanine, arginine, glutamic acid, ethanolamine sarcosine, and tryptophan. Control participants had higher levels of ornithine and taurine. These findings indicate that a specific profile of amino acids and derivatives characterizes pre-frail/frail older persons with T2DM. The dissection of these pathways may provide novel insights into the metabolic perturbations involved in the disabling cascade in older persons with T2DM.

Keywords: aging; metabolomics; systems biology; personalized medicine; metabolism; frailty; sarcopenia; muscle wasting; precision medicine; metabolic profiling

1. Introduction

Type 2 diabetes mellitus (T2DM) is a chronic condition frequently occurring in old age [1,2]. T2DM is associated with higher risk of negative outcomes, including disability and mortality [3]. T2DM-related complications are especially prevalent in older adults and account for the increasing costs of T2DM [4]. Frailty defines a geriatric syndrome characterized by reduced ability to cope with life stressors and increased risk of adverse events (e.g., falls, delirium, loss of independence, mortality) [5,6]. T2DM and frailty are intimately related and share common features, including complex pathophysiology and heterogeneous phenotypes [7], that challenge their management [5,8].

Muscle failure, both in its metabolic and functional manifestations, is a hallmark of T2DM and frailty [7,9]. The progressive and generalized loss of muscle mass, strength, and function with age, termed sarcopenia, fuels a self-reinforcing cycle in which structural, metabolic, and endocrine perturbations in muscle exacerbate T2DM-related signs and symptoms [10]. T2DM further promotes the decline in muscle mass and function [11,12] which, in turn, aggravates functional impairment [13].

The central role of muscle wasting in frailty and T2DM may guide the identification of novel biomarkers and possibly new treatment targets for the two conditions [14–16]. In this context, circulating amino acids are promising candidates given their sensor-transducer-effector role in systemic metabolism, muscle homeostasis, and physical function [17–20]. Moreover, amino acids are involved in processes critical to the development and progression of frailty and T2DM, such as inflammation, glucose homeostasis, and redox regulation [21–23].

Targeted metabolomics allowed identifying specific amino acid profiles that were associated with insulin resistance and risk of developing T2DM in independent cohorts across US, Europe, and China [24–27]. A plasma amino acid signature, together with specific circulating lipid species, was linked to glucose dyshomeostasis and impaired insulin sensitivity in older adults from the Baltimore Longitudinal Study of Aging (BLSA) [28]. In addition, distinct patterns of circulating amino acids were associated with frailty and/or muscle-related parameters (mass, turnover, performance) in older individuals at risk for frailty [29–32]. Finally, within the "BIOmarkers associated with Sarcopenia and PHysical frailty in EldeRly pErsons" (BIOSPHERE) study, a combination of serum amino acids and derivatives was identified that characterized the metabotype of older adults with physical frailty and sarcopenia (PF&S) [17].

Here, we sought to define the circulating amino acid profile of frail/pre-frail older adults with T2DM (F-T2DM). Our approach, described in the context of the "Metabolic biomarkers of frailty in older people with type 2 diabetes mellitus" (MetaboFrail) study, coupled targeted metabolomics with a chemometric modeling strategy [16]. Through this innovative biomarker discovery strategy, we identified a specific profile of serum amino acids in F-T2DM older people. These findings may offer new insights into the metabolic perturbations associated with the disabling cascade in older persons with T2DM.

2. Materials and Methods

2.1. Study Population

MetaboFrail was developed as an ancillary study of the "Multi-modal Intervention in Diabetes in Frailty" (MID-Frail) project [16,33,34]. The latter was a cluster-randomized multicenter clinical trial that evaluated the effectiveness of a multicomponent intervention (mainly based on resistance exercise and lifestyle counseling) on improving physical performance compared with usual care in F-T2DM older adults from seven European countries (ClinicalTrials.gov identifier: NCT01654341) [16,33]. For the present study, a subgroup of MID-Frail participants recruited in Spanish and French study centers were enrolled. The main eligibility criteria were: (a) age at screening 70 years or older; (b) T2DM diagnosis from at least two years; and (c) being pre-frail or frail according to Fried's criteria [35]. The main exclusion criteria were: (a) poor cognition operationalized as a Mini Mental State Examination score <20 [36]; (b) severe disability defined as a Barthel index score <60 [37]; critical conditions and/or major illnesses with a life expectancy <6 months; (c) inability or unwillingness to provide informed consent. Control participants were enrolled at the Università Cattolica del Sacro Cuore (Rome, Italy) and had the following characteristics: 70+ years of age, no T2DM, and no functional impairment. The study protocol was approved by local ethics committees according to both national and international laws. Prior to enrolment, all participants provided written informed consent. The study was conducted in agreement with legal requirements and international norms (Declaration of Helsinki, 1964).

2.2. *Blood Collection and Determination of Serum Concentrations of Amino Acids and Derivatives*

Blood samples were collected after overnight fasting. For serum separation, blood samples were kept on ice for about 30 min until clotting and were subsequently centrifuged at 1000× g for 10 min at 4 °C. Serum samples were eventually aliquoted and stored at −80 °C until analysis.

Concentrations of 37 amino acids and derivatives were determined in serum by ultraperformance liquid chromatography/mass spectrometry (UPLC/MS), as described previously [17]. Briefly, 50 µL of sample was added to 100 µL 10% (w/v) sulfosalicylic acid containing an internal standard mix (50 µM; Cambridge Isotope Laboratories, Inc., Tewksbury, MA, USA) and centrifuged at 1000× g for 15 min. Ten µL of the resulting supernatant were mixed with 70 µL of borate buffer and 20 µL of AccQ Tag reagents (Waters Corporation, Milford, MA, USA) and heated at 55 °C for 10 min. Samples were eventually loaded onto a CORTECS UPLC C18 column 1.6 µm 2.1 × 150 mm (Waters Corporation) for chromatographic separation (ACQUITY H-Class, Waters Corporation, Milford, MA, USA). Elution was performed at 500 µL/min flow rate with a linear gradient (9 min) from 99:1 to 1:99 water 0.1% formic acid/acetonitrile 0.1% formic acid. Analytes were detected on an ACQUITY QDa single quadrupole mass spectrometer equipped with electrospray source operating in positive mode (Waters Corporation, Milford, MA, USA). Amino acid controls (MCA laboratory of the Queen Beatrix Hospital, Winterswijk, The Netherlands) were used to monitor the analytic process.

2.3. *Statistical Analysis*

The normal distribution of data was ascertained through the Kolmogorov-Smirnov test. Comparisons between F-T2DM and control participants for normally distributed continuous variables were performed by t-test statistics. The non-parametric test Mann-Whitney U was applied to assess differences for non-normally distributed continuous data. Differences in categorical variables between groups were determined via χ^2 statistics. Descriptive analyses were performed using the GraphPrism 5.03 software (GraphPad Software, Inc., San Diego, CA), with statistical significance set at $p < 0.05$.

2.4. *Partial Least Squares-Discriminant Analysis and Double Cross-Validation Procedures*

In order to unveil possible differences in circulating amino acid patterns between F-T2DM and control participants, a multivariate classification strategy based on partial least squares-discriminant analysis (PLS-DA) modeling was adopted [38]. PLS-DA is a classification method particularly suited for dealing with highly correlated predictors, as it is based on projecting the predictors (measured variables) onto a reduced subspace of latent variables (LVs; directions in space) of highest covariance with the responses, i.e., providing the maximum separation between classes. In order to validate the results of PLS-DA modeling and rule out the possibility that good results were obtained because of chance correlation, a procedure based on repeated double cross-validation (DCV) and permutation tests was used [39,40]. DCV consists of spitting the samples to obtain two cross-validation loops, an internal loop for model building/model selection and an outer loop that mimics external (test set) validation. The DCV procedure is repeated a sufficient number of times such that estimates do to depend on one specific sample splitting. This allows evaluating the consistency of model parameters and the confidence intervals for model predictions. To assess the statistical significance of the obtained predictions, the figures of merit which summarize the classification accuracy in repeated DCV [i.e., number of misclassifications (NMC), area under the receiver operating characteristic curve (AUROC), and discriminant (DQ2)] are compared with their distribution under the null hypothesis, which is estimated non-parametrically through permutation tests with 1000 randomizations. A more detailed description of the procedure can be found elsewhere [41]. PLS-DA and DCV were run under Matlab R2015b environment by means of in-house written functions (freely downloadable at: https://www.chem.uniroma1.it/romechemometrics/research/algorithms/plsda/).

3. Results

3.1. Study Population

The present investigation included 66 F-T2DM older adults and 30 age and sex-matched robust, non-diabetic controls. The main characteristics of the two groups are reported in Table 1. F-T2DM and control participants were comparable for age, sex distribution, and number of diseases. F-T2DM older adults showed higher body mass index relative to controls. As expected, a significant difference was found in physical functional between groups, as indicated by the scores on the short physical performance battery (SPPB).

Table 1. Main characteristics of study participants.

	F-T2DM (n = 66)	Controls (n = 30)	p
Age, years (mean ± SD)	76.5 ± 14.5	74.6 ± 4.3	0.46
Sex (female), n (%)	32 (48)	16 (53)	0.82
BMI, kg/m^2 (mean ± SD)	29.2 ± 4.9	26.7 ± 2.4	0.01
SPPB score (mean ± SD)	8.6 ± 2.9	11.3 ± 0.9	<0.0001
Number of diseases (mean ± SD) §	2.8 ± 1.0	2.9 ± 2.0	0.86

§ Includes hypertension, coronary artery disease, prior stroke, peripheral vascular disease, diabetes, chronic obstructive pulmonary disease, and osteoarthritis; Abbreviations: BMI, body mass index; F-T2DM, frail/pre-frail older adults with type 2 diabetes mellitus; SD, standard deviation; SPPB, short physical performance battery.

3.2. Identification of Circulating Amino Acid Profiles

In the present study, we aimed at identifying profiles of circulating amino acids that discriminate older persons with F-T2DM from functionally intact non-diabetic peers. Among the available statistical options, we selected a PLS-DA-based strategy for its ability to handle multiple interdependent variables. The best PLS-DA model was built using two LVs. As indicated by the stringent DCV applied, the classification performance of the model was almost perfect. Indeed, the proportion of correct classification of participants was 96.6 ± 1.5% over the calibration sets (95.0 ± 2.2% for cases and 100.0 ± 0.0% for controls), 96.6 ± 1.5% (95.0 ± 2.2% for cases and 100.0 ± 0.0% for controls) in the internal DCV loop (i.e., the one used for model selection), and 95.9 ± 1.3% (94.1 ± 1.9% for cases and 100.0 ± 0.0% for controls) in the outer DCV loop, which accounts for the results of repeated external validation.

The remarkable classification performance of the PLS-DA model can be appreciated by inspecting the projection of study participants over the space spanned by the two LVs (Figure 1).

A sharp separation between F-T2DM participants and controls is evident. To ensure the reliability of our findings against the possibility of chance correlations, DCV results of the PLS-DA model were compared with the distributions of specific figures of merit under the null hypothesis. As depicted in Figure 2, for all of the figures considered (i.e., NMC, AUROC, and DQ2), values obtained from the unpermuted dataset fell outside the corresponding null hypothesis distribution, indicating a p value <0.05.

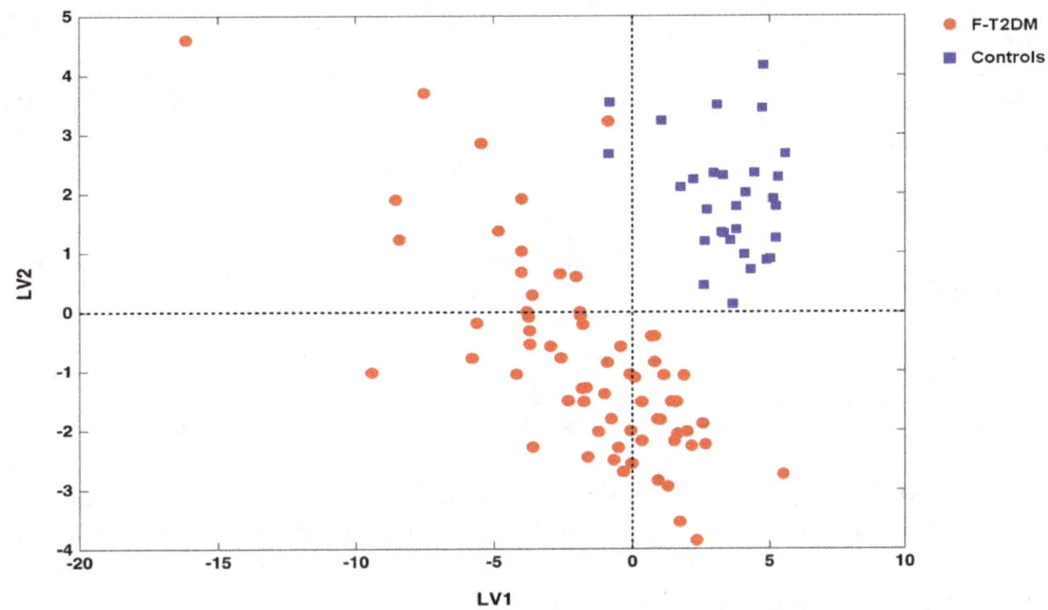

Figure 1. Scores plot showing the separation of frail/pre-frail older adults with type 2 diabetes mellitus (F-T2DM) from control participants according to the serum concentrations of amino acids and derivatives in the space spanned by the two latent variables (LV1 and LV2), as determined by partial least squares-discriminant analysis.

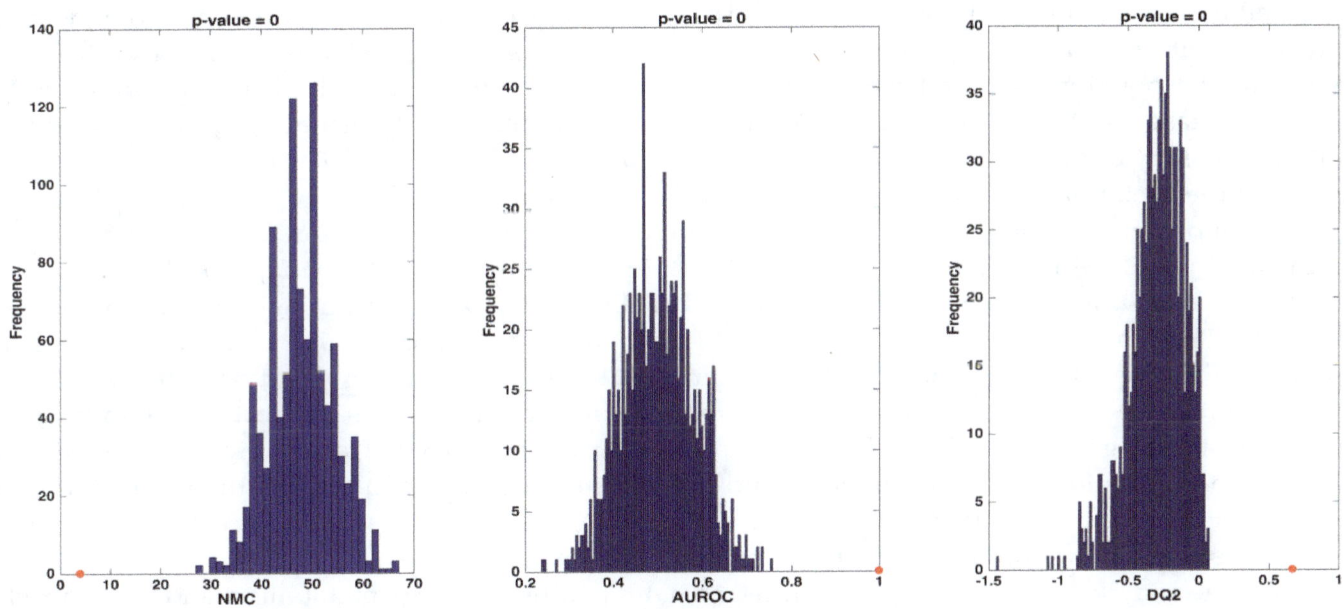

Figure 2. Distribution of values of number of misclassifications (NMC), area under the receiver operating characteristic curve (AUROC), and discriminant Q2 (DQ2) under their respective null hypothesis as estimated by permutation tests (blue histograms) and the corresponding values obtained by the partial least squares-discriminant analysis model on unpermuted data (red circles). Values obtained on the real dataset (red circles) fall outside of the corresponding null hypothesis distribution (blue histograms), corresponding to a $p < 0.05$.

The identification of the metabolites with the greatest discriminating power was accomplished by inspecting variable importance in projection (VIP) indices. Table 2 reports variables with a VIP value higher than 1.

Table 2. Serum concentrations of discriminant biomolecules as resulted from partial least squares-discriminant analysis.

Analytes	F-T2DM (n = 66)	Controls (n = 30)
3-methylhistidine	7.8 ± 4.2	5.2 ± 2.5
Alanine	542.3 ± 165.8	384.3 ± 98.3
Arginine	168.3 ± 91.2	103.7 ± 31.2
Ethanolamine	11.5 ± 3.4	9.0 ± 2.2
Glutamic acid	130.0 ± 66.8	54.3 ± 21.3
Ornithine	103.2 ± 37.6	109.4 ± 25.0
Sarcosine	2.5 ± 0.9	1.6 ± 0.6
Taurine	100.4 ± 49.0	189.5 ± 47.2
Tryptophan	66.2 ± 23.4	62.0 ± 13.1

Data are shown as mean ± standard deviation. Concentrations are expressed in μmol/L.

F-T2DM participants showed higher serum levels of 3-methyl histidine, alanine, arginine, ethanolamine, glutamic acid, sarcosine, and tryptophan. Instead, controls were characterized by higher circulating levels of ornithine and taurine. Serum concentrations of non-discriminant analytes in the two participant groups are listed in Table S1.

4. Discussion

Over the last few years, analytical platforms have been developed together with sophisticated computational algorithms to allow the study of complex diseases in unprecedented detail [42]. This new healthcare paradigm, called personalized or precision medicine, incorporates "omics" technologies to unveil the inner biological properties of morbid conditions [42] and devise innovative diagnostics and interventions tailored to the needs of single individuals [42,43]. Metabolomics, by virtue of its privileged position at the interface between biological pathways and clinical manifestations of healthy/disease conditions [44], are improving our understanding of "normal" physiology and the pathophysiology of many disorders, including frailty and T2DM [15,45,46]. These premises led to the design of the MetaboFrail study [16].

In the present investigation, we applied targeted metabolomics to characterize the circulating amino acid profile of functionally impaired older persons with T2DM. Our major finding was that a specific pattern of amino acids discriminated F-T2DM older people from age- and sex-matched controls. The amino acid signature of F-T2DM participants included higher circulating levels of 3-methyl histidine, alanine, arginine, ethanolamine, glutamic acid, sarcosine, and tryptophan.

The presence of 3-methyl histidine among the most relevant predictors supports the involvement of muscle wasting in frailty [30]. Indeed, 3-methyl histidine derives from the post-translational methylation of histidine moieties of actin and myosin [47,48]. Hence, 3-methyl histidine has been proposed as a biomarker of myofibrillar proteolysis and skeletal muscle loss [49]. Interestingly, 3-methyl histidine is also a marker of increased protein catabolism in T2DM [50].

Alanine and glutamic acid are crucial intermediates of muscle energy metabolism and liver-muscle metabolic interchange under both physiologic and pathologic conditions [51–53]. Perturbations in alanine and glutamate circulating pool may be indicative of skeletal muscle dysfunction, and are commonly encountered in age-related chronic conditions and models of muscle atrophy [54,55]. Notably, both alanine and glutamic acid levels were positively associated with insulin resistance and risk of T2DM in several independent study cohorts [56–58].

Arginine metabolism involves the cooperation of various organs, including kidneys, muscles, gut, and liver [59]. Major pathways in arginine metabolism include muscle protein breakdown and its de novo synthesis from citrulline [59]. Arginine is involved in nitric oxide as well as urea and polyamine synthesis, and research focus has recently been directed towards the determination of the pathophysiological role of arginine and its metabolites in aging and age-related chronic diseases [60]. Noticeably, our findings mirror the higher levels of arginine and lower concentrations of its urea-cycle companion ornithine found in Chinese adults with T2DM [61]. Higher concentrations of another intermediate of urea-cycle, i.e., citrulline, defined the serum amino acid profile of older people with PF&S [17]. Further investigations on arginine/nitrogen interorgan networks are needed to explain the results found in F-T2DM older adults.

Sarcosine, the N-methylated derivative of glycine, is an important intermediate of one-carbon metabolism [62]. Recent studies have investigated the association between sarcosine levels and age-related conditions in humans with conflicting results [63–66]. In a comparative metabolomics analysis, circulating sarcosine was found to be reduced with aging and increased by dietary restriction in both rodents and humans [67]. Conversely, elevated urine sarcosine levels were associated with incident T2DM [68], and higher serum concentrations of sarcosine characterized the metabotype of older adults with PF&S [17]. Collectively, these findings suggest that perturbations in folate/one-carbon metabolism may play a role in frailty and T2DM as well as in other age-related conditions.

Ethanolamine is a crucial intermediate of the CDP-ethanolamine pathway, the main route of phosphatidylethanolamine synthesis, and modulates lipid metabolism and the turnover of biological membranes [69]. Recently, a critical role for skeletal muscle phospholipid metabolism has been described in the regulation of both insulin sensitivity and contractile function [70]. Moreover, the ethanolamine/phosphatidylethanolamine synthesis dyad is directly involved in autophagy regulation, thereby modulating anti-aging properties of this cellular process [71]. Interestingly, perturbations in the CDP-ethanolamine pathway were associated with altered mitochondrial biogenesis in mouse models of muscle atrophy [71], while higher circulating levels of ethanolamine were found in older adults with PF&S [17].

Tryptophan is an essential amino acid that exerts multiple roles in growth, mood, behavior, and immune responses [72]. Tryptophan is metabolized via two major pathways, the tryptophan-kynurenine and the tryptophan-methoxyndole pathways, that lead to the production of NAD, serotonin, and melatonin [72]. Alterations in tryptophan metabolism have been described in the context of frailty and T2DM [73,74]. In particular, tryptophan and its associated metabolites have been associated with insulin resistance and incident T2DM in independent cohorts [74,75]. Moreover, higher circulating levels of tryptophan were associated with low muscle quality in a large cohort of men and women enrolled in the BLSA [32].

Non-frail non-T2DM controls were characterized by higher serum levels of taurine. Taurine is the most abundant free amino acid in several organs, including the skeletal muscle that contains approximately 70% of total body taurine [76]. Taurine has multiple regulatory effects and its role in osmoregulation, modulation of inflammatory response, protection against oxidative stress, and stimulation of cellular quality control processes is widely acknowledged [76,77]. Taurine deficiency is commonly encountered in people with T2DM [78,79], and its supplementation has been proposed as a strategy against T2DM complications, including retinopathy, nephropathy, neuropathy, atherosclerosis, and cardiomyopathy [80]. Recently, taurine supplementation has also been proposed as a possible remedy against sarcopenia [81]. The causes of taurine depletion in F-T2DM older adults are multifaceted and may include decreased dietary intake, reduced intestinal absorption, renal wasting, and inflammation [77].

Unexpectedly, branched-chain amino acids (BCAAs) were not found to be discriminant by the PLS-DA classification model. BCAAs are metabolic rheostats that modulate whole-body and tissular metabolism [20]. Recent evidence suggests that BCAAs may have a Janus-like behavior in F-T2DM older adults. Indeed, while BCAA-induced activation of the mammalian target of rapamycin (mTOR) in skeletal myocytes may contrast sarcopenia and functional decline in advanced age [20,31], other studies found an association between higher circulating levels of BCAAs and insulin resistance or T2DM in older adults [24–27]. The low discriminant power of BCAAs in MetaboFrail might therefore reflect the dual effect of BCAAs in F-T2DM older people.

Although innovative, the present investigation has some limitations that should be mentioned. The study sample was quite small while the dataset comprised numerous variables. To cope with this issue, we adopted a PLS-DA-based strategy which is particularly suited for handling matrices populated by highly correlated variables. The MetaboFrail study enrolled older adults from three European countries; thus, a validation study in other ethnic groups is warranted. Eating habits may affect circulating amino acid levels, but diet was not objectively assessed in our study sample. However, it has recently been reported that differences in blood amino acid concentrations do not necessarily mirror those of amino acid intakes [82]. As commonly occurs in biomarker discovery studies, although a large number of candidates were investigated, we could not evaluate all possible mediators involved in frailty and T2DM.

In conclusion, in the present investigation, we showed the existence of a specific amino acid signature in F-T2DM older persons. Our novel approach enabled us to obtain new insights into the pathophysiology of the two conditions. In particular, a relevant role for perturbations in muscle metabolism and muscle-liver interorgan communication was highlighted. The longitudinal implementation of our analytical strategy could allow validating novel sets of biomarkers and identifying new targets for interventions.

Author Contributions: Conceptualization, A.P. (Anna Picca), E.M., and R.C.; methodology, A.P. (Aniello Primiano), G.C., and J.G.; software, A.B. and F.M.; validation, A.P. (Anna Picca), E.M., and R.C.; formal analysis, A.B. and F.M.; investigation, A.P. (Anna Picca), E.M., and R.C.; resources, A.J.S., G.G., L.R.-M., and R.B.; data curation, A.P. (Anna Picca) and R.C.; writing—original draft preparation, E.M. and R.C.; writing—review and editing, A.P. (Anna Picca), F.M., I.B.-M., L.P., O.L., R.C., and S.C.R.; supervision, A.J.S., G.G., L.R.-M., and R.B.; funding acquisition, A.J.S., G.G., L.R.-M., and R.B. All authors have read and agreed to the published version of the manuscript.

Acknowledgments: The authors thank Luca Mariotti for his precious technical and administrative support.

References

1. Sinclair, A.; Dunning, T.; Rodriguez-Mañas, L. Diabetes in older people: New insights and remaining challenges. *Lancet Diabetes Endocrinol.* **2015**, *3*, 275–285. [CrossRef]
2. Cho, N.H.; Shaw, J.E.; Karuranga, S.; Huang, Y.; da Rocha Fernandes, J.D.; Ohlrogge, A.W.; Malanda, B. IDF Diabetes Atlas: Global estimates of diabetes prevalence for 2017 and projections for 2045. *Diabetes Res. Clin. Pract.* **2018**, *138*, 271–281. [CrossRef] [PubMed]
3. GBD 2017 Disease and Injury Incidence and Prevalence Collaborators; James, S.L.; Abate, D.; Abate, K.H.; Abay, S.M.; Abbafati, C.; Abbasi, N.; Abbastabar, H.; Abd-Allah, F.; Abdela, J.; et al. Global, regional, and national incidence, prevalence, and years lived with disability for 354 diseases and injuries for 195 countries and territories, 1990–2017: A systematic analysis for the Global Burden of Disease Study 2017. *Lancet* **2018**, *392*, 1789–1858. [CrossRef]
4. Kalyani, R.R.; Golden, S.H.; Cefalu, W.T. Diabetes and Aging: Unique Considerations and Goals of Care. *Diabetes Care* **2017**, *40*, 440–443. [CrossRef] [PubMed]
5. Cesari, M.; Calvani, R.; Marzetti, E. Frailty in Older Persons. *Clin. Geriatr. Med.* **2017**, *33*, 293–303. [CrossRef] [PubMed]
6. Clegg, A.; Young, J.; Iliffe, S.; Rikkert, M.O.; Rockwood, K. Frailty in elderly people. *Lancet* **2013**, *381*, 752–762. [CrossRef]

7. El Assar, M.; Laosa, O.; Rodríguez Mañas, L. Diabetes and frailty. *Curr. Opin. Clin. Nutr. Metab. Care* **2019**, *22*, 52–57. [CrossRef]
8. LeRoith, D.; Biessels, G.J.; Braithwaite, S.S.; Casanueva, F.F.; Draznin, B.; Halter, J.B.; Hirsch, I.B.; McDonnell, M.E.; Molitch, M.E.; Murad, M.H.; et al. Treatment of Diabetes in Older Adults: An Endocrine Society* Clinical Practice Guideline. *J. Clin. Endocrinol. Metab.* **2019**, *104*, 1520–1574. [CrossRef]
9. Sinclair, A.J.; Rodriguez-Mañas, L. Diabetes and Frailty: Two Converging Conditions? *Can. J. Diabetes* **2016**, *40*, 77–83. [CrossRef]
10. Larsson, L.; Degens, H.; Li, M.; Salviati, L.; Lee, Y., II; Thompson, W.; Kirkland, J.L.; Sandri, M. Sarcopenia: Aging-Related Loss of Muscle Mass and Function. *Physiol. Rev.* **2019**, *99*, 427–511. [CrossRef]
11. Guerrero, N.; Bunout, D.; Hirsch, S.; Barrera, G.; Leiva, L.; Henríquez, S.; De la Maza, M.P. Premature loss of muscle mass and function in type 2 diabetes. *Diabetes Res. Clin. Pract.* **2016**, *117*, 32–38. [CrossRef] [PubMed]
12. Park, S.W.; Goodpaster, B.H.; Strotmeyer, E.S.; Kuller, L.H.; Broudeau, R.; Kammerer, C.; de Rekeneire, N.; Harris, T.B.; Schwartz, A.V.; Tylavsky, F.A.; et al. Accelerated Loss of Skeletal Muscle Strength in Older Adults With Type 2 Diabetes: The Health, Aging, and Body Composition Study. *Diabetes Care* **2007**, *30*, 1507–1512. [CrossRef] [PubMed]
13. Landi, F.; Calvani, R.; Cesari, M.; Tosato, M.; Martone, A.M.; Bernabei, R.; Onder, G.; Marzetti, E. Sarcopenia as the Biological Substrate of Physical Frailty. *Clin. Geriatr. Med.* **2015**, *31*, 367–374. [CrossRef] [PubMed]
14. Calvani, R.; Marini, F.; Cesari, M.; Tosato, M.; Anker, S.D.; von Haehling, S.; Miller, R.R.; Bernabei, R.; Landi, F.; Marzetti, E.; et al. Biomarkers for physical frailty and sarcopenia: State of the science and future developments. *J. Cachexia. Sarcopenia Muscle* **2015**, *6*, 278–286. [CrossRef] [PubMed]
15. Picca, A.; Coelho-Junior, H.J.; Cesari, M.; Marini, F.; Miccheli, A.; Gervasoni, J.; Bossola, M.; Landi, F.; Bernabei, R.; Marzetti, E.; et al. The metabolomics side of frailty: Toward personalized medicine for the aged. *Exp. Gerontol.* **2019**, *126*, 110692. [CrossRef] [PubMed]
16. Calvani, R.; Rodriguez-Mañas, L.; Picca, A.; Marini, F.; Biancolillo, A.; Laosa, O.; Pedraza, L.; Gervasoni, J.; Primiano, A.; Miccheli, A.; et al. The "Metabolic biomarkers of frailty in older people with type 2 diabetes mellitus" (MetaboFrail) study: Rationale, design and methods. *Exp. Gerontol.* **2020**, *129*, 110782. [CrossRef] [PubMed]
17. Calvani, R.; Picca, A.; Marini, F.; Biancolillo, A.; Gervasoni, J.; Persichilli, S.; Primiano, A.; Coelho-Junior, H.; Bossola, M.; Urbani, A.; et al. A Distinct Pattern of Circulating Amino Acids Characterizes Older Persons with Physical Frailty and Sarcopenia: Results from the BIOSPHERE Study. *Nutrients* **2018**, *10*, 1691. [CrossRef]
18. Pasini, E.; Corsetti, G.; Aquilani, R.; Romano, C.; Picca, A.; Calvani, R.; Dioguardi, F.S. Protein-Amino Acid Metabolism Disarrangements: The Hidden Enemy of Chronic Age-Related Conditions. *Nutrients* **2018**, *10*, 391. [CrossRef]
19. Lu, Y.; Karagounis, L.G.; Ng, T.P.; Carre, C.; Narang, V.; Wong, G.; Tan, C.T.Y.; Zin Nyunt, M.S.; Gao, Q.; Abel, B.; et al. Systemic and Metabolic Signature of Sarcopenia in Community-Dwelling Older Adults. *J. Gerontol. Ser. A* **2019**. [CrossRef]
20. Neinast, M.; Murashige, D.; Arany, Z. Branched Chain Amino Acids. *Annu. Rev. Physiol.* **2019**, *81*, 139–164. [CrossRef]
21. Zhenyukh, O.; Civantos, E.; Ruiz-Ortega, M.; Sánchez, M.S.; Vázquez, C.; Peiró, C.; Egido, J.; Mas, S. High concentration of branched-chain amino acids promotes oxidative stress, inflammation and migration of human peripheral blood mononuclear cells via mTORC1 activation. *Free Radic. Biol. Med.* **2017**, *104*, 165–177. [CrossRef] [PubMed]
22. Yoon, M.-S. The Emerging Role of Branched-Chain Amino Acids in Insulin Resistance and Metabolism. *Nutrients* **2016**, *8*, 405. [CrossRef] [PubMed]
23. Yang, Q.; Vijayakumar, A.; Kahn, B.B. Metabolites as regulators of insulin sensitivity and metabolism. *Nat. Rev. Mol. Cell Biol.* **2018**, *19*, 654–672. [CrossRef] [PubMed]
24. Wang, T.J.; Larson, M.G.; Vasan, R.S.; Cheng, S.; Rhee, E.P.; McCabe, E.; Lewis, G.D.; Fox, C.S.; Jacques, P.F.; Fernandez, C.; et al. Metabolite profiles and the risk of developing diabetes. *Nat. Med.* **2011**, *17*, 448–453. [CrossRef] [PubMed]
25. Wang-Sattler, R.; Yu, Z.; Herder, C.; Messias, A.C.; Floegel, A.; He, Y.; Heim, K.; Campillos, M.; Holzapfel, C.; Thorand, B.; et al. Novel biomarkers for pre-diabetes identified by metabolomics. *Mol. Syst. Biol.* **2012**, *8*, 615. [CrossRef] [PubMed]

26. Floegel, A.; Stefan, N.; Yu, Z.; Mühlenbruch, K.; Drogan, D.; Joost, H.-G.; Fritsche, A.; Häring, H.-U.; Hrabě de Angelis, M.; Peters, A.; et al. Identification of serum metabolites associated with risk of type 2 diabetes using a targeted metabolomic approach. *Diabetes* **2013**, *62*, 639–648. [CrossRef]
27. Chen, T.; Ni, Y.; Ma, X.; Bao, Y.; Liu, J.; Huang, F.; Hu, C.; Xie, G.; Zhao, A.; Jia, W.; et al. Branched-chain and aromatic amino acid profiles and diabetes risk in Chinese populations. *Sci. Rep.* **2016**, *6*, 20594. [CrossRef]
28. Semba, R.D.; Gonzalez-Freire, M.; Moaddel, R.; Sun, K.; Fabbri, E.; Zhang, P.; Carlson, O.D.; Khadeer, M.; Chia, C.W.; Salem, N.; et al. Altered Plasma Amino Acids and Lipids Associated With Abnormal Glucose Metabolism and Insulin Resistance in Older Adults. *J. Clin. Endocrinol. Metab.* **2018**, *103*, 3331–3339. [CrossRef]
29. Adachi, Y.; Ono, N.; Imaizumi, A.; Muramatsu, T.; Andou, T.; Shimodaira, Y.; Nagao, K.; Kageyama, Y.; Mori, M.; Noguchi, Y.; et al. Plasma Amino Acid Profile in Severely Frail Elderly Patients in Japan. *Int. J. Gerontol.* **2018**, *12*, 290–293. [CrossRef]
30. Kochlik, B.; Stuetz, W.; Pérès, K.; Féart, C.; Tegner, J.; Rodriguez-Mañas, L.; Grune, T.; Weber, D. Associations of Plasma 3-Methylhistidine with Frailty Status in French Cohorts of the FRAILOMIC Initiative. *J. Clin. Med.* **2019**, *8*, 1010. [CrossRef]
31. Lustgarten, M.S.; Price, L.L.; Chale, A.; Phillips, E.M.; Fielding, R.A. Branched chain amino acids are associated with muscle mass in functionally limited older adults. *J. Gerontol. A Biol. Sci. Med. Sci.* **2014**, *69*, 717–724. [CrossRef] [PubMed]
32. Moaddel, R.; Fabbri, E.; Khadeer, M.A.; Carlson, O.D.; Gonzalez-Freire, M.; Zhang, P.; Semba, R.D.; Ferrucci, L. Plasma Biomarkers of Poor Muscle Quality in Older Men and Women from the Baltimore Longitudinal Study of Aging. *J. Gerontol. A Biol. Sci. Med. Sci.* **2016**, *71*, 1266–1272. [CrossRef] [PubMed]
33. Rodríguez-Mañas, L.; Bayer, A.J.; Kelly, M.; Zeyfang, A.; Izquierdo, M.; Laosa, O.; Hardman, T.C.; Sinclair, A.J.; Moreira, S.; Cook, J.; et al. An evaluation of the effectiveness of a multi-modal intervention in frail and pre-frail older people with type 2 diabetes–the MID-Frail study: Study protocol for a randomised controlled trial. *Trials* **2014**, *15*, 34. [CrossRef] [PubMed]
34. Rodriguez-Mañas, L.; Laosa, O.; Vellas, B.; Paolisso, G.; Topinkova, E.; Oliva-Moreno, J.; Bourdel-Marchasson, I.; Izquierdo, M.; Hood, K.; Zeyfang, A.; et al. Effectiveness of a multimodal intervention in functionally impaired older people with type 2 diabetes mellitus. *J. Cachexia. Sarcopenia Muscle* **2019**. [CrossRef]
35. Fried, L.P.; Tangen, C.M.; Walston, J.; Newman, A.B.; Hirsch, C.; Gottdiener, J.; Seeman, T.; Tracy, R.; Kop, W.J.; Burke, G.; et al. Frailty in older adults: Evidence for a phenotype. *J. Gerontol. A Biol. Sci. Med. Sci.* **2001**, *56*, M146–M156. [CrossRef] [PubMed]
36. Folstein, M.F.; Folstein, S.E.; McHugh, P.R. "Mini-mental state". A practical method for grading the cognitive state of patients for the clinician. *J. Psychiatr. Res.* **1975**, *12*, 189–198. [CrossRef]
37. Mahoney, F.I.; Barthel, D.W. Functional Evaluation: The barthel index. *Md. State Med. J.* **1965**, *14*, 61–65.
38. Ståhle, L.; Wold, S. Partial least squares analysis with cross-validation for the two-class problem: A Monte Carlo study. *J. Chemom.* **1987**, *1*, 185–196. [CrossRef]
39. Westerhuis, J.A.; Hoefsloot, H.C.J.; Smit, S.; Vis, D.J.; Smilde, A.K.; van Velzen, E.J.J.; van Duijnhoven, J.P.M.; van Dorsten, F.A. Assessment of PLSDA cross validation. *Metabolomics* **2008**, *4*, 81–89. [CrossRef]
40. Smit, S.; van Breemen, M.J.; Hoefsloot, H.C.J.; Smilde, A.K.; Aerts, J.M.F.G.; de Koster, C.G. Assessing the statistical validity of proteomics based biomarkers. *Anal. Chim. Acta* **2007**, *592*, 210–217. [CrossRef]
41. Marzetti, E.; Landi, F.; Marini, F.; Cesari, M.; Buford, T.W.; Manini, T.M.; Onder, G.; Pahor, M.; Bernabei, R.; Leeuwenburgh, C.; et al. Patterns of Circulating Inflammatory Biomarkers in Older Persons with Varying Levels of Physical Performance: A Partial Least Squares-Discriminant Analysis Approach. *Front. Med.* **2014**, *1*, 27. [CrossRef] [PubMed]
42. Chen, R.; Snyder, M. Promise of Personalized Omics to Precision Medicine. *Wiley Interdiscip. Rev. Syst. Biol. Med.* **2013**, *5*, 73. [CrossRef] [PubMed]
43. Loscalzo, J.; Barabasi, A.-L. Systems biology and the future of medicine. *Wiley Interdiscip. Rev. Syst. Biol. Med.* **2011**, *3*, 619–627. [CrossRef] [PubMed]
44. Guijas, C.; Montenegro-Burke, J.R.; Warth, B.; Spilker, M.E.; Siuzdak, G. Metabolomics activity screening for identifying metabolites that modulate phenotype. *Nat. Biotechnol.* **2018**, *36*, 316–320. [CrossRef] [PubMed]
45. Karczewski, K.J.; Snyder, M.P. Integrative omics for health and disease. *Nat. Rev. Genet.* **2018**, *19*, 299–310. [CrossRef] [PubMed]

46. Wishart, D.S. Metabolomics for Investigating Physiological and Pathophysiological Processes. *Physiol. Rev.* **2019**, *99*, 1819–1875. [CrossRef] [PubMed]
47. Johnson, P.; Perry, S.V. Biological activity and the 3-methylhistidine content of actin and myosin. *Biochem. J.* **1970**, *119*, 293–298. [CrossRef]
48. Asatoor, A.M.; Armstrong, M.D. 3-methylhistidine, a component of actin. *Biochem. Biophys. Res. Commun.* **1967**, *26*, 168–174. [CrossRef]
49. Sheffield-Moore, M.; Dillon, E.L.; Randolph, K.M.; Casperson, S.L.; White, G.R.; Jennings, K.; Rathmacher, J.; Schuette, S.; Janghorbani, M.; Urban, R.J.; et al. Isotopic decay of urinary or plasma 3-methylhistidine as a potential biomarker of pathologic skeletal muscle loss. *J. Cachexia. Sarcopenia Muscle* **2014**, *5*, 19–25. [CrossRef]
50. Marchesini, G.; Forlani, G.; Zoli, M.; Vannini, P.; Pisi, E. Muscle protein breakdown in uncontrolled diabetes as assessed by urinary 3-methylhistidine excretion. *Diabetologia* **1982**, *23*, 456–458. [CrossRef]
51. Wagenmakers, A.J. Protein and amino acid metabolism in human muscle. *Adv. Exp. Med. Biol.* **1998**, *441*, 307–319. [PubMed]
52. Jang, C.; Hui, S.; Zeng, X.; Cowan, A.J.; Wang, L.; Chen, L.; Morscher, R.J.; Reyes, J.; Frezza, C.; Hwang, H.Y.; et al. Metabolite Exchange between Mammalian Organs Quantified in Pigs. *Cell Metab.* **2019**, *30*, 594–606.e3. [CrossRef] [PubMed]
53. Gancheva, S.; Jelenik, T.; Álvarez-Hernández, E.; Roden, M. Interorgan Metabolic Crosstalk in Human Insulin Resistance. *Physiol. Rev.* **2018**, *98*, 1371–1415. [CrossRef] [PubMed]
54. Jagoe, R.T.; Engelen, M.P.K.J. Muscle wasting and changes in muscle protein metabolism in chronic obstructive pulmonary disease. *Eur. Respir. J.* **2003**, *22*, 52s–63s. [CrossRef] [PubMed]
55. Ilaiwy, A.; Quintana, M.T.; Bain, J.R.; Muehlbauer, M.J.; Brown, D.I.; Stansfield, W.E.; Willis, M.S. Cessation of biomechanical stretch model of C2C12 cells models myocyte atrophy and anaplerotic changes in metabolism using non-targeted metabolomics analysis. *Int. J. Biochem. Cell Biol.* **2016**, *79*, 80–92. [CrossRef]
56. Lu, Y.; Wang, Y.; Liang, X.; Zou, L.; Ong, C.N.; Yuan, J.M.; Koh, W.P.; Pan, A. Serum amino acids in association with prevalent and incident type 2 diabetes in a Chinese population. *Metabolites* **2019**, *9*, 14. [CrossRef]
57. Seibert, R.; Abbasi, F.; Hantash, F.M.; Caulfield, M.P.; Reaven, G.; Kim, S.H. Relationship between insulin resistance and amino acids in women and men. *Physiol. Rep.* **2015**, *3*, e12392. [CrossRef]
58. Cheng, S.; Rhee, E.P.; Larson, M.G.; Lewis, G.D.; McCabe, E.L.; Shen, D.; Palma, M.J.; Roberts, L.D.; Dejam, A.; Souza, A.L.; et al. Metabolite profiling identifies pathways associated with metabolic risk in humans. *Circulation* **2012**, *125*, 2222–2231. [CrossRef]
59. Wu, G.; Morris, S.M. Arginine metabolism: Nitric oxide and beyond. *Biochem. J.* **1998**, *336*, 1–17. [CrossRef]
60. Mangoni, A.A.; Rodionov, R.N.; Mcevoy, M.; Zinellu, A.; Carru, C.; Sotgia, S. New horizons in arginine metabolism, ageing and chronic disease states. *Age Ageing* **2019**, *48*, 776–782. [CrossRef]
61. Cao, Y.-F.; Li, J.; Zhang, Z.; Liu, J.; Sun, X.-Y.; Feng, X.-F.; Luo, H.-H.; Yang, W.; Li, S.-N.; Yang, X.; et al. Plasma Levels of Amino Acids Related to Urea Cycle and Risk of Type 2 Diabetes Mellitus in Chinese Adults. *Front. Endocrinol.* **2019**, *10*, 50. [CrossRef] [PubMed]
62. Ducker, G.S.; Rabinowitz, J.D. One-Carbon Metabolism in Health and Disease. *Cell Metab.* **2017**, *25*, 27–42. [CrossRef] [PubMed]
63. Koutros, S.; Meyer, T.E.; Fox, S.D.; Issaq, H.J.; Veenstra, T.D.; Huang, W.Y.; Yu, K.; Albanes, D.; Chu, L.W.; Andriole, G.; et al. Prospective evaluation of serum sarcosine and risk of prostate cancer in the prostate, lung, colorectal and ovarian cancer screening trial. *Carcinogenesis* **2013**, *34*, 2281–2285. [CrossRef] [PubMed]
64. De Vogel, S.; Ulvik, A.; Meyer, K.; Ueland, P.M.; Nygård, O.; Vollset, S.E.; Tell, G.S.; Gregory, J.F.; Tretli, S.; Bjørge, T. Sarcosine and other metabolites along the choline oxidation pathway in relation to prostate cancer—A large nested case-control study within the JANUS cohort in Norway. *Int. J. Cancer* **2014**, *134*, 197–206. [CrossRef] [PubMed]
65. Hasokawa, M.; Shinohara, M.; Tsugawa, H.; Bamba, T.; Fukusaki, E.; Nishiumi, S.; Nishimura, K.; Yoshida, M.; Ishida, T.; Hirata, K.; et al. Identification of biomarkers of stent restenosis with serum metabolomic profiling using gas chromatography/mass spectrometry. *Circ. J.* **2012**, *76*, 1864–1873. [CrossRef]
66. Tsai, C.H.; Huang, H.C.; Liu, B.L.; Li, C.I.; Lu, M.K.; Chen, X.; Tsai, M.C.; Yang, Y.W.; Lane, H.Y. Activation of N-methyl-D-aspartate receptor glycine site temporally ameliorates neuropsychiatric symptoms of Parkinson's disease with dementia. *Psychiatry Clin. Neurosci.* **2014**, *68*, 692–700. [CrossRef]

67. Walters, R.O.; Arias, E.; Diaz, A.; Burgos, E.S.; Guan, F.; Tiano, S.; Mao, K.; Green, C.L.; Qiu, Y.; Shah, H.; et al. Sarcosine Is Uniquely Modulated by Aging and Dietary Restriction in Rodents and Humans. *Cell Rep.* **2018**, *25*, 663–676. [CrossRef]
68. Svingen, G.F.T.; Schartum-Hansen, H.; Pedersen, E.R.; Ueland, P.M.; Tell, G.S.; Mellgren, G.; Njølstad, P.R.; Seifert, R.; Strand, E.; Karlsson, T.; et al. Prospective associations of systemic and urinary choline metabolites with incident type 2 diabetes. *Clin. Chem.* **2016**, *62*, 755–765. [CrossRef]
69. van der Veen, J.N.; Kennelly, J.P.; Wan, S.; Vance, J.E.; Vance, D.E.; Jacobs, R.L. The critical role of phosphatidylcholine and phosphatidylethanolamine metabolism in health and disease. *Biochim. Biophys. Acta Biomembr.* **2017**, *1859*, 1558–1572. [CrossRef]
70. Funai, K.; Lodhi, I.J.; Spears, L.D.; Yin, L.; Song, H.; Klein, S.; Semenkovich, C.F. Skeletal muscle phospholipid metabolism regulates insulin sensitivity and contractile function. *Diabetes* **2016**, *65*, 358–370. [CrossRef]
71. Rockenfeller, P.; Koska, M.; Pietrocola, F.; Minois, N.; Knittelfelder, O.; Sica, V.; Franz, J.; Carmona-Gutierrez, D.; Kroemer, G.; Madeo, F. Phosphatidylethanolamine positively regulates autophagy and longevity. *Cell Death Differ.* **2015**, *22*, 499–508. [CrossRef] [PubMed]
72. Le Floc'h, N.; Otten, W.; Merlot, E. Tryptophan metabolism, from nutrition to potential therapeutic applications. *Amino Acids* **2011**, *41*, 1195–1205. [CrossRef] [PubMed]
73. Marcos-Pérez, D.; Sánchez-Flores, M.; Maseda, A.; Lorenzo-López, L.; Millán-Calenti, J.C.; Strasser, B.; Gostner, J.M.; Fuchs, D.; Pásaro, E.; Valdiglesias, V.; et al. Frailty Status in Older Adults Is Related to Alterations in Indoleamine 2,3-Dioxygenase 1 and Guanosine Triphosphate Cyclohydrolase I Enzymatic Pathways. *J. Am. Med. Dir. Assoc.* **2017**, *18*, 1049–1057. [CrossRef] [PubMed]
74. Chen, T.; Zheng, X.; Ma, X.; Bao, Y.; Ni, Y.; Hu, C.; Rajani, C.; Huang, F.; Zhao, A.; Jiia, W.; et al. Tryptophan Predicts the Risk for Future Type 2 Diabetes. *PLoS ONE* **2016**, *11*, e0162192. [CrossRef] [PubMed]
75. Yu, E.; Papandreou, C.; Ruiz-Canela, M.; Guasch-Ferre, M.; Clish, C.B.; Dennis, C.; Liang, L.; Corella, D.; Fitó, M.; Razquin, C.; et al. Association of tryptophan metabolites with incident type 2 diabetes in the PREDIMED trial: A case–cohort study. *Clin. Chem.* **2018**, *64*, 1211–1220. [CrossRef]
76. Huxtable, R.J. Physiological actions of taurine. *Physiol. Rev.* **1992**, *72*, 101–163. [CrossRef]
77. Lambert, I.H.; Kristensen, D.M.; Holm, J.B.; Mortensen, O.H. Physiological role of taurine—From organism to organelle. *Acta Physiol.* **2015**, *213*, 191–212. [CrossRef]
78. De Luca, G.; Calpona, P.R.; Caponetti, A.; Romano, G.; Di Benedetto, A.; Cucinotta, D.; Di Giorgio, R.M. Taurine and osmoregulation: Platelet taurine content, uptake, and release in type 2 diabetic patients. *Metabolism* **2001**, *50*, 60–64. [CrossRef]
79. Franconi, F.A.; Bennardini, F.R.; Giuseppe, A.; Miceli, S.M.; Ciuti, M.; Mian, M. Plasma and platelet taurine are reduced in subjects with mellitus: Effects of taurine. *Am. J. Clin. Nutr.* **1995**, *61*, 1115–1119. [CrossRef]
80. Ito, T.; Schaffer, S.W.; Azuma, J. The potential usefulness of taurine on diabetes mellitus and its complications. *Amino Acids* **2012**, *42*, 1529–1539. [CrossRef]
81. Scicchitano, B.M.; Sica, G. The Beneficial Effects of Taurine to Counteract Sarcopenia. *Curr. Protein Pept. Sci.* **2018**, *19*, 673–680. [CrossRef] [PubMed]
82. Schmidt, J.A.; Rinaldi, S.; Scalbert, A.; Ferrari, P.; Achaintre, D.; Gunter, M.J.; Appleby, P.N.; Key, T.J.; Travis, R.C. Plasma concentrations and intakes of amino acids in male meat-eaters, fish-eaters, vegetarians and vegans: A cross-sectional analysis in the EPIC-Oxford cohort. *Eur. J. Clin. Nutr.* **2016**, *70*, 306–312. [CrossRef] [PubMed]

8

Lactate Stimulates a Potential for Hypertrophy and Regeneration of Mouse Skeletal Muscle

Yoshitaka Ohno [1], Koki Ando [1], Takafumi Ito [1], Yohei Suda [1], Yuki Matsui [1], Akiko Oyama [1], Hikari Kaneko [1], Shingo Yokoyama [1], Tatsuro Egawa [2] and Katsumasa Goto [1,3,*]

1 Laboratory of Physiology, School of Health Sciences, Toyohashi SOZO University, Toyohashi 440-8511, Japan; yohno@sozo.ac.jp (Y.O.); r1482701@sc.sozo.ac.jp (K.A.); r1482703@sc.sozo.ac.jp (T.I.); r1482716@sc.sozo.ac.jp (Y.S.); r1482724@sc.sozo.ac.jp (Y.M.); r1382605@sc.sozo.ac.jp (A.O.); r1382606@sc.sozo.ac.jp (H.K.); s-yokoyama@sozo.ac.jp (S.Y.)

2 Laboratory of Sports and Exercise Medicine, Graduate School of Human and Environmental Studies, Kyoto University, Kyoto 606-8501, Japan; egawa.tatsuro.4u@kyoto-u.ac.jp

3 Department of Physiology, Graduate School of Health Sciences, Toyohashi SOZO University, Toyohashi 440-8511, Japan

* Correspondence: gotok@sepia.ocn.ne.jp

Abstract: The effects of lactate on muscle mass and regeneration were investigated using mouse skeletal muscle tissue and cultured C2C12 cells. Male C57BL/6J mice were randomly divided into (1) control, (2) lactate (1 mol/L in distilled water, 8.9 mL/g body weight)-administered, (3) cardio toxin (CTX)-injected (CX), and (4) lactate-administered after CTX-injection (LX) groups. CTX was injected into right tibialis anterior (TA) muscle before the oral administration of sodium lactate (five days/week for two weeks) to the mice. Oral lactate administration increased the muscle weight and fiber cross-sectional area, and the population of Pax7-positive nuclei in mouse TA skeletal muscle. Oral administration of lactate also facilitated the recovery process of CTX-associated injured mouse TA muscle mass accompanied with a transient increase in the population of Pax7-positive nuclei. Mouse myoblast-derived C2C12 cells were differentiated for five days to form myotubes with or without lactate administration. C2C12 myotube formation with an increase in protein content, fiber diameter, length, and myo-nuclei was stimulated by lactate. These observations suggest that lactate may be a potential molecule to stimulate muscle hypertrophy and regeneration of mouse skeletal muscle via the activation of muscle satellite cells.

Keywords: lactate; skeletal muscle; hypertrophy; regeneration; muscle satellite cell

1. Introduction

Muscle satellite cells are known as skeletal muscle-specific stem cells that reside between the basal lamina and sarcolemma of mature myo-fibers [1]. Muscle satellite cells, which express the paired box transcription factor 7 (Pax7), are normally quiescent but become activated in response to exercise or injury [2–4]. Activated muscle satellite cells proliferate and undergo differentiation into myoblasts. Then the myoblasts differentiate and fuse into preexisting myofibers or fuse to form new myofibers, which result in skeletal muscle hypertrophy or regeneration [5–7].

Muscle satellite cells are considered to play a crucial role in exercise-associated muscle hypertrophy in human skeletal muscles [6,8] even though the studies using rodent models indicated that satellite cells may not contribute to exercise-associated hypertrophy of skeletal muscle [9,10]. Furthermore, exercise-associated stimuli, such as mechanical and heat stresses, are proposed to be potential stimuli to activate the regenerative process of injured skeletal muscle [11–13]. However, the mechanism of exercise-induced hypertrophy and regeneration of skeletal muscle is not fully elucidated.

Recent studies demonstrate that the number of biologically active molecules, so-called myokines, are released from resting as well as contracting skeletal muscle cells [14]. It is generally accepted that intensive exercise induces the release of lactate from contracting skeletal muscle. Extracellular lactate is re-uptaken by skeletal muscle to utilize it for an energy source [15,16]. On the other hand, the previous study using C2C12 skeletal muscle cells showed that a high level of extracellular lactate changed the expression of follistatin and myostatin [17], which regulate the proliferation of muscle satellite cells [18]. Furthermore, we recently demonstrated extracellular lactate-associated C2C12 myotube hypertrophy by activating the anabolic intracellular signals, such as p42/44 extracellular signal-regulated kinase-1/2 (ERK1/2) pathway [19], which stimulates muscle cell proliferation and differentiation [20–22]. Judging from published results, we hypothesize that increasing extracellular lactate level, which is generally induced by intensive exercise, may induce muscle hypertrophy as well as regeneration of injured skeletal muscle by activating muscle satellite cells.

In the present study, we investigated the effects of oral lactate administration on hypertrophy and regeneration in mouse skeletal muscle. Since previous studies have reported that an increase of satellite cells, which is caused by extracellular stimuli including electrical and heat stimulation [11,23], facilitated muscle regeneration, we evaluated the population of satellite cells following lactate administration. The effects of lactate on the formation of myotubes were also investigated by using cultured C2C12 cells.

2. Materials and Methods

2.1. Animal Experiments

All animal experimental procedures were conducted in accordance with the Guide for the Care and Use of Laboratory Animals, as adopted and promulgated by the National Institutes of Health (Bethesda, MD, USA). The Animal Use Committee of Toyohashi SOZO University (A2016003, A2017002) approved the procedures of animal experiments in this study. Male C57BL/6J mice aged 8-week old were used. To investigate the effects of lactate on skeletal muscle hypertrophy or regeneration, mice were randomly divided into control (C) and lactate-administered (L) groups (n = 24), or cardio-toxin (CTX)-injected (CX) and lactate-administered after CTX injection (LX) groups (n = 28). All mice were housed in a clean room controlled at approximately 23 °C with a 12/12 h light-dark cycle. Solid diet and water were provided ad libitum.

Muscle injury-regeneration cycle was induced by injecting 0.1 mL cardiotoxin (CTX, 10 μmol/L in physiological saline, Sigma-Aldrich, St. Louis, MO, USA) of Naja naja atra venom into right tibialis anterior (TA) muscles in the CX and LX groups. After epilation of right hind limb with a commercial hair remover for human, injection of CTX into right TA muscle was performed using a 27-gauge needle. During this procedure, all mice were under anesthesia with intraperitoneal injection of sodium pentobarbital (50 mg/kg) [23].

In the L and LX group, sodium lactate (1 mol/L in distilled water, 8.9 mL/g body weight, Otsuka Pharmaceutical Factory, Inc., Naruto, Tokushima, Japan) was administered to the mice by using an oral sonde 5 days a week for 2 weeks after CTX injection. The dose (or amount) of lactate was selected considering the previous rat study [18]. The same volume of ultrapure water was administered to the C and CX groups. In a pilot study, the changes of blood lactate concentration, which was collected from the tail vein of mice after oral lactate administration, were evaluated using the Lactate Pro2 blood lactate test meter (ARKRAY, Inc., Kyoto, Japan). Before the administration of lactate, the blood lactate concentration of mice (n = 7) was 2.9 ± 0.2 mmol/L (Table 1). Two hours after the lactate administration, blood lactate level significantly increased up to 4.1 ± 0.3 mmol/L. Similar to this observation, the oral administration of lactic acid to rats led to a rise in the blood level [24].

Table 1. Blood lactate concentration of mice following orally administered sodium lactate.

	Pre	2 h	6 h	24 h
Concentration, mmol/L	2.9 ± 0.2	4.1 ± 0.3 †	2.9 ± 0.3 §	3.0 ± 0.4

Pre: before oral lactate administration (base line); 2 h, 6 h, and 24 h: 2, 6, and 24 h after the lactate administration. Values are means ± SEM. $n = 7$. † and §: $p < 0.05$ vs. Pre and 2 h, respectively.

Mice were sacrificed by cervical dislocation under anesthesia with intraperitoneal injection of sodium pentobarbital (50 mg/kg) 1 and 2 weeks after CTX injection. Immediately after the sacrification, right TA muscle was excised. Dissected TA muscles were rapidly weighed and frozen in isopentane cooled in liquid nitrogen. All samples were then stored at −80 °C until analyses.

Serial transverse cryo-sections (8-μm thick) of the samples were cut at −20 °C and immediately mounted onto glass slides. Sections were stained to analyze the cross-sectional area (fiber CSA) of muscle fibers by hematoxylin and eosin (H&E), and the profiles of Pax7-positive nuclei by a standard immuno-histochemical technique [23]. Monoclonal anti-Pax7 antibody (Developmental Studies Hybridoma Bank, Iowa, IA, USA) was used for the detection of muscle satellite cells [3]. The sections were fixed in 4% paraformaldehyde, and were then post-fixed in ice-cooled methanol. After blocking by using 1% Roche blocking reagent (Roche Diagnostic, Penzberg, Germany), sections were incubated with the primary antibodies for Pax7 and rabbit polyclonal anti-laminin (Z0097, DakoCytomation, Glostrup, Denmark). Following an incubation period at 4 °C, sections were incubated with secondary antibodies for Cy3-conjugated anti-mouse IgG (Jackson Immuno Research, West Grove, PA, USA) and with fluorescein isothiocyanate-conjugated anti-rabbit IgG (Sigma-Aldrich) at room temperature. Nuclear counterstaining was performed in a solution of 4′,6-diamidino-2-phenylindole dihydrochloride (DAPI, Sigma-Aldrich). The number of Pax7-positive nuclei located within the laminin-positive basal membrane per muscle fiber (approximately 250 fibers) from each muscle was calculated. Using H&E stained sections, mean fiber CSA was measured from approximately 250 fibers of each muscle using the National Institutes of Health Image J 1.38X (NIH, Bethesda, MD, USA) software for Windows.

2.2. *Cell Culture Experiments*

Mouse myoblast-derived C2C12 cells (6×10^4 cells/well) were cultured on 6-well culture plates, coated with type I collagen (Biocoat, Corning, NY, USA). Cells were maintained in 2 mL of growth medium that consisted of Dulbecco's modified Eagle's medium (DMEM, Thermo Fisher Scientific, Yokohama, Japan) supplemented with 10% heat-inactivated fetal bovine serum containing high glucose (4.5 g/L glucose, 4.0 mM L-glutamine, without sodium pyruvate) for proliferation. During the third day of the proliferation phase (at ~80% confluence), the culture medium was then changed to the same amount of differentiation medium, which consisted of DMEM supplemented with 2% heat-inactivated horse serum containing low glucose (1.0 g/L glucose, 4.0 mM L-glutamine, and 110 mg/L sodium pyruvate) for differentiation, as was described previously [19]. Every 2 days, cells were replenished with fresh differentiation medium and cultures were maintained for 5 days. All cells were maintained at 37 °C, under a humidified atmosphere with 5% CO_2 and 95% air.

Sodium lactate was administered into the conditioned medium throughout the differentiation phase. The concentration of lactate was set at 20 mM in the conditioned culture medium, which took into account previous studies using skeletal muscle cells [19,25]. Ultrapure water alone was added to the conditioning medium for the control group ($n = 6$ well in each group).

The images of myotubes at the 5th day of the differentiation phase were visualized at x40 magnification using a calibrated color imaging camera (DP12, Olympus, Tokyo, Japan) set up to a phase contrast light microscope (CK40, Olympus). In order to measure the myotube diameter, we used a modified method of a previous study [26]. We first randomly selected fields of view from 6 wells of each condition. Using Image J, the diameters of at least 100 myotubes in each well were measured at three randomly selected portions taken along the length of the myotube. Then, the average diameter of a myotube was calculated as the mean of three measurements. The myotubes were also used for the evaluation of myotube length and the myo-nuclei number as described below. Cells were fixed with 4% paraformaldehyde. After blocking, cells were incubated with the primary antibodies for skeletal myosin (M4276, Sigma-Aldrich). Cells were then incubated with the secondary antibodies for Cy3-conjugated anti-mouse IgG. Then nuclei were counterstained with DAPI. Since a muscle cell containing 3 or more nuclei was considered to be a myotube [27], the myotube length and myonuclei number in differentiated myotubes (>2 myonuclei) were measured using Image J.

In addition, the myotubes at the 5th day of differentiation were used to analyze muscular protein content as described below. In order to extract protein from C2C12 cells, the cells were lysed in a cell lysis reagent (CelLytic^{TM}-M, Sigma-Aldrich), in accordance with the previously reported method [19]. The cells in each well were rinsed twice in 1 mL of ice-cooled phosphate-buffered saline. The cells of each well were then scraped into 0.3 mL of cell lysis reagent on ice. The cell lysate was sonicated and centrifuged at 20,000 g at 4 °C for 10 min. The supernatant was collected for the analysis of protein content. Protein content in the supernatant was determined using the Bradford technique (protein Assay kit, Bio-Rad, Hercules, CA, USA) and bovine serum albumin (Sigma-Aldrich) as the standard.

2.3. Animal Experiments

All values were expressed as means ± SEM. In animal experiments, the statistically significant level of blood lactate concentration was analyzed using one-way analysis of variance (ANOVA) followed by the Tukey-Kramer test. Other significant levels were tested using a two-way (lactate administration and time) ANOVA for multiple comparisons followed by the Tukey-Kramer test. When a significant interaction between main factors was observed, one-way ANOVA followed by the Tukey-Kramer test was performed. Statistically significant levels in cell experiments were evaluated using unpaired Student's t-test following F-test. The significance level was accepted at $p < 0.05$.

3. Results

3.1. Effect of Lactate on Skeletal Muscle Hypertrophy

The body weight, TA muscle weight, and fiber CSA in response to oral lactate administration were shown in Figure 1. There was no significant difference in body weight between groups. A significant increase in the absolute TA muscle weight and the muscle weight relative to body weight was observed in the lactate-administered L group (Figure 1A, $p < 0.05$). Similarly, the fiber CSA in the L group was significantly larger than that in the C group (Figure 1B, $p < 0.05$).

There was no significant change in the population number of Pax7-positive nuclei a fiber of TA muscle in the C group during the experimental period. In the L group, the population of Pax7-positive nuclei was significantly increased (200% and 138% at 1 and 2 weeks after lactate administration, respectively), compared with that in the C group (Figure 1C, $p < 0.05$).

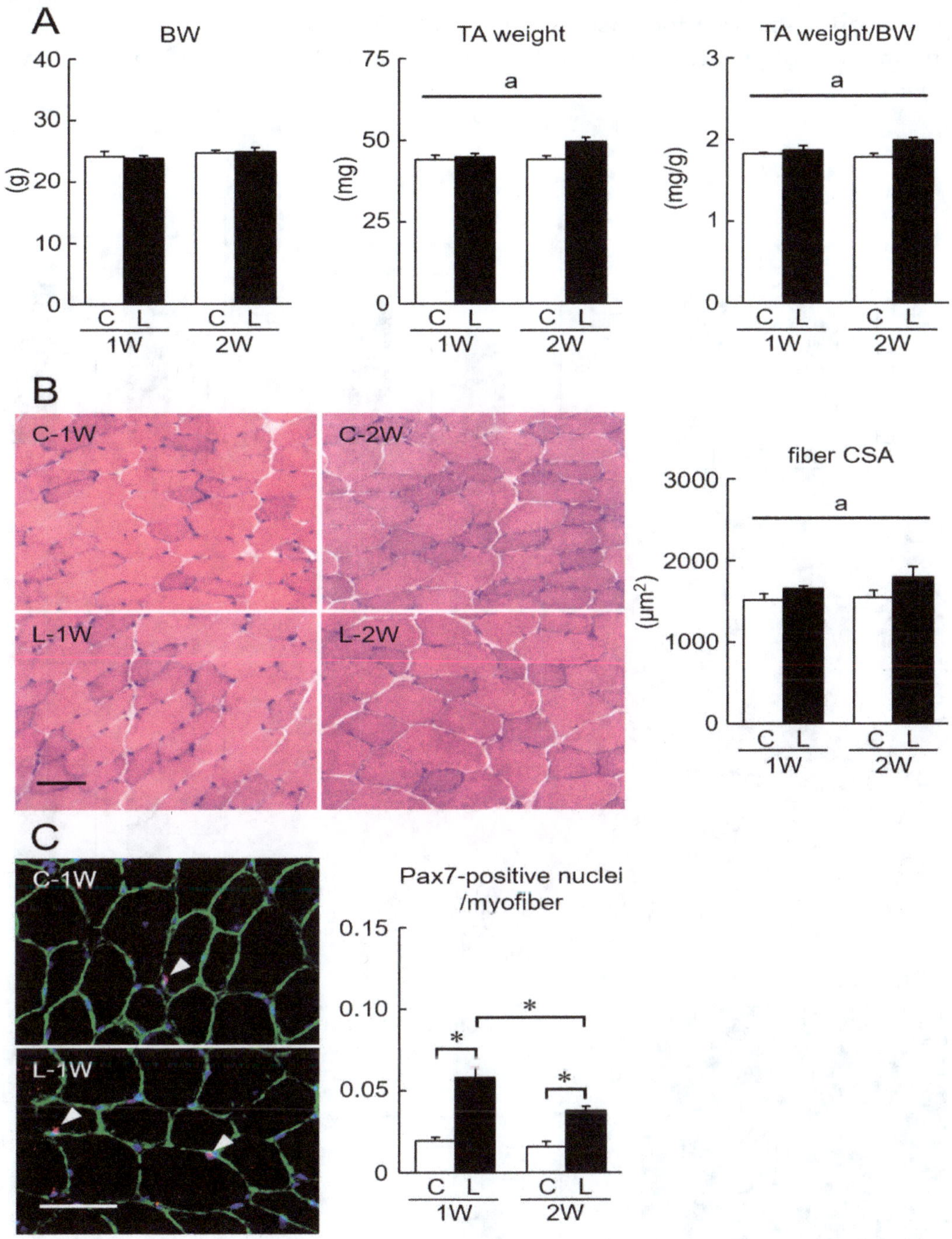

Figure 1. (**A**) Effects of oral lactate administration on body weight (BW) and tibialis anterior (TA) weight in mice. Effect of oral lactate administration on the TA muscle fiber cross-sectional area (CSA) (**B**) and the number of Pax7-positive nuclei per muscle fiber (**C**). Representative images of histochemical and immuno-histochemical staining in TA muscle are shown. Arrowheads indicate the Pax7-positive nuclei. Scale bar = 50 μm. TA weight/BW: relative TA weight to BW. C: control group. L: lactate-administered group. 1W and 2W: 1 and 2 weeks of lactate administration, respectively. Values are means ± SEM. $n = 6$ per group. a: Significant main effect of lactate, $p < 0.05$. *: $p < 0.05$.

3.2. Effect of Lactate on Skeletal Muscle Regeneration

Many regenerating fibers with centrally located nuclei in CTX-injected TA muscle were observed 1 and 2 weeks after the injection (Figure 2B). There was no significant change in body weight of not only CX but also LX groups during the experimental period (Figure 2A). Both TA muscle weight (24% and 29% of absolute and relative levels, respectively) and fiber CSA (44%) 2 weeks after CTX injection increased, compared with those 1 week after the injection. Two weeks after CTX injection, lactate administration-associated increase in the absolute TA muscle weight was observed ($p < 0.05$). A significant main effect of lactate administration was observed in the relative muscle weight as well as fiber CSA ($p < 0.05$).

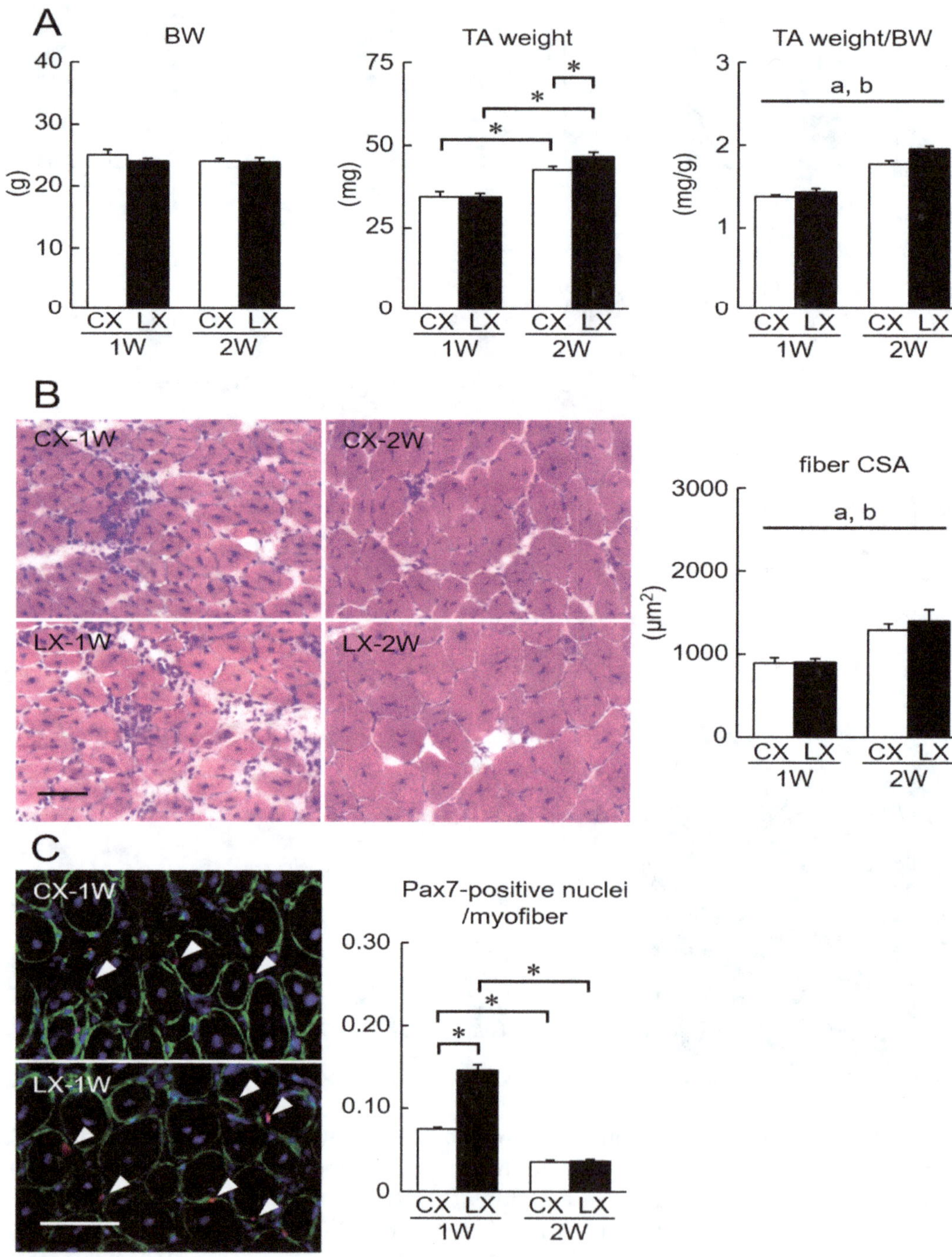

Figure 2. (**A**) Effects of oral lactate administration on BW and TA weight in cardio-toxin (CTX)-injected mice. Effect of oral lactate administration on CTX-injected TA muscle fiber CSA (**B**) and the number of Pax7-positive nuclei per muscle fiber (**C**). Representative images of histochemical and immuno-histochemical staining in CTX-injected TA muscle are shown. Arrowheads indicate the Pax7-positive nuclei. Scale bar = 50 μm. CX: CTX-injected group. LX: lactate-administered after the CTX-injection group. 1W and 2W: 1 and 2 weeks after CTX injection, respectively. See Figure 1 for other abbreviations. Values are means ± SEM. $n = 7$ per group. a and b: Significant main effect of lactate and time, respectively. $p < 0.05$. *: $p < 0.05$.

One week after CTX injection, the population of Pax7-positive nuclei was increased (0.08/myofiber), compared with that in the C group (0.02/myofiber). Furthermore, the additional increase in the population of Pax7-positive nuclei was observed in the lactate-administered LX group, when compared with the CX group, 1 week after CTX injection ($p < 0.05$).

3.3. *Effects of Lactate on Myotube Formation*

We examined the effects of lactate on myotube formation of C2C12 cells. The typical images of myotubes, on the 5th day of differentiation, with or without lactate in the medium were shown in Figure 3. In the lactate-administered cells, myotubes have a wider diameter, longer length, and more myonuclei compared with the control. A significant increase in the myotube diameter and muscular protein content was induced by lactate (Figure 3A,B, $p < 0.05$). Lactate administration also increased myotube length as well as myo-nuclei number (Figure 3C, $p < 0.05$).

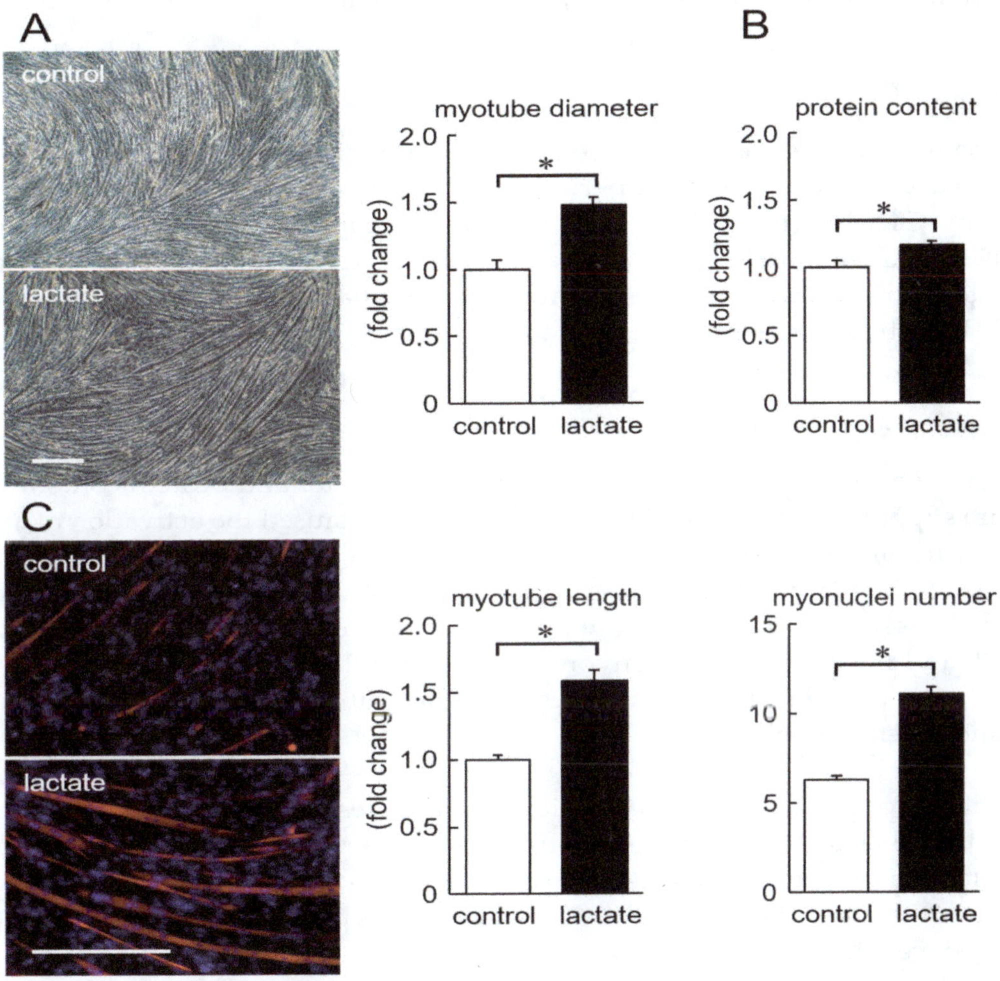

Figure 3. Myo-tube diameter (**A**), muscular protein content (**B**), myo-tube length, and myonuclei number (**C**) of C2C12 cells in response to lactate. Scale bar = 300 μm. Values are means ± SEM. $n = 6$ wells per group. *: $p < 0.05$.

4. Discussion

The present study demonstrated that oral lactate administration induced muscle hypertrophy accompanied with an increase of Pax7-positive nuclei in mouse TA muscle. In injured TA muscle, the increase of muscle mass and Pax7-positive nuclei population was stimulated by lactate administration. Furthermore, lactate-induced myotube formation including higher protein content, wider diameter, longer length, and more myo-nuclei were observed in C2C12 cells.

4.1. Muscle Hypertrophy

In the present study, oral lactate administration increased TA muscle weight and fiber CSA in mice. This is the first report showing the effect of lactate on skeletal muscle mass in animals. Furthermore, the population of Pax7-positive nuclei in TA muscle was increased by lactate administration. Since the previous study using C2C12 skeletal muscle cells reported that extracellular lactate increased follistatin and decreased myostatin expressions involved in the proliferation of satellite cells [17,18], oral lactate administration-associated increase of blood lactate concentration may enhance the proliferation of muscle satellite cells. Recently, we demonstrated an extracellular lactate-associated increase in the diameter of C2C12 myo-tubes [19]. These observations suggest that lactate administration, which could increase blood lactate levels, stimulated the hypertrophy of skeletal muscle with the activation of muscle satellite cells. Training with a blood flow restriction, which is exercise with vascular occlusion, is known to increase muscle size [28,29] and the blood lactate level [29,30] in humans. Therefore, there is a possibility that the blood lactate level may contribute to muscle size following occlusion training.

4.2. Muscle Regeneration

In the present study, increase in muscle weight and fiber CSA in CTX-injected TA muscle was observed during a 2-week experimental period. In addition, the population of Pax7-positive nuclei was increased by CTX injection. These phenomena are consistent with the previously reported data in mice [23]. Larger muscle mass and Pax7-positive nuclei population were also observed in lactate-administered mouse, which suggests that lactate stimulates the regenerative potential of injured skeletal muscle by activating muscle satellite cells.

4.3. Myotube Formation

In the present study, lactate increased the myotube diameter and protein content in C2C12 cells. These results are supported by the previous report that lactate caused the activation of anabolic signals for hypertrophy and myogenesis in skeletal muscle cells [18]. Our previous data also showed that extracellular lactate increased the diameter of C2C12 myotubes in a dose-dependent manner [19]. In addition, the present study demonstrated that extracellular lactate caused the extension of the myotube length and the increase of the myonuclei number. Therefore, it was suggested that lactate may stimulate the fusion of myoblasts, which results in myotube formation. This contributes to muscle hypertrophy and regeneration [5–7].

It has been a debatable argument that various metabolites, including lactate, may be involved in exercise-associated skeletal muscle hypertrophy [31]. In the present study, cell culture experiments demonstrated lactate induces an increase in muscle mass even though no myotube contraction is observed. On the other hand, lactate may also stimulate the hypertrophic effects of physical activity on skeletal muscle, since mice moved freely immediately after the administration of lactate in the present study. Additional results are needed to elucidate the difference and interaction between lactate and muscle contraction in skeletal muscle hypertrophy.

5. Conclusions

The present study demonstrated oral lactate administration-associated hypertrophy and regeneration of mouse skeletal muscle. Extracellular lactate might contribute to the regulation of skeletal muscle plasticity.

Author Contributions: Conceptualization, Y.O., T.E., and K.G. Investigation, Y.O., K.A., T.I., Y.S., Y.M., A.O., H.K., and S.Y. Formal analysis, Y.O., K.A., T.I., Y.S., Y.M., A.O., and H.K. Writing—original draft preparation, Y.O., T.E., and K.G. Funding acquisition, Y.O and K.G.

References

1. Mauro, A. Satellite cell of skeletal muscle fibers. *J. Biophys. Biochem. Cytol.* **1961**, *9*, 493–495. [CrossRef] [PubMed]
2. Bazgir, B.; Fathi, R.; Rezazadeh Valojerdi, M.; Mozdziak, P.; Asgari, A. Satellite cells contribution to exercise mediated muscle hypertrophy and repair. *Cell J.* **2017**, *18*, 473–484. [PubMed]
3. Seale, P.; Sabourin, L.A.; Girgis-Gabardo, A.; Mansouri, A.; Gruss, P.; Rudnicki, M.A. Pax7 is required for the specification of myogenic satellite cells. *Cell* **2000**, *102*, 777–786. [CrossRef]
4. Tidball, J.G. Inflammatory processes in muscle injury and repair. *Am. J. Physiol. Regul. Integr. Comp. Physiol.* **2005**, *288*, R345–R353. [CrossRef] [PubMed]
5. Bischoff, R. Analysis of muscle regeneration using single myofibers in culture. *Med. Sci. Sports Exerc.* **1989**, *21*, S164–S172. [CrossRef] [PubMed]
6. Petrella, J.K.; Kim, J.S.; Mayhew, D.L.; Cross, J.M.; Bamman, M.M. Potent myofiber hypertrophy during resistance training in humans is associated with satellite cell-mediated myonuclear addition: A cluster analysis. *J. Appl. Physiol.* **2008**, *104*, 1736–1742. [CrossRef]
7. Relaix, F.; Zammit, P.S. Satellite cells are essential for skeletal muscle regeneration: The cell on the edge returns centre stage. *Development* **2012**, *139*, 2845–2856. [CrossRef]
8. Bellamy, L.M.; Joanisse, S.; Grubb, A.; Mitchell, C.J.; McKay, B.R.; Phillips, S.M.; Baker, S.; Parise, G. The acute satellite cell response and skeletal muscle hypertrophy following resistance training. *PLoS ONE* **2014**, *9*, e109739. [CrossRef] [PubMed]
9. Jackson, J.R.; Mula, J.; Kirby, T.J.; Fry, C.S.; Lee, J.D.; Ubele, M.F.; Campbell, K.S.; McCarthy, J.J.; Peterson, C.A.; Dupont-Versteegden, E.E. Satellite cell depletion does not inhibit adult skeletal muscle regrowth following unloading-induced atrophy. *Am. J. Physiol. Cell Physiol.* **2012**, *303*, C854–C861. [CrossRef]
10. McCarthy, J.J.; Mula, J.; Miyazaki, M.; Erfani, R.; Garrison, K.; Farooqui, A.B.; Srikuea, R.; Lawson, B.A.; Grimes, B.; Keller, C.; et al. Effective fiber hypertrophy in satellite cell-depleted skeletal muscle. *Development* **2011**, *138*, 3657–3666. [CrossRef] [PubMed]
11. Kojima, A.; Goto, K.; Morioka, S.; Naito, T.; Akema, T.; Fujiya, H.; Sugiura, T.; Ohira, Y.; Beppu, M.; Aoki, H.; et al. Heat stress facilitates the regeneration of injured skeletal muscle in rats. *J. Orthop. Sci.* **2007**, *12*, 74–82. [CrossRef]
12. Matsuba, Y.; Goto, K.; Morioka, S.; Naito, T.; Akema, T.; Hashimoto, N.; Sugiura, T.; Ohira, Y.; Beppu, M.; Yoshioka, T. Gravitational unloading inhibits the regenerative potential of atrophied soleus muscle in mice. *Acta Physiol.* **2009**, *196*, 329–339. [CrossRef] [PubMed]
13. Morioka, S.; Goto, K.; Kojima, A.; Naito, T.; Matsuba, Y.; Akema, T.; Fujiya, H.; Sugiura, T.; Ohira, Y.; Beppu, M.; et al. Functional overloading facilitates the regeneration of injured soleus muscles in mice. *J. Physiol. Sci.* **2008**, *58*, 397–404. [CrossRef] [PubMed]
14. So, B.; Kim, H.J.; Kim, J.; Song, W. Exercise-induced myokines in health and metabolic diseases. *Integr. Med. Res.* **2014**, *3*, 172–179. [CrossRef]
15. Brooks, G.A. Cell-cell and intracellular lactate shuttles. *J. Physiol.* **2009**, *587*, 5591–5600. [CrossRef] [PubMed]
16. Gladden, L.B. Lactate metabolism: A new paradigm for the third millennium. *J. Physiol.* **2004**, *558*, 5–30. [CrossRef]
17. Gilson, H.; Schakman, O.; Kalista, S.; Lause, P.; Tsuchida, K.; Thissen, J.P. Follistatin induces muscle hypertrophy through satellite cell proliferation and inhibition of both myostatin and activing. *Am. J. Physiol. Endocrinol. Metab.* **2009**, *297*, E157–E164. [CrossRef] [PubMed]
18. Oishi, Y.; Tsukamoto, H.; Yokokawa, T.; Hirotsu, K.; Shimazu, M.; Uchida, K.; Tomi, H.; Higashida, K.; Iwanaka, N.; Hashimoto, T. Mixed lactate and caffeine compound increases satellite cell activity and anabolic signals for muscle hypertrophy. *J. Appl. Physiol.* **2015**, *118*, 742–749. [CrossRef] [PubMed]
19. Ohno, Y.; Oyama, A.; Kaneko, H.; Egawa, T.; Yokoyama, S.; Sugiura, T.; Ohira, Y.; Yoshioka, T.; Goto, K. Lactate is a potential hypertrophic stimulus for myotubes via activation of MEK/ERK pathway. *Acta Physiol.* **2018**, *223*, e13042. [CrossRef]
20. Coolican, S.A.; Samuel, D.S.; Ewton, D.Z.; McWade, F.J.; Florini, J.R. The mitogenic and myogenic actions of insulin-like growth factors utilize distinct signaling pathways. *J. Biol. Chem.* **1997**, *272*, 6653–6662. [CrossRef]
21. Li, J.; Johnson, S.E. ERK2 is required for efficient terminal differentiation of skeletal myoblasts. *Biochem. Biophys. Res. Commun.* **2006**, *345*, 1425–1433. [CrossRef]

22. Wu, Z.; Woodring, P.J.; Bhakta, K.S.; Tamura, K.; Wen, F.; Feramisco, J.R.; Karin, M.; Wang, J.Y.; Puri, P.L. p38 and extracellular signal-regulated kinases regulate the myogenic program at multiple steps. *Mol. Cell. Biol.* **2000**, *20*, 3951–3964. [CrossRef]
23. Fujiya, H.; Ogura, Y.; Ohno, Y.; Goto, A.; Nakamura, A.; Ohashi, K.; Uematsu, D.; Aoki, H.; Musha, H.; Goto, K. Microcurrent electrical neuromuscular stimulation facilitates regeneration of injured skeletal muscle in mice. *J. Sports Sci. Med.* **2015**, *14*, 297–303.
24. Morotomi, M.; Sakai, K.; Yazawa, K.; Suegara, N.; Kawai, Y.; Mutai, M. Effect and fate of orally administered lactic acid in rats. *J. Nutr. Sci. Vitaminol.* **1981**, *27*, 117–128. [CrossRef]
25. Hashimoto, T.; Hussien, R.; Oommen, S.; Gohil, K.; Brooks, G.A. Lactate sensitive transcription factor network in L6 cells: Activation of MCT1 and mitochondrial biogenesis. *FASEB J.* **2007**, *21*, 2602–2612. [CrossRef]
26. Williamson, D.L.; Butler, D.C.; Always, S.E. AMPK inhibits myoblast differentiation through a PGC-1alpha-dependent mechanism. *Am. J. Physiol. Endocrinol. Metab.* **2009**, *297*, E304–E314. [CrossRef]
27. Ge, X.; Zhang, Y.; Park, S.; Cong, X.; Gerrard, D.E.; Jiang, H. Stac3 inhibits myoblast differentiation into myotubes. *PLoS ONE* **2014**, *9*, e95926. [CrossRef]
28. Abe, T.; Kearns, C.F.; Sato, Y. Muscle size and strength are increased following walk training with restricted venous blood flow from the leg muscle, Kaatsu-walk training. *J. Appl. Physiol.* **2006**, *100*, 1460–1466. [CrossRef]
29. Takarada, Y.; Takazawa, H.; Sato, Y.; Takebayashi, S.; Tanaka, Y.; Ishii, N. Effects of resistance exercise combined with moderate vascular occlusion on muscular function in humans. *J. Appl. Physiol.* **2000**, *88*, 2097–2106. [CrossRef]
30. Takarada, Y.; Nakamura, Y.; Aruga, S.; Onda, T.; Miyazaki, S.; Ishii, N. Rapid increase in plasma growth hormone after low-intensity resistance exercise with vascular occlusion. *J. Appl. Physiol.* **2000**, *88*, 61–65. [CrossRef]
31. Dankel, S.J.; Mattocks, K.T.; Jessee, M.B.; Buckner, S.L.; Mouser, J.G.; Loenneke, J.P. Do metabolites that are produced during resistance exercise enhance muscle hypertrophy? *Eur. J. Appl. Physiol.* **2017**, *117*, 2125–2135. [CrossRef]

9

Phytomedicine in Joint Disorders

Dorin Dragos [1,2], Marilena Gilca [3], Laura Gaman [3], Adelina Vlad [4], Liviu Iosif [5], Irina Stoian [3,5,*] and Olivera Lupescu [6,7]

1 Medical Semiology Department, Faculty of General Medicine, "Carol Davila" University of Medicine and Pharmacy, B-dul "Eroilor Sanitari" nr. 8, Sector 6, 76241 Bucharest, Romania; dordrag@drdorindragos.ro
2 Nephrology Clinic, University Emergency Hospital Bucharest, 050098 Bucharest, Romania
3 Biochemistry Department, Faculty of General Medicine, "Carol Davila" University of Medicine and Pharmacy, B-dul "Eroilor Sanitari" nr. 8, Sector 6, 76241 Bucharest, Romania; marilenagilca@gmail.com (M.G.); glauraelena@gmail.com (L.G.)
4 Physiology Department, Faculty of General Medicine, "Carol Davila" University of Medicine and Pharmacy, B-dul "Eroilor Sanitari" nr. 8, Sector 6, 76241 Bucharest, Romania; adelina_munteanu@yahoo.com
5 R&D IRIST LABMED SRL, Str. Miraslau, nr. 24, Sector 3, 031235 Bucharest, Romania; iristlabmed@gmail.com
6 Orthopaedic and Trauma Clinic 2, Faculty of General Medicine, "Carol Davila" University of Medicine and Pharmacy, 020022 Bucharest, Romania; olivera_lupescu@yahoo.com
7 Clinical Emergency Hospital Bucharest, 014461 Bucharest, Romania
* Correspondence: irina.stoian@umf.ro or irina_stoian64@yahoo.com

Abstract: Chronic joint inflammatory disorders such as osteoarthritis and rheumatoid arthritis have in common an upsurge of inflammation, and oxidative stress, resulting in progressive histological alterations and disabling symptoms. Currently used conventional medication (ranging from pain-killers to biological agents) is potent, but frequently associated with serious, even life-threatening side effects. Used for millennia in traditional herbalism, medicinal plants are a promising alternative, with lower rate of adverse events and efficiency frequently comparable with that of conventional drugs. Nevertheless, their mechanism of action is in many cases elusive and/or uncertain. Even though many of them have been proven effective in studies done in vitro or on animal models, there is a scarcity of human clinical evidence. The purpose of this review is to summarize the available scientific information on the following joint-friendly medicinal plants, which have been tested in human studies: *Arnica montana, Boswellia* spp., *Curcuma* spp., *Equisetum arvense, Harpagophytum procumbens, Salix* spp., *Sesamum indicum, Symphytum officinalis, Zingiber officinalis, Panax notoginseng*, and *Whitania somnifera*.

Keywords: osteoarthritis; rheumatoid arthritis; medicinal plants; herbs

1. Introduction

Chronic joint inflammatory disorders such as osteoarthritis and rheumatoid arthritis have in common an upsurge of inflammation, and oxidative stress, resulting in progressive histological alterations and disabling symptoms.

Osteoarthritis, one of the most common musculoskeletal disorders, affecting approximately 15% of the population [1], is characterized by irreversible destruction of articular cartilage and bone erosion, induced by pro-inflammatory cytokines, e.g., interleukin 1 (IL-1), interleukin 6 (IL-6), and tumor necrosis factor α (TNF-α). These mediators increased the collagenase or matrix metaloproteinase (MMP) synthesis and the degradation of collagen type II, and decreased the synthesis of collagenase inhibitors, collagen and proteoglycans [2]. Degradation of collagen type II by collagenase-1 and collagenase-3 (also called MMP-13) represents one of the biochemical hallmarks of osteoarthritis [3].

Factors that increase the risk of OA are advanced age, sex, overweight, increased body mass index (BMI), genetics, ethnicity, diet, trauma, certain physical or occupational activities that imply biomechanical stress (e.g., pressure, load-bearing) across the joints [4–6]. Monitoring the OA evolution and therapy involves pain and physical function assessment for shorter studies, as well as joint imaging for longer studies (1 year or more). Pain is evaluated with visual analog scales (VAS), while the functional impairment with Western Ontario and McMaster Universities OA Index (WOMAC) [7]. Other useful assessment tools of functional impairment are Lequesne Functional Severity Index [8] and Karnofski Performance Scale Index [9].

Rheumatoid arthritis (RA) is a chronic progressive systemic autoimmune disease affecting 1% of the population and generating disability and increased risk for cardiovascular disease, lymphoma, and death [10], typically associated with high levels of oxidative stress and inflammatory mediators. RA is currently treated with a wide variety of medicines ranging from steroidal/nonsteroidal anti-inflammatory drugs (NSAID and pain killers), to potent biological agents targeting specific immune and inflammatory pathways, such as TNF-alpha (TNF-α) inhibitors and interleukin-1 receptor antagonists [11]. Among nonsteroidal anti-inflammatory drugs, acetaminophen is most frequently used in very high doses (4000 mg/day). Concerning the pain killers, tramadol is highly recommended, but also other opioids (e.g., morphine) [12]. Etanercept, infliximab and rituximab represent few examples of TNF-α inhibitors used for the treatment of severe RA [13,14]. Anakinra (an IL-1 receptor antagonist) [15] and methotrexat are other therapeutic choices for RA [16].

The biologic therapies have proven to be highly successful and effective in the majority of RA cases, including the severe ones.

Unfortunately, the use of standard drugs in arthropathies is accompanied by numerous and frequently serious side effects [17]: gastrointestinal ulcerations, hemorrhagic events, and nephrotoxicity induced by NSAID [18]; infusion hypersensitivity reactions, and auto-immune responses (e.g., lupus-like syndrome) triggered by TNFα inhibitors [19]; increased risk of severe infection, affecting mainly the respiratory tract, caused by biological drugs (anakinra, rituximab, or abatacept) [20]; fatal cytopenia induced by methotrexate [21]; etc.

Hence the renewed interest in medicines of botanical origin, which lack severe adverse effects and have a millennia-proven efficacy [22]. These remedies may be have a beneficial effect not only on the symptoms but also on the course of the disease [23].

The purpose of this review is to summarize the available scientific information obtained from medical databases and literature on medicinal plants that have been reported to have anti-arthritic activity in vitro, in animal models and also in human clinical studies.

A literature search was performed using the following phrases "medicinal plants or herb and osteoarthritis or arthritis or rheumatoid arthritis", "*specific herb Latin name* or *specific herb English name* and osteoarthritis or arthritis or rheumatoid arthritis" (e.g., *Curcuma longa* or turmeric and osteoarthritis or arthritis or rheumatoid arthritis), in PubMed database. Only medicinal plants studied in human clinical studies were selected, and presented in alphabetical order of their Latin names. For all the plants included in the paper, we have analyzed in vitro studies, animal studies, and human clinical studies using herbal extracts, and potentially active phytochemicals. The corresponding papers were retrieved and evaluated in terms of the relevance for the present paper topic. Supplementary information was also obtained by a manual search in various books, including books of traditional medicine.

Several herbal extracts presented in the present paper (see Table 1) showed benefits in terms of pain and physical mobility, with low risk of side effects in arthritic subjects. These results warranting further investigation.

2. Anti-Arthritic Medicinal Plants

2.1. *Arnica montana, family (fam.) Asteraceae*

Traditional knowledge. This plant has been used for centuries in traditional herbalism as a remedy for trauma-, strain- and/or inflammation-related conditions of the locomotor system [24], and is one of the natural remedies most often used for rheumatologic conditions [25].

Animal studies. An orally administered *Arnica* extract was shown (on the collagen induced arthritis rat model) to alleviate both the histological and radiological changes in the affected joints, in parallel with a decrease in NO, TNF-α, IL-1β, IL-6, and IL-12 concentrations, anti-type II collagen antibodies level, and an improvement of the oxidative status (higher antioxidant levels and milder peroxidative injury) [24].

Human clinical studies. In an open multicenter trial, a gel prepared form *Arnica montana* fresh plant was tested in knee OA and proven to alleviate symptoms, improve functionality, and to be well tolerated. Rare adverse events were reported. Allergy might be a concern, as is fitting for a true Asteraceae herb [26]. A double-blind study on 204 patients comparing *Arnica montana* with ibuprofen in topical applications for hand OA found no difference in terms of efficiency and side effects (less frequent for *Arnica*) [27], a result corroborated by another study [28]. The equipotency of *Arnica* with NSAID in the local treatment of hand OA was acknowledged also by a Cochrane review [29].

Active phytochemicals. The anti-arthritic efficiency is attributed by some authors to a synergism of phenolic and flavonoid compounds, the dominant active principles, detected in a methanol extract, which was found efficient on a collagen-induced arthritis (CIA) rat model [24].

2.2. *Boswellia spp., fam. Burseraceae*

Traditional knowledge. Used for centuries in Ayurveda medicine (where it is called sallaki) *Boswellia serrata* (BS) yields a gum resin, known as frankincense, efficacious in the treatment of inflammatory disorders [30], particularly arthritis. Nowadays, many anti-arthritic combinations contain BS.

In vitro studies. A BS preparation enriched in active principles was able to hinder cartilage breakdown by metalloproteinase-3 (MMP-3) and to block Intercellular Adhesion Molecule 1 (ICAM-1) and thereby the inflammatory reaction [31]. In another study, a *B. frereana* preparation decreased the synthesis/ activation of several inflammation-related mediators and enzymes (MMP-9 and MMP-13, cycloxygenase-2, nitric oxide, prostaglandin E2), thus thwarting collagen and cartilage dissolution [32].

A poly-herbal formulation containing *Zingiber officinale* root, *Tinospora cordifolia* stem, *Phyllanthus emblica* fruit and oleoresin of BS has been shown to halt cartilage degradation in the knee (decreased release of glycosaminoglycans and aggrecan) associated with anti-inflammatory activity (as assessed by lower levels of nitric oxide) [33].

Another combination including three herbs (*Uncaria tomentosa*, *Boswellia* spp., and *Lepidium meyenii*) and an amino acid (L-leucine) has been shown to hamper inflammation and protect the articular cartilage. Tested on OA chondrocytes, it blocked the IL-1β-triggered activation of NF-κB and consequently abrogated the activity of inflammation-related enzymes (iNOS, MMP-9 and MMP-13), leading to a decreased rate of NO production and of cartilage matrix deterioration (less glycosaminoglycans-GAGs-released); simultaneously, enhanced production of structural proteins (including aggrecan and type II collagen) was detected [23].

Animal studies. Using the rat model of collagen induced arthritis, an extract of BS was able to suppress pro-inflammatory mediators and to improve the antioxidant status, as reflected by lactoperoxidase, myeloperoxidase, catalase, superoxide dismutase (SOD), glutathione (GSH), nitric oxide (NO) [22]. A mixture of *Withania somnifera*, BS, *Zingiber officinale* and *Curcuma longa* was tested on a rat model of adjuvant induced arthritis and proven to relieve inflammation and arthritis, and also to diminish the production of TNF-α and NO [34].

Human clinical studies. A Cochrane systematic review concluded that preparations from BS "show trends of benefits" (when used for the treatment of OA) coupled with a low burden of side effects, citing two high-quality and two moderate-quality studies demonstrating superiority compared to placebo in reducing pain and increasing functionality, and a moderate-quality study indicating a favorable adverse events profile [35]. Indeed, a couple of double-blind, randomized, placebo-controlled studies done on patients with knee OA demonstrated that phytopreparations from BS gum resin are able to reduce pain and increase functionality after only a few days (a week or so at most) with no serious adverse effects [31,36]. A phytosomal *Boswellia* preparation has been shown to be beneficial in the treatment of knee OA when added to the standard management of this condition (ameliorating the functional status (higher Karnofski Scale Index) and the symptoms (lower WOMAC (Western Ontario and McMaster Universities questionnaire) Score) [37]). It also hasten functional recovery and diminished pain and objective physical and humoral signs of inflammations in persons with arthritis of the hand induced by work-related overstraining [38]. A combination of *Curcuma longa* and BS was proven to be safe and efficient in patients with osteoarthritis, alleviating symptoms and objective signs, even better than celecoxib (a selective COX-2 inhibitor) and being practically devoid of side effects [39]. However other studies failed to confirm the efficiency of BS in the treatment of active RA [40].

Active phytochemicals. The role of bioactive principles is revendicated by the boswellic acids [41,42], a family of pentacyclic triterpenes, among which the main contenders were, initially, 11-keto-β-boswellic acid and acetyl-11-keto-β-boswellic acid. Oral or local administration of boswellic acids in a bovine serum albumin-induced arthritis model ameliorated the electrophoretic pattern of the synovial fluid proteins and decreased the infiltration of leucocytes into the knee joint [43]. These compounds were considered until recently to inhibit leukotriene synthesis by suppressing lipoxygenase-5 (LOX-5) in vitro and in animal models [30,44]. Other mechanisms were also invoked such as suppression of NF-κB activation, reduction of the production of pro-inflammatory cytokines (TNF-α, IL-1, IL-2, IL-4, IL-6 and IFN-γ), and reduced cleavage of C3 into the active components C3a and C3b, hampering the activation of the classic path of the complement [45]. These were showed in various in vivo experiments, with various arthritic or non-arthritic inflammation models (e.g., hypersensitivity reaction in mice) [46]. More recently, concerns were raised regarding both the action intensity of 11-keto-β-boswellic acid and acetyl-11-keto-β-boswellic acid, and their bioavailability, the latter being too poor to provide concentrations high enough for bioactivity [47]. Nonetheless, another member of the family was proposed as active principle, namely β-boswellic acid, able to reach much higher levels in plasma, enough to efficiently exert its inhibitory action on microsomal prostaglandin E synthase-1 and on the serine protease cathepsin G, which might be the substrate of the inflammation-suppressing aptitude of BS preparations [17].

2.3. *Curcuma spp., fam. Zingiberaceae*

Traditional knowledge. Several members of the *Curcuma* genus are used in traditional medicine, most important being *Curcuma longa* (CL), turmeric. Its rhizome has a centuries-long use as a dietary spice as well as an Ayurveda herb prized for its anti-inflammatory properties, hence its utility in arthritic conditions including RA [48].

Animal studies. In an animal arthritis model a preparation from CL lacking essential oil strongly suppressed joint inflammation and periarticular damage in correlation with decreased activation of NF-κB and of the ensuing cascade of events (involving mediators of inflammation and injury such as chemokines, cyclooxygenase 2, and receptor activator of nuclear factor kappa-B ligand (RANKL)) [49]. The ability to prevent the destructive changes in joints and periarticular bone seems to be comparable to that of betamethasone [50,51]. Liposomal encapsulation may help overcome the poor bioavailability problem generated by the low water-solubility [52]. The osteoclast-osteoblast balance is tipped in favor of bone building, while halting the OA progression [52]. In a rat-model of experimentally induced arthritis, a combination of ginger and turmeric rhizomes was superior to indomethacin (a potent NSAID) regarding the ability to alleviate both joint histopathological changes, and the extra-articular manifestations, including systemic inflammation (leukocytosis, thrombocytosis, and hyperglobulinemia), malnutrition (decreased body weight gain, and hypoalbuminemia), and iron deficiency anemia, with no prejudice to kidney function and reduced risk of cardiovascular disease (favorable lipid and oxidative profile) [53].

Human clinical studies. A mixture of *Curcuma longa* and *Boswellia serrata* has been shown to be more efficient than a standard dose of celecoxib (a selective COX-2 inhibitor) in the treatment of osteoarthritis, improving both objectively and subjectively the condition of the patients, with no toxicity detectable by clinical examination and laboratory tests (hemogram, liver and renal function tests) [39]. *Curcuma domestica* extracts have been shown to be useful in knee osteoarthritis, reducing the pain and preserving functionality with an efficiency equivalent to ibuprofen, but with fewer gastrointestinal side effects [54]. A recent meta-analysis found relevant scientific evidence for the efficacy of turmeric as a therapeutic option in arthritis, but concluded that more studies are necessary in order to definitively pin it down [55].

Active phytochemicals. The active ingredient is diferuloylmethane, a yellow phenolic pigment commonly known as curcumin, which has a multifaceted beneficial action in various fields of pathology (diabetes, cancer, inflammation, oxidative stress) due to its ability to favorably influence a variety of signaling pathways and mediators [56]. In a rat model of arthritis, it has been shown to ameliorate the joint inflammation (evaluated by the neutrophil infiltrate density), in the first six hours after the arthritis-inducing event (zymosan infiltration) being even more effective than a low dose of prednisone [57].

The reduction of the systemic oxidative stress as reflected by enhanced serum SOD activity, increased GSH level, and decreased malondialdehyde level was considered part of the mechanism of action [58]. The blockage of glial activation resulting in decreased synthesis and secretion of inflammatory mediators in the spinal cord, corroborated by similar results in studies on cultures of astrocytes and microglia can be responsible for arthritic pain reduction [59].

β-Elemene, found in *Curcuma Wenyujin*, an herb used in Traditional Chinese Medicine for the treatment of rheumatoid arthritis, may be another phytochemical active in arthropathies. This compound antiproliferative activity (useful in neoplastic diseases) may explain the suppressive effect on accumulation of fibroblast-like synoviocytes. One in vitro study showed that the underlying mechanism may be represented by the apoptosis induction via increased production of reactive oxygen species and activation of p38 mitogen-activated protein kinase (MAPK) [60].

2.4. *Equisetum arvense, fam. Equisetaceae*

Traditional knowledge. Equisetum arvense, also known as horsetail, has a long history of use in European ethnomedicine as an anti-inflammatory remedy [61].

Animal studies. An animal model of arthritis induced through an antigen challenge was used to prove the downregulating effects of *Equisetum giganteum* on lymphocyte proliferation. B and T lymphocytes are both affected by the immunomodulatory action of this plant, which is nevertheless free of cytotoxicity [62].

Human clinical studies. The beneficial effect of horsetail in RA was substantiated by a study that pointed out the decrease in TNF-α as one of the contributing mechanisms [63].

Active phytochemicals. Kynurenic acid was proposed as a putative mediator of the anti-inflammatory and antalgic effect of several herbs beneficial in RA, horsetail among them [64]. The anti-inflammatory potential of kynurenic acid was showed until now only in non-arthritic animal models (e.g., acute experimental colitis in rat) [65]. Kynurenic acid is also an endogenous oxidative metabolite of tryptophan, with glutamate-receptor antagonist activity, which may explain partially its analgesic properties. One in vitro study showed that kynurenic acid is able to inhibit the proliferation of synoviocytes [66]. Its level was significantly lower in human subjects with RA than that in those with OA [67], fact which suggests the beneficial potential of kynurenic acid supplementation in RA patients.

2.5. *Harpagophytum procumbens, fam. Pedaliaceae*

Traditional knowledge. Harpagophytum procumbens (HP), also known as devil's claw, a medicinal plant native to Africa, is a "celebrity" among anti-osteoarthritis natural remedies, being approved by German Commission E for the treatment of degenerative diseases of the musculoskeletal system [68].

In vitro studies. HP extracts showed chondroprotective activity, several mechanisms being potentially responsible for this: decreased synthesis of inflammatory mediators (e.g., TNF-α, and interleukin-1β), and inhibition of matrix metalloproteinases and elastase [69].

Animal studies. A dried aqueous extract of HP has been shown to have a significant dose-dependent analgesic and anti-inflammatory activity in rats at 5 and 10 mg/kg. Nevertheless, carrageenan-induced paw edema was not affected by the isolated harpagoside constituent. This signifies that harpagoside may not have an anti-inflammatory effect, at least in the dosage used in this study [70,71]. This suggests that other HP constituents may be responsible for the anti-inflammatory effect.

Human clinical studies. Several human clinical studies showed that various HP tuber extracts (equivalent to 50–60 mg harpagoside daily, administered for a variable period between 8 and 16 weeks, depending on the study) significantly improved the clinical picture of subjects with knee and hip osteoarthritis in terms of pain, movement limitation, and joint crepitus [72–74]. The severity of pain and other symptoms was assessed by the WOMAC questionnaire, VAS, Lequesne Index, physician exam and/or pain-relieving medication dose.

Active phytochemicals. The major phytochemicals responsible for the anti-osteoarthritis effect are the iridoid glycosides (harpagoside, harpagide, and procumbide), which are found in a higher amount in tubers and root. Although, it is worthy to mention that the whole-plant extracts seem to have a better therapeutic effect than those obtained from isolated parts [75]. Harpagoside inhibited in vitro the synthesis of various pro-inflammatory mediators via suppression of iNOS and COX-2 expression through inhibition of NF-κB activation [76], but showed no anti-inflammatory activity in one animal model of inflammation (carrageenan-induced paw edema) [70]. The scientists suggested that other phytochemicals than harpagoside may be contributors to the anti-inflammatory effect of HP [70,77].

2.6. *Panax notoginseng, fam. Araliaceae*

Traditional knowledge. Panax notoginseng (PN), known as sanqi in Chinese, has a long history of clinical use for the treatment of traumatic injuries, swellings and pains [78].

In vitro studies. An n-butanol extract of PN inhibited the synthesis of pro-inflammatory mediators (TNF-alpha, IL-1, inducible NOS, and MMP-13) in vitro [79].

Animal studies. PN in combination with other two herbs (*Rehmannia glutinosa* and *Eleutherococcus senticosus*), had a suppressive effect on collagen-induced arthritis in mice, through inhibition of TNF-alpha, IL-1, iNOS, and MMP-13 synthesis [80].

Human clinical studies. The same combination of PN with *Rehmannia glutinosa* and *Eleutherococcus senticosus*, administered as capsules, 4 capsules of 400 mg daily for six weeks (containing ginsenoside Rb1, 19.49 $\pm$ 3.89 mg/g, stachyose 0.87 $\pm$ 0.17 mg/g and eleutheroside E 0.07 $\pm$ 0.014 mg/g) improved the physical function and pain according to the Korean version of WOMAC questionnaire in 57 patients with knee OA, and was considered effective for symptomatic relief [2].

Active phytochemicals. Saponins are considered the main osteo-active phytochemicals from PN. PN saponins promoted the autograft tendon healing in bone tunnel [81], and amplified the effect of routine therapy (diclofenac sodium, Leflunomide and prednisone) in terms of joint swelling, tenderness, and pain index, as well as time of morning stiffness, VAS and immunological parameters, in patients with RA [82].

2.7. *Salix spp., fam. Salicaceae*

Traditional knowledge. Various species from the genus *Salix*, or willow, were already in common use for pain relief in antiquity [83,84], being first mentioned in the Ebers papyrus (about 1550 BC) [85], and afterwards by all the great masters of medicine in antiquity, middle ages, and modern times [86].

In vitro studies. The inflammation-suppressing effect of willow bark extract (WBE) relies, at least partially, on its ability to antagonize the activated monocytes, by blocking the activity of pro-inflammatory cytokines (TNFα), enzymes (COX-2), and mediators (NF-κB) [87].

Animal studies. The mechanism of the anti-inflammatory action of WBE was examined on two animal models of arthritis, an acute and a chronic one. WBE decreased the inflammatory infiltrate and exudate and blocked the cytokine surge with a potency at least equivalent to that of acetylsalicylic acid (ASA), was better than ASA in reducing leukotrienes levels and in inhibiting COX-2, and as good as ASA in decreasing prostaglandins levels. WBE influenced favorably the oxidative stress increasing GSH and decreasing malondialdehyde levels more efficiently than ASA or celecoxib (a selective COX-2 inhibitor). Despite being more potent than ASA, on a molar basis, the salicin amount in WBE is much less than the salicylate content of ASA, suggesting that active principles other than salicin might play a role in the anti-inflammatory and antioxidative action of WBE, the polyphenols being among the candidates, at least regarding the protection against free radicals [88]. The ability to mitigate pro-inflammatory cytokines and oxidative stress was corroborated by still another study on the collagen induced arthritis animal model [89].

Human clinical studies. The first clinical trial of aspirin, albeit uncontrolled and non-randomized, was conducted in the 18th century by the English Reverend Edward Stone—the good fellow, struck by the quinine-like bitterness of aspirin, surmised an antifebrile activity and, indeed, was able to cure fever in 50 patients [86]. A two-week, double-blind, randomized, placebo-controlled trial demonstrated the ability of willow bark extract (in a dose equivalent to 240 mg salicin/day) to control the symptoms of patients with OA, especially to reduce pain, although with rather subdued efficiency [90]. The same dose of willow bark extract was used in two other six-week, randomized, controlled, double-blind trials in patients with OA and RA, respectively, the herbal preparation being compared with a potent NSAID (diclofenac) and with placebo. The two trials yielded sobering results, as in neither was willow bark extract significantly better than placebo in pain relief [91]. In a six-week, open, multicentric observational study with reference treatment, WBE was evaluated as better as conventional therapy by physicians and patients alike, in terms of both therapeutic efficiency and side effects, when used for hip and knee degenerative disease [92].

A systematic review concluded that there is moderate evidence for the efficiency of WBE in low back pain, but insufficient data for OA and RA, suggesting that higher doses should be tested [84].

In a longer (six months) observational study on 436 patients with OA and back pain, WBE significantly decreased pain and was well tolerated [93].

Active phytochemicals. Although traditionally salicin was considered as the active principle, there are opinions that this substance cannot explain the whole range of effects of WBE, and that other phytochemicals might be involved, such as polyphenols and flavonoids, which showed inhibitory activity on COX-2 and decreased synthesis of pro-inflammatory mediators in vitro, in human monocytes and differentiated macrophages [87,88,94–96].

2.8. Sesamum indicum, fam. Pedaliaceae

Traditional knowledge. Sesame oil (SO) extracted from *Sesamum indicum* (SI) has been used in various Asian traditional medicines to alleviate pain in inflammatory conditions of the joints, teeth, skin, etc. [97].

Animal studies. SO was tested in a rat model of adjuvant (Freund's adjuvant)-induced arthritis and was able to dampen the biochemical consequences of oxidative stress: lower plasmatic levels of thiobarbituric acid reactive substances and reduced gamma-glutamyltransferase activity in the joints and spleen [98]. In a rat model of acute gout-like arthritis, SO strongly hindered the inflammatory reaction, thinning the inflammatory infiltrate, lowering the levels of inflammatory mediators (TNF-α, IL-1β, IL-6), impeding the activity of nuclear factor-κB (NF-κB) (at least in the mast cells) and complement system activation [97]. In another rat model of OA, SO alleviated joint pain by inhibiting oxidative aggression (decline in the peroxidation of lipids and in the production of superoxide anion and peroxynitrite, and a surge in glutathione and glutathione peroxidase levels) in the muscles associated with nuclear factor erythroid-2-related factor [1]. SO is active in experimentally induced arthritis through its minor constituents (devoid of these minor constituents it is inactive), decreasing not only the clinically visible joint inflammation, but also its serum markers (oxidative stress related molecules, RA markers, inflammatory eicosanoids and cytokines) and the activity of hydrolytic enzymes; additionally, bone loss was also diminished [99].

Human clinical studies. In a study on patients with knee OA, oral administration of sesame together with standard therapy produced better outcomes in terms of objective and subjective manifestations compared to standard therapy alone [100]. In a placebo controlled trial on patients with knee OA, sesame seed administration was associated with a statistically significant drop in serum levels of malondialdehyde and of high-sensitivity C-reactive protein (hs-CRP) after two months of treatment. and significantly lowered levels of IL-6 after treatment [101].

Active phytochemicals. The ability of SI to protect from the dire consequences of inflammation and oxidative stress (aging, cancer, cardiovascular disease, to name only a few) seems to be due to the lignans. It contains sesamin and its hydroxylated counterpart, sesamolin. Similar biological activity has a phenolic compound, sesamol (3,4-methylene-dioxy-phenol) which results from the degradation of sesamolin [102]. Sesamol has been proven to mitigate joint inflammation, cartilage degradation, and periarticular bone resorbtion in adjuvant-induced arthritis animal model. This action was paralleled by a drop in the level of pro-inflammatory cytokines and in the activity of tissue-destructive enzymes [103]. In addition, a restoration of the oxidant homeostasis reflected in decreased oxidative stress markers and a boost in the activity of protective enzymes were noticed [103]. The hydroperoxides-scavenging capacity of sesamol makes it able to arrest the oxidation state of iron and consequently the conversion of inactive LOX (Fe^{2+}) to active LOX (Fe^{3+}), which leads to the inhibition of this inflammation-promoting enzyme [102].

In a study done on porcine cartilage explant exposed to the pro-inflammatory action of TNF-α and oncostatin M (as an animal RA model), sesamin has been proven to preclude the cytokine-induced cartilage degeneration by slowing down the degradation of constitutive glycosaminoglycans and collagen [104].

2.9. Symphytum officinalis, fam. Boraginaceae

Traditional knowledge. Symphytum officinalis, also known as comfrey, is a medicinal plant traditionally used in Europe for the treatment of inflammatory disorders [105,106].

In vitro studies. An extract of comfrey significantly inhibited the respiratory burst of polymorphonuclear leukocytes, suggesting an anti-inflammatory potential [107].

Animal studies. Comfrey extracts showed anti-inflammatory activity, by *inhibiting carrageenan-induced* rat paw oedema [108,109].

Human clinical studies. A study on people aged 50–80 with OA of the knee proved that topically applied comfrey preparation decreased pain, although was unable to decrease the burden of inflammatory molecules or the rate of cartilage breakdown, the only noticeable adverse effect being local rash [110].

Similar results yielded another study on a similar population of years-long sufferers from OA of the knee: a comfrey-containing ointment improved the quality of life by decreasing pain and increasing knee-mobility [111].

Active phytochemicals. Phenolic acids (e.g., rosmarinic acid), glycopeptides and amino acids are considered to be, at least in part, responsible for the anti-inflammatory potential of comfrey root extracts, in various vitro models [108,112]. Rosmarinic acid inhibited prostaglandin synthesis, and carrageenan- and gelatine-induced erythrocyte aggregation [113].

2.10. *Zingiber officinalis, fam. Zingiberaceae*

Traditional knowledge. Zingiber officinalis (ZO), also known as ginger, is a common spice used in Asian cuisine, and a traditional remedy for joint diseases in ethnomedicine [48].

In vitro studies. ZO is thought to have anti-inflammatory effects, possibly by inhibiting COX-1, COX-2 and LOX [114–116]. Nevertheless, the squeezed ginger extract paradoxically increased the synthesis of pro-inflammatory cytokines (TNF-α, IL-6, and monocyte chemotactic protein-1) in RAW 264 cell culture [117].

Animal studies. The oral administration of the squeezed ginger extract had a dual effect on TNF-α synthesis in mice, in peritoneal cells: ZO extract initially augmented it, but after repeated administrations decreased it [117]. In addition, it augmented the serum corticosterone level, and this may contribute to the anti-inflammatory effect of ZO.

Human clinical studies. A recent study found that ZO powder supplementation (1 g/day) for three months can reduce the serum level of nitric oxide and high-sensitivity reactive protein hs-CRP in patients with knee OA. The inflammatory markers started to decrease after three weeks of treatment [118]. Several other studies showed clinical improvement in OA patients with ZO extract, as evaluated by the pain score with VAS, reduction in intake of rescue medication, having mostly mild gastrointestinal adverse events, and similar or even better efficacy and satisfaction score than the standard treatment prescribed by the orthopedic specialist [119–121].

Another study found that the oral daily administration of one ZO preparation (340 mg EV.EXT 35 *Zingiber officinalis* extract) and glucosamine (1000 mg) for four weeks, in 21 patients with confirmed knee and hip OA, significantly reduced the arthritic pain on standing and moving, according to VAS scale evaluation. Moreover, this treatment had a similar efficacy as diclofenac (100 mg/day) plus glucosamine (1000 mg/day), but a higher safety, due to the decrease of gastrointestinal pain and increase of gastroprotective prostaglandin (PGE1, PGE2, and PGF2α) levels in the stomach mucosa [122]. However, one cross-over study (a wash-out period of one week followed by three treatment periods of three weeks duration each) found no significant difference between placebo and ginger extract in OA patients [123].

Active phytochemicals. Pungent constituents of ZO were thought to contribute to the anti-inflammatory activity of this medicinal plant. For instance, 1-dehydro-[10]-gingerdione inhibited κB kinase β activity required for NF-κB activation and suppressed NF-κB-regulated expression of inflammatory genes in lipopolysaccharide S-activated macrophage [124]. 6-Dehydrogingerdione attenuated iNOS, COX-2, IL-1β, IL-6, and TNF-α gene expression in vitro, in RAW 264.7 macrophages. [114]. Other compounds from ZO (10-gingerol, 8-shogaol and 10-shogaol) showed the capacity to decrease COX-2 activity in vitro [115].

2.11. *Whitania somnifera, fam. Solanaceae*

Withania somnifera (WS), also known as ashwagandha, is a potent anti-osteoarthritic and anti-inflammatory plant used in Ayurveda [125].

In vitro. One study showed that the WS extract inhibited liposaccharyde S induced synthesis of pro-inflammatory cytokines (TNF-alpha, IL-1beta and IL-12) in peripheral and synovial fluid mononuclear cells from rheumatoid arthritis subjects in vitro, but had no effect on IL-6 synthesis [126]. The WS extract also showed inhibitory effects on collagenase activity against the degradation of the bovine Achilles tendon type I collagen, that may be useful in joint disease treatment [127].

Animal studies. WS root powder had protective effect on bone collagen in experimental induced arthritis model in rats [128].

Human clinical studies. A randomized, double blind placebo controlled study showed that the aqueous extract of WS produced significant reduction of scores for pain, stiffness and disability in human subjects with knee joint pain [129].

Active phytochemicals. Withaferin A, belonging to the steroid class of phytochemicals, is thought to be one of contributor compounds to the beneficial effects of WS in OA subjects [126]. Whitaferin A reverted to near normal levels the increase in paw volume, lysosomal enzymes, lipid peroxidation, and TNFα in an monosodium urate crystal-induced arthritis in mice [130]. Withaferin A supressess NF-κB activation by targeting a crucial cysteine 179 in IκB kinase β, and by inhibition of the NF-κB Essential Modulator/ IκB kinase β association complex formation, according to molecular docking and molecular dynamics simulations studies [131,132].

Table 1. Medicinal plants with therapeutic potential in ostheoarthritis and rheumatoid arthritis (Legend: AM, animal model; CAT, catalase; COX, cyclooxygenase; GPx, glutathione peroxidase; GSH, glutathione; GST, glutathione-S-transferase; HS, human study; IL, interleukine; iNOS, inducible nitric oxide synthase; LOX, lipooxygenase; PGE1-S, prostaglandin E2 synthase; ROS, reactive oxygen species; SOD, superoxide dismutase; MAPK, mitogen-activated protein kinase; MCP-1, monocyte chemoattractant protein-1; MIP-1α, monocyte inflammatory protein-1; MMP, matrix metaloproteinase; NO, nitric oxide; TNF, tumoral necrosis factor; (−), decreased synthesis/decreased activation/inhibition of various mediators, enzymes, transcription factors, and processes; (+), increased synthesis/increased activation of various mediators, enzymes, transcription factors, and processes). Note: References in the table correspond only to the mechanism of action.

Plant	Active Phytochemicals	Mechanism of Action	References
Arnica montana	phenols, flavonoids	(−) NO, TNF-α, IL-1β, IL-6, IL-12, anti-type II collagen antibodies, (+) antioxidants (AM)	[24]
Boswelia spp.	boswelic acids	(−) PGE1-S, cathepsin G, LOX-5, MMP-9, MMP-13, COX-2, NO, PGE1, TNF-α, IL-1, IL-2, IL-4, IL-6, IFN-γ (in vitro, AM)	[17,30,31,41]
		(−) leukocyte infiltration in knee (AM)	[43]
Curcuma spp.	curcuminoids	(+) SOD, GSH, (−) MDA (HS)	[58]
		(−) neutrophil infiltrate in knee, (AM), (−) IL-1β, TNFα, MCP-1, and MIP-1α (in vitro, AM)	[57,59]
	β-elemene	(+) p38 MAPK (in vitro)	[60]
Equisetum arvense	kynurenic acid	(−) synoviocyte proliferation (in vitro)	[64,66]
Harpagophytum procumbens	iridoid glycosides	(−) iNOS and COX-2 (in vitro)	[76]
Panax notoginseng	saponins	(−) TNF-alpha, IL-1, iNOS, MMP-13 (AM)	[79,80]
Salix spp.	salicin, polyphenols, flavonoids	(−) TNFα, COX-2, IL-1, IL-6 (in vitro)	[87,95]
Sesamum indicum	sesamin, sesamol, sesamolin	(−) thiobarbituric acid reactive substances, LOX (in vitro), TNF-α, IL-1β, IL-6, hyaluronidase, MMP-13, MMP-3, MMP-9, exoglycosidases, cathepsin D, phosphatases, COX-2, PGE2, ROS, H2O2, MDA (AM), IL-6 (HS)	[1,97,98,101–103]
		(+) GSH, GPx (AM)	
Symphitum officinalis	rosmarinic acids, glycopeptides, amino acids	(−) PG (in vitro)	[108,112,113]
Zingiber officinalis	gingerdione derivatives, 10-gingerol, 8,10-shogaol	(−) COX-1, COX-2, LOX, iNOS, TNF-α, IL-1β, IL-6, MCP-1, κB kinase β (in vitro, AM), NO (HS)	[114,115,117,118,124]
		(+) cortisone (AM)	
Whitania somnifera	whitaferin A	(−)TNF-alpha, IL-1β, IL-12, collagenase (in vitro), NF kB (docking studies)	[126,127,131,132]

3. Concluding Remarks

Several medicinal plant extracts showed trends of clinical and biochemical benefits with low risk of side effects in arthritic patients that warrant further investigation, including imagistic and histological evaluation. The search for effective herbal supplements as a complementary therapy of degenerative arthropathies is a complex issue and implies a long process, in the end of which the conclusions are difficult to be drawn, due to the differences in terms of study design and protocols [133]. The available studies did not evaluate the effect of plant extracts on disease progression, or whether it halts the aggravation of arthropathies. For this purpose, studies of longer duration should be performed.

Almost no studies confirmed in humans the biological mechanisms of herbal extracts found in vitro or in animal studies, the majority of the available ones being focused only on the evaluation of the symptomatic relief induced by the herbal treatment.

Despite their advantages, herbal treatments raise several concerns, such as drug–herbal interactions, low bioavailability, lack of standardization, insufficient regulatory guidelines at national and international levels, and therefore possibility of adulteration [134–137].

More evidence of medicinal plant efficacy, safety and mechanisms of action are needed before herbal treatment can gain a place in therapeutic guidelines of OA and RA.

Author Contributions: Dorin Dragos and Marilena Gilca equally contributed to this work as first authors. All the authors have contributed to all of the following steps: (1) the conception of the study, search of literature, and acquisition of data; (2) analysis and interpretation of data retrieved from the literature; and (3) writing the draft of the manuscript and revision of the article. All authors have read and approved the final manuscript.

References

1. Hsu, D.-Z.; Chu, P.-Y.; Jou, I.-M. Daily sesame oil supplement attenuates joint pain by inhibiting muscular oxidative stress in osteoarthritis rat model. *J. Nutr. Biochem.* **2016**, *29*, 36–40. [CrossRef] [PubMed]
2. Park, S.-H.; Kim, S.-K.; Shin, I.-H.; Kim, H.-G.; Choe, J.-Y. Effects of AIF on Knee Osteoarthritis Patients: Double-blind, Randomized Placebo-controlled Study. *Korean J. Physiol. Pharmacol.* **2009**, *13*, 33–37. [CrossRef] [PubMed]
3. Peat, G.; McCarney, R.; Croft, P. Knee pain and osteoarthritis in older adults: A review of community burden and current use of primary health care. *Ann. Rheum. Dis.* **2001**, *60*, 91–97. [CrossRef] [PubMed]
4. McWilliams, D.F.; Leeb, B.F.; Muthuri, S.G.; Doherty, M.; Zhang, W. Occupational risk factors for osteoarthritis of the knee: A meta-analysis. *Osteoarthr. Cartil.* **2011**, *19*, 829–839. [CrossRef]
5. Smith, R.L.; Carter, D.R.; Schurman, D.J. Pressure and shear differentially alter human articular chondrocyte metabolism: A review. *Clin. Orthop. Relat. Res.* **2004**, *427*, S89–S95.
6. Murphy, N.J.; Eyles, J.P.; Hunter, D.J. Hip Osteoarthritis: Etiopathogenesis and Implications for Management. *Adv. Ther.* **2016**, *33*, 1921–1946. [CrossRef]
7. Dougados, M. Monitoring osteoarthritis progression and therapy. *Osteoarthr. Cartil.* **2004**, *12* (Suppl. A), S55–S60. [CrossRef] [PubMed]
8. Lequesne, M.G.; Mery, C.; Samson, M.; Gerard, P. Indexes of severity for osteoarthritis of the hip and knee. Validation—Value in comparison with other assessment tests. *Scand. J. Rheumatol. Suppl.* **1987**, *65*, 85–89. [CrossRef] [PubMed]
9. Johnson, M.J.; Bland, J.M.; Davidson, P.M.; Newton, P.J.; Oxberry, S.G.; Abernethy, A.P.; Currow, D.C. The relationship between two performance scales: New York Heart Association Classification and Karnofsky Performance Status Scale. *J. Pain Symptom Manag.* **2014**, *47*, 652–658. [CrossRef] [PubMed]
10. Yang, C.L.H.; Or, T.C.T.; Ho, M.H.K.; Lau, A.S.Y. Scientific Basis of Botanical Medicine as Alternative Remedies for Rheumatoid Arthritis. *Clin. Rev. Allergy Immunol.* **2013**, *44*, 284–300. [CrossRef] [PubMed]
11. Smolen, J.S.; Landewe, R.; Breedveld, F.C.; Buch, M.; Burmester, G.; Dougados, M.; Emery, P.; Gaujoux-Viala, C.; Gossec, L.; Nam, J.; et al. EULAR recommendations for the management of rheumatoid arthritis with synthetic and biological disease-modifying antirheumatic drugs: 2013 update. *Ann. Rheum. Dis.* **2014**, *73*, 492–509. [CrossRef] [PubMed]
12. Hochberg, M.C.; Altman, R.D.; April, K.T.; Benkhalti, M.; Guyatt, G.; McGowan, J.; Towheed, T.; Welch, V.; Wells, G.; Tugwell, P. American College of Rheumatology 2012 recommendations for the use of nonpharmacologic and pharmacologic therapies in osteoarthritis of the hand, hip, and knee. *Arthritis Care Res.* **2012**, *64*, 465–474. [CrossRef]

13. Hyrich, K.L.; Watson, K.D.; Silman, A.J.; Symmons, D.P.M. Predictors of response to anti-TNF-alpha therapy among patients with rheumatoid arthritis: Results from the British Society for Rheumatology Biologics Register. *Rheumatology* **2006**, *45*, 1558–1565. [CrossRef] [PubMed]
14. Soliman, M.M.; Hyrich, K.L.; Lunt, M.; Watson, K.D.; Symmons, D.P.M.; Ashcroft, D.M. Effectiveness of rituximab in patients with rheumatoid arthritis: Observational study from the British Society for Rheumatology Biologics Register. *J. Rheumatol.* **2012**, *39*, 240–246. [CrossRef] [PubMed]
15. Cavalli, G.; Dinarello, C.A. Treating rheumatological diseases and co-morbidities with interleukin-1 blocking therapies. *Rheumatology* **2015**, *54*, 2134–2144. [CrossRef] [PubMed]
16. Nishina, N.; Kaneko, Y.; Kameda, H.; Kuwana, M.; Takeuchi, T. Reduction of plasma IL-6 but not TNF-alpha by methotrexate in patients with early rheumatoid arthritis: A potential biomarker for radiographic progression. *Clin. Rheumatol.* **2013**, *32*, 1661–1666. [CrossRef] [PubMed]
17. Abdel-Tawab, M.; Werz, O.; Schubert-Zsilavecz, M. *Boswellia serrata*: An overall assessment of in vitro, preclinical, pharmacokinetic and clinical data. *Clin. Pharmacokinet.* **2011**, *50*, 349–369. [CrossRef] [PubMed]
18. McAlindon, T.E.; Bannuru, R.R.; Sullivan, M.C.; Arden, N.K.; Berenbaum, F.; Bierma-Zeinstra, S.M.; Hawker, G.A.; Henrotin, Y.; Hunter, D.J.; Kawaguchi, H.; et al. OARSI guidelines for the non-surgical management of knee osteoarthritis. *Osteoarthr. Cartil.* **2014**, *22*, 363–388. [CrossRef] [PubMed]
19. Matucci, A.; Cammelli, D.; Cantini, F.; Goletti, D.; Marino, V.; Milano, G.M.; Scarpa, R.; Tocci, G.; Maggi, E.; Vultaggio, A. Influence of anti-TNF immunogenicity on safety in rheumatic disease: A narrative review. *Expert Opin. Drug Saf.* **2016**, *15*, 3–10. [CrossRef] [PubMed]
20. Cabral, V.P.; Andrade, C.A.; Passos, S.R.; Martins, M.F.; Hökerberg, Y.H. Severe infection in patients with rheumatoid arthritis taking anakinra, rituximab, or abatacept: A systematic review of observational studies. *Rev. Bras. Reumatol.* **2016**, *56*, 543–550. [CrossRef] [PubMed]
21. Mameli, A.; Barcellona, D.; Marongiu, F. Fatal Cytopenia Induced by Low-Dose Methotrexate in Elderly With Rheumatoid Arthritis. Identification of Risk Factors. *Am. J. Ther.* **2017**, *24*, e106–e107. [CrossRef]
22. Umar, S.; Umar, K.; Sarwar, A.H.M.G.; Khan, A.; Ahmad, N.; Ahmad, S.; Katiyar, C.K.; Husain, S.A.; Khan, H.A. *Boswellia serrata* extract attenuates inflammatory mediators and oxidative stress in collagen induced arthritis. *Phytomedicine* **2014**, *21*, 847–856. [CrossRef]
23. Akhtar, N.; Miller, M.J.; Haqqi, T.M. Effect of a Herbal-Leucine mix on the IL-1β-induced cartilage degradation and inflammatory gene expression in human chondrocytes. *BMC Complement. Altern. Med.* **2011**, *11*, 66. [CrossRef] [PubMed]
24. Sharma, S.; Arif, M.; Nirala, R.K.; Gupta, R.; Thakur, S.C. Cumulative therapeutic effects of phytochemicals in *Arnica montana* flower extract alleviated collagen-induced arthritis: Inhibition of both pro-inflammatory mediators and oxidative stress. *J. Sci. Food Agric.* **2016**, *96*, 1500–1510. [CrossRef] [PubMed]
25. Álvarez-Hernández, E.; César Casasola-Vargas, J.; Lino-Pérez, L.; Burgos-Vargas, R.; Vázquez-Mellado, J. Frecuencia de uso de medicinas complementarias y alternativas en sujetos que acuden por primera vez al servicio de reumatología. Análisis de 800 casos. *Reumatol. Clín.* **2006**, *2*, 183–189. [CrossRef]
26. Knuesel, O.; Weber, M.; Suter, A. *Arnica montana* gel in osteoarthritis of the knee: An open, multicenter clinical trial. *Adv. Ther.* **2002**, *19*, 209–218. [CrossRef] [PubMed]
27. Widrig, R.; Suter, A.; Saller, R.; Melzer, J. Choosing between NSAID and *Arnica* for topical treatment of hand osteoarthritis in a randomised, double-blind study. *Rheumatol. Int.* **2007**, *27*, 585–591. [CrossRef]
28. Ross, S.M. Osteoarthritis. *Holist. Nurs. Pract.* **2008**, *22*, 237–239. [CrossRef] [PubMed]
29. Cameron, M.; Chrubasik, S. Topical herbal therapies for treating osteoarthritis. *CDSR* **2013**, *2013*, CD010538. [CrossRef]
30. Ammon, H.P.T. Boswellic acids (components of frankincense) as the active principle in treatment of chronic inflammatory diseases. *Wien. Med. Wochenschr.* **2002**, *152*, 373–378. (In German) [CrossRef] [PubMed]
31. Sengupta, K.; Krishnaraju, A.V.; Vishal, A.A.; Mishra, A.; Trimurtulu, G.; Sarma, K.V.S.; Raychaudhuri, S.K.; Raychaudhuri, S.P. Comparative efficacy and tolerability of 5-Loxin and AflapinAgainst osteoarthritis of the knee: A double blind, randomized, placebo controlled clinical study. *Int. J. Med. Sci.* **2010**, *7*, 366–377. [CrossRef] [PubMed]
32. Blain, E.J.; Ali, A.Y.; Duance, V.C. *Boswellia frereana* (frankincense) suppresses cytokine-induced matrix metalloproteinase expression and production of pro-inflammatory molecules in articular cartilage. *Phyther. Res.* **2009**, *24*, 905–912. [CrossRef] [PubMed]

33. Sumantran, V.N.; Joshi, A.K.; Boddul, S.; Koppikar, S.J.; Warude, D.; Patwardhan, B.; Chopra, A.; Chandwaskar, R.; Wagh, U.V. Antiarthritic Activity of a Standardized, Multiherbal, Ayurvedic Formulation containing *Boswellia serrata*: In Vitro Studies on Knee Cartilage from Osteoarthritis Patients. *Phyther. Res.* **2011**, *25*, 1375–1380. [CrossRef] [PubMed]
34. Dey, D.; Chaskar, S.; Athavale, N.; Chitre, D. Inhibition of LPS-Induced TNF-α and NO Production in Mouse Macrophage and Inflammatory Response in Rat Animal Models by a Novel Ayurvedic Formulation, BV-9238. *Phyther. Res.* **2014**, *28*, 1479–1485. [CrossRef]
35. Cameron, M.; Chrubasik, S. Oral herbal therapies for treating osteoarthritis. *CDSR* **2014**, *2014*, CD002947. [CrossRef]
36. Vishal, A.A.; Mishra, A.; Raychaudhuri, S.P. A double blind, randomized, placebo controlled clinical study evaluates the early efficacy of aflapin in subjects with osteoarthritis of knee. *Int. J. Med. Sci.* **2011**, *8*, 615–622. [CrossRef] [PubMed]
37. Belcaro, G.; Dugall, M.; Luzzi, R.; Ledda, A.; Pellegrini, L.; Cesarone, M.R.; Hosoi, M.; Errichi, M.; Francis, S.; Cornelli, U. FlexiQule (*Boswellia* extract) in the supplementary management of osteoarthritis: A supplement registry. *Minerva Med.* **2014**, *105*, 9–16.
38. Belcaro, G.; Feragalli, B.; Cornelli, U.; Dugall, M. Hand "stress" arthritis in young subjects: Effects of Flexiqule (pharma-standard *Boswellia* extract). A preliminary case report. *Minerva Gastroenterol. Dietol.* **2015**, in press.
39. Kizhakkedath, R. Clinical evaluation of a formulation containing *Curcuma longa* and *Boswellia serrata* extracts in the management of knee osteoarthritis. *Mol. Med. Rep.* **2013**, *8*, 1542–1548. [CrossRef] [PubMed]
40. Sander, O.; Herborn, G.; Rau, R. Is H15 (resin extract of *Boswellia serrata*, "incense") a useful supplement to established drug therapy of chronic polyarthritis? Results of a double-blind pilot study. *Z. Rheumatol.* **1998**, *57*, 11–16. [CrossRef] [PubMed]
41. Wang, H.; Zhang, C.; Wu, Y.; Ai, Y.; Lee, D.Y.-W.; Dai, R. Comparative pharmacokinetic study of two boswellic acids in normal and arthritic rat plasma after oral administration of *Boswellia serrata* extract or Huo Luo Xiao Ling Dan by LC-MS. *Biomed. Chromatogr.* **2014**, *28*, 1402–1408. [CrossRef] [PubMed]
42. Hamidpour, R.; Hamidpour, S.; Hamidpour, M.; Shahlari, M. Frankincense (Rǔ Xiāng; *Boswellia* Species): From the Selection of Traditional Applications to the Novel Phytotherapy for the Prevention and Treatment of Serious Diseases. *J. Tradit. Complement. Med.* **2013**, *3*, 221–226. [CrossRef] [PubMed]
43. Sharma, M.L.; Bani, S.; Singh, G.B. Anti-arthritic activity of boswellic acids in bovine serum albumin (BSA)-induced arthritis. *Int. J. Immunopharmacol.* **1989**, *11*, 647–652. [CrossRef]
44. Singh, S.; Khajuria, A.; Taneja, S.C.; Johri, R.K.; Singh, J.; Qazi, G.N. Boswellic acids: A leukotriene inhibitor also effective through topical application in inflammatory disorders. *Phytomedicine* **2008**, *15*, 400–407. [CrossRef] [PubMed]
45. Ammon, H.P.T. Modulation of the immune system by *Boswellia serrata* extracts and boswellic acids. *Phytomedicine* **2010**, *17*, 862–867. [CrossRef] [PubMed]
46. Khajuria, A.; Gupta, A.; Suden, P.; Singh, S.; Malik, F.; Singh, J.; Gupta, B.D.; Suri, K.A.; Srinivas, V.K.; Ella, K.; et al. Immunomodulatory activity of biopolymeric fraction BOS 2000 from *Boswellia serrata*. *Phyther. Res.* **2008**, *22*, 340–348. [CrossRef] [PubMed]
47. Sengupta, K.; Kolla, J.N.; Krishnaraju, A.V.; Yalamanchili, N.; Rao, C.V.; Golakoti, T.; Raychaudhuri, S.; Raychaudhuri, S.P. Cellular and molecular mechanisms of anti-inflammatory effect of Aflapin: A novel *Boswellia serrata* extract. *Mol. Cell. Biochem.* **2011**, *354*, 189–197. [CrossRef] [PubMed]
48. Sharma, R.; Dash, B. *Caraka Samhita*, 2006th ed.; Chowkhamba Sanskrit Series Office: Varanasi, India, 2006.
49. Funk, J.L.; Frye, J.B.; Oyarzo, J.N.; Kuscuoglu, N.; Wilson, J.; McCaffrey, G.; Stafford, G.; Chen, G.; Lantz, R.C.; Jolad, S.D.; et al. Efficacy and mechanism of action of turmeric supplements in the treatment of experimental arthritis. *Arthritis Rheum.* **2006**, *54*, 3452–3464. [CrossRef] [PubMed]
50. Taty Anna, K.; Elvy Suhana, M.R.; Das, S.; Faizah, O.; Hamzaini, A.H. Anti-inflammatory effect of *Curcuma longa* (turmeric) on collagen-induced arthritis: An anatomico-radiological study. *Clin. Ter.* **2011**, *162*, 201–207. [PubMed]
51. Kamarudin, T.A.; Othman, F.; Mohd Ramli, E.S.; Md Isa, N.; Das, S. Protective effect of curcumin on experimentally induced arthritic rats: Detailed histopathological study of the joints and white blood cell count. *EXCLI J.* **2012**, *11*, 226–236. [PubMed]

52. Chang, H.-I.; Su, Y.-H.; Lin, Y.-J.; Chen, P.-J.; Shi, C.-S.; Chen, C.-N.; Yeh, C.-C. Evaluation of the protective effects of curcuminoid (curcumin and bisdemethoxycurcumin)-loaded liposomes against bone turnover in a cell-based model of osteoarthritis. *Drug Des. Dev. Ther.* **2015**, *9*, 2285–2300. [CrossRef] [PubMed]
53. Ramadan, G.; El-Menshawy, O. Protective effects of ginger-turmeric rhizomes mixture on joint inflammation, atherogenesis, kidney dysfunction and other complications in a rat model of human rheumatoid arthritis. *Int. J. Rheum. Dis.* **2013**, *16*, 219–229. [CrossRef] [PubMed]
54. Kuptniratsaikul, V.; Dajpratham, P.; Taechaarpornkul, W.; Buntragulpoontawee, M.; Lukkanapichonchut, P.; Chootip, C.; Saengsuwan, J.; Tantayakom, K.; Laongpech, S. Efficacy and safety of *Curcuma* domestica extracts compared with ibuprofen in patients with knee osteoarthritis: A multicenter study. *Clin. Interv. Aging* **2014**, *9*, 451–458. [CrossRef] [PubMed]
55. Daily, J.W.; Yang, M.; Park, S. Efficacy of Turmeric Extracts and Curcumin for Alleviating the Symptoms of Joint Arthritis: A Systematic Review and Meta-Analysis of Randomized Clinical Trials. *J. Med. Food* **2016**, *19*, 717–729. [CrossRef] [PubMed]
56. Ghosh, S.; Banerjee, S.; Sil, P.C. The beneficial role of curcumin on inflammation, diabetes and neurodegenerative disease: A recent update. *Food Chem. Toxicol.* **2015**, *83*, 111–124. [CrossRef] [PubMed]
57. Nonose, N.; Pereira, J.A.; Machado, P.R.M.; Rodrigues, M.R.; Sato, D.T.; Martinez, C.A.R. Oral administration of curcumin (*Curcuma longa*) can attenuate the neutrophil inflammatory response in zymosan-induced arthritis in rats. *Acta Cir. Bras.* **2014**, *29*, 727–734. [CrossRef] [PubMed]
58. Panahi, Y.; Alishiri, G.H.; Parvin, S.; Sahebkar, A. Mitigation of Systemic Oxidative Stress by Curcuminoids in Osteoarthritis: Results of a Randomized Controlled Trial. *J. Diet. Suppl.* **2016**, *13*, 209–220. [CrossRef] [PubMed]
59. Chen, J.-J.; Dai, L.; Zhao, L.-X.; Zhu, X.; Cao, S.; Gao, Y.-J. Intrathecal curcumin attenuates pain hypersensitivity and decreases spinal neuroinflammation in rat model of monoarthritis. *Sci. Rep.* **2015**, *5*, 10278. [CrossRef]
60. Zou, S.; Wang, C.; Cui, Z.; Guo, P.; Meng, Q.; Shi, X.; Gao, Y.; Yang, G.; Han, Z. β-Elemene induces apoptosis of human rheumatoid arthritis fibroblast-like synoviocytes via reactive oxygen species-dependent activation of p38 mitogen-activated protein kinase. *Pharmacol. Rep.* **2016**, *68*, 7–11. [CrossRef]
61. Gründemann, C.; Lengen, K.; Sauer, B.; Garcia-Käufer, M.; Zehl, M.; Huber, R. *Equisetum arvense* (common horsetail) modulates the function of inflammatory immunocompetent cells. *BMC Complement. Altern. Med.* **2014**, *14*, 283. [CrossRef]
62. Farinon, M.; Lora, P.S.; Francescato, L.N.; Bassani, V.L.; Henriques, A.T.; Xavier, R.M.; de Oliveira, P.G. Effect of Aqueous Extract of Giant Horsetail (*Equisetum giganteum* L.) in Antigen-Induced Arthritis. *Open Rheumatol. J.* **2013**, *7*, 129–133. [CrossRef] [PubMed]
63. Jiang, X.; Qu, Q.; Li, M.; Miao, S.; Li, X.; Cai, W. Horsetail mixture on rheumatoid arthritis and its regulation on TNF-α and IL-10. *Pak. J. Pharm. Sci.* **2014**, *27*, 2019–2023. [PubMed]
64. Zgrajka, W.; Turska, M.; Rajtar, G.; Majdan, M.; Parada-Turska, J. Kynurenic acid content in anti-rheumatic herbs. *Ann. Agric. Environ. Med.* **2013**, *20*, 800–802. [PubMed]
65. Varga, G.; Erces, D.; Fazekas, B.; Fulop, M.; Kovacs, T.; Kaszaki, J.; Fulop, F.; Vecsei, L.; Boros, M. *N*-Methyl-D-aspartate receptor antagonism decreases motility and inflammatory activation in the early phase of acute experimental colitis in the rat. *Neurogastroenterol. Motil.* **2010**, *22*, 217–225. [CrossRef] [PubMed]
66. Parada-Turska, J.; Rzeski, W.; Zgrajka, W.; Majdan, M.; Kandefer-Szerszen, M.; Turski, W. Kynurenic acid, an endogenous constituent of rheumatoid arthritis synovial fluid, inhibits proliferation of synoviocytes in vitro. *Rheumatol. Int.* **2006**, *26*, 422–426. [CrossRef]
67. Parada-Turska, J.; Zgrajka, W.; Majdan, M. Kynurenic acid in synovial fluid and serum of patients with rheumatoid arthritis, spondyloarthropathy, and osteoarthritis. *J. Rheumatol.* **2013**, *40*, 903–909. [CrossRef] [PubMed]
68. Blumenthal, M.; Busse, W.R. *The Complete German Commission E Monographs*; American Botanical Council: Austin, TX, USA, 1998.
69. Fiebich, B.; Heinrich, M.; Hiller, K.; Kammerer, N. Inhibition of TNF-α synthesis in LPS-stimulated primary human monocytes by *Harpagophytum* extract SteiHap 69. *Phytomedicine* **2001**, *8*, 28–30. [CrossRef]
70. Lanhers, M.; Fleurentin, J.; Mortier, F.; Al, E. Antiinflammatory and analgesic effects of an aqueous extract of *Harpagophytum procumbens*. *Planta Med.* **1992**, *58*, 117–123. [CrossRef] [PubMed]

71. Akhtar, N.; Haqqi, T.M. Current nutraceuticals in the management of osteoarthritis: A review. *Ther. Adv. Musculoskelet. Dis.* **2012**, *4*, 181–207. [CrossRef] [PubMed]
72. Wegener, T.; Lupke, N. Treatment of patients with arthrosis of hip or knee with an aqueous extract of devil's claw (*Harpagophytum procumbens* DC.). *Phytother. Res.* **2003**, *17*, 1165–1172. [CrossRef] [PubMed]
73. Chantre, P.; Cappelaere, A.; Leblan, D.; Al, E. Efficacy and tolerance of *Harpagophytum procumbens* versus diacerhein in treatment of osteoarthritis. *Phytomedicine* **2000**, *7*, 177–183. [CrossRef]
74. Chrubasik, S.; Thanner, J.; Kunzel, O.; Al, E. Comparison of outcome measures during treatment with the proprietary *Harpagophytum* extract Doloteffin in patients with pain in the lower back, knee, or hip. *Phytomedicine* **2002**, *9*, 181–194. [CrossRef] [PubMed]
75. *Harpagophytum procumbens* (devil's claw). Monograph. *Altern. Med. Rev.* **2008**, *13*, 248–252.
76. Huang, T.H.-W.; Tran, V.H.; Duke, R.K.; Tan, S.; Chrubasik, S.; Roufogalis, B.D.; Duke, C.C. Harpagoside suppresses lipopolysaccharide-induced iNOS and COX-2 expression through inhibition of NF-κB activation. *J. Ethnopharmacol.* **2006**, *104*, 149–155. [CrossRef] [PubMed]
77. Kaszkin, M.; Beck, K.; Koch, E.; Al, E. Downregulation of iNOS expression in rat mesangial cells by special extracts of *Harpagophytum procumbens* derives from harpagoside-dependent and independent effects. *Phytomedicine* **2004**, *11*, 585–595. [CrossRef]
78. Liu, Z.; Liu, L. *Essentials of Chinese Medicine*; Liu, Z., Liu, L., Eds.; Springer: London, UK, 2009.
79. Chang, S.-H.; Choi, Y.; Park, J.-A.; Jung, D.-S.; Shin, J.; Yang, J.-H.; Ko, S.-Y.; Kim, S.-W.; Kim, J.-K. Anti-inflammatory effects of BT-201, an *n*-butanol extract of *Panax notoginseng*, observed in vitro and in a collagen-induced arthritis model. *Clin. Nutr.* **2007**, *26*, 785–791. [CrossRef] [PubMed]
80. Chang, S.-H.; Sung, H.-C.; Choi, Y.; Ko, S.-Y.; Lee, B.-E.; Baek, D.-H.; Kim, S.-W.; Kim, J.-K. Suppressive effect of AIF, a water extract from three herbs, on collagen-induced arthritis in mice. *Int. Immunopharmacol.* **2005**, *5*, 1365–1372. [CrossRef] [PubMed]
81. Zhang, L.; Li, Z.; Sun, J.; Ma, J.; Zhang, S.; Liu, J.; Zhu, J. Effect of *Panax Notoginseng* Saponins on autograft tendon healing in bone tunnel: Interface histological characteristics. *Zhongguo Gu Shang* **2011**, *24*, 132–136. [PubMed]
82. Zhang, J.; Wang, J.; Wang, H. Clinical study on effect of total *Panax notoginseng* saponins on immune related inner environment imbalance in rheumatoid arthritis patients. *Zhongguo Zhong Xi Yi Jie He Za Zhi/Chin. J. Integr. Tradit. West. Med.* **2007**, *27*, 589–592.
83. Appelboom, T. Arthropathy in art and the history of pain management—Through the centuries to cyclooxygenase-2 inhibitors. *Rheumatology* **2002**, *41* (Suppl. 1), 28–34. [CrossRef] [PubMed]
84. Vlachojannis, J.E.; Cameron, M.; Chrubasik, S. A systematic review on the effectiveness of willow bark for musculoskeletal pain. *Phyther. Res.* **2009**, *23*, 897–900. [CrossRef] [PubMed]
85. Mackowiak, P.A. Brief History of Antipyretic Therapy. *Clin. Infect. Dis.* **2000**, *31*, S154–S156. [CrossRef]
86. Vane, J.R. The fight against rheumatism: From willow bark to COX-1 sparing drugs. *J. Physiol. Pharmacol.* **2000**, *51*, 573–586. [PubMed]
87. Bonaterra, G.A.; Heinrich, E.U.; Kelber, O.; Weiser, D.; Metz, J.; Kinscherf, R. Anti-inflammatory effects of the willow bark extract STW 33-I (Proaktiv®) in LPS-activated human monocytes and differentiated macrophages. *Phytomedicine* **2010**, *17*, 1106–1113. [CrossRef] [PubMed]
88. Khayyal, M.; El-Ghazaly, M.; Abdallah, D.; Okpanyi, S.; Kelber, O.; Weiser, D. Mechanisms Involved in the Anti-inflammatory Effect of a Standardized Willow Bark Extract. *Arzneimittelforschung* **2011**, *55*, 677–687. [CrossRef] [PubMed]
89. Sharma, S.; Sahu, D.; Das, H.R.; Sharma, D. Amelioration of collagen-induced arthritis by *Salix nigra* bark extract via suppression of pro-inflammatory cytokines and oxidative stress. *Food Chem. Toxicol.* **2011**, *49*, 3395–3406. [CrossRef] [PubMed]
90. Schmid, B.; Lüdtke, R.; Selbmann, H.K.; Kötter, I.; Tschirdewahn, B.; Schaffner, W.; Heide, L. Efficacy and tolerability of a standardized willow bark extract in patients with osteoarthritis: Randomized placebo-controlled, double blind clinical trial. *Phytother. Res.* **2001**, *15*, 344–350. [CrossRef] [PubMed]
91. Biegert, C.; Wagner, I.; Lüdtke, R.; Kötter, I.; Lohmüller, C.; Günaydin, I.; Taxis, K.; Heide, L. Efficacy and safety of willow bark extract in the treatment of osteoarthritis and rheumatoid arthritis: Results of 2 randomized double-blind controlled trials. *J. Rheumatol.* **2004**, *31*, 2121–2130.
92. Beer, A.-M.; Wegener, T. Willow bark extract (*Salicis cortex*) for gonarthrosis and coxarthrosis—Results of a cohort study with a control group. *Phytomedicine* **2008**, *15*, 907–913. [CrossRef] [PubMed]

93. Uehleke, B.; Müller, J.; Stange, R.; Kelber, O.; Melzer, J. Willow bark extract STW 33-I in the long-term treatment of outpatients with rheumatic pain mainly osteoarthritis or back pain. *Phytomedicine* **2013**, *20*, 980–984. [CrossRef] [PubMed]
94. Nahrstedt, A.; Schmidt, M.; Jäggi, R.; Metz, J.; Khayyal, M.T. Willow bark extract: The contribution of polyphenols to the overall effect. *Wien. Med. Wochenschr.* **2007**, *157*, 348–351. [CrossRef] [PubMed]
95. Drummond, E.M.; Harbourne, N.; Marete, E.; Martyn, D.; Jacquier, J.; O'Riordan, D.; Gibney, E.R. Inhibition of Proinflammatory Biomarkers in THP1 Macrophages by Polyphenols Derived From Chamomile, Meadowsweet and Willow bark. *Phyther. Res.* **2013**, *27*, 588–594. [CrossRef] [PubMed]
96. Shara, M.; Stohs, S.J. Efficacy and Safety of White Willow Bark (*Salix alba*) Extracts. *Phyther. Res.* **2015**, *29*, 1112–1116. [CrossRef] [PubMed]
97. Hsu, D.-Z.; Chen, S.-J.; Chu, P.-Y.; Liu, M.-Y. Therapeutic effects of sesame oil on monosodium urate crystal-induced acute inflammatory response in rats. *Springerplus* **2013**, *2*, 659. [CrossRef] [PubMed]
98. Sotnikova, R.; Ponist, S.; Navarova, J.; Mihalova, D.; Tomekova, V.; Strosova, M.; Bauerova, K. Effects of sesame oil in the model of adjuvant arthritis. *Neuro Endocrinol. Lett.* **2009**, *30* (Suppl. 1), 22–24.
99. Yadav, N.V.; Sadashivaiah; Ramaiyan, B.; Acharya, P.; Belur, L.; Talahalli, R.R. Sesame Oil and Rice Bran Oil Ameliorates Adjuvant-Induced Arthritis in Rats: Distinguishing the Role of Minor Components and Fatty Acids. *Lipids* **2016**, *51*, 1385–1395. [CrossRef] [PubMed]
100. Eftekhar Sadat, B.; Khadem Haghighian, M.; Alipoor, B.; Malek Mahdavi, A.; Asghari Jafarabadi, M.; Moghaddam, A. Effects of sesame seed supplementation on clinical signs and symptoms in patients with knee osteoarthritis. *Int. J. Rheum. Dis.* **2013**, *16*, 578–582. [CrossRef] [PubMed]
101. Khadem Haghighian, M.; Alipoor, B.; Malek Mahdavi, A.; Eftekhar Sadat, B.; Asghari Jafarabadi, M.; Moghaddam, A. Effects of sesame seed supplementation on inflammatory factors and oxidative stress biomarkers in patients with knee osteoarthritis. *Acta Med. Iran.* **2015**, *53*, 207–213. [PubMed]
102. Yashaswini, P.S.; Rao, A.G.A.; Singh, S.A. Inhibition of lipoxygenase by sesamol corroborates its potential anti-inflammatory activity. *Int. J. Biol. Macromol.* **2017**, *94*, 781–787. [CrossRef] [PubMed]
103. Hemshekhar, M.; Thushara, R.M.; Jnaneshwari, S.; Devaraja, S.; Kemparaju, K.; Girish, K.S. Attenuation of adjuvant-induced arthritis by dietary sesamol via modulation of inflammatory mediators, extracellular matrix degrading enzymes and antioxidant status. *Eur. J. Nutr.* **2013**, *52*, 1787–1799. [CrossRef] [PubMed]
104. Khansai, M.; Boonmaleerat, K.; Pothacharoen, P.; Phitak, T.; Kongtawelert, P. Ex vivo model exhibits protective effects of sesamin against destruction of cartilage induced with a combination of tumor necrosis factor-alpha and oncostatin M. *BMC Complement. Altern. Med.* **2016**, *16*. [CrossRef] [PubMed]
105. Cavero, R.Y.; Calvo, M.I. Medicinal plants used for musculoskeletal disorders in Navarra and their pharmacological validation. *J. Ethnopharmacol.* **2015**, *168*, 255–259. [CrossRef] [PubMed]
106. Di Lorenzo, C.; Dell'Agli, M.; Badea, M.; Dima, L.; Colombo, E.; Sangiovanni, E.; Restani, P.; Bosisio, E. Plant food supplements with anti-inflammatory properties: A systematic review (II). *Crit. Rev. Food Sci. Nutr.* **2013**, *53*, 507–516. [CrossRef] [PubMed]
107. Gilca, M.; Gaman, L.; Lixandru, D.; Stoian, I. Estimating the yin-yang nature of Western herbs: A potential tool based on antioxidation-oxidation theory. *Afr. J. Tradit. Complement. Altern. Med.* **2014**, *11*, 210–216. [CrossRef] [PubMed]
108. Hiermann, A.; Writzel, M. Antiphlogistic glycopeptide from the roots of *Symphytum officinale*. *Pharm. Pharmacol. Lett.* **1998**, *8*, 154–157.
109. Mascolo, N.; Autore, G.; Capasso, F.; Menghini, A.; Fasulo, M.P. Biological screening of Italian medicinal plants for anti-inflammatory activity. *Phyther. Res.* **1987**, *1*, 28–31. [CrossRef]
110. Laslett, L.L.; Quinn, S.J.; Darian-Smith, E.; Kwok, M.; Fedorova, T.; Körner, H.; Steels, E.; March, L.; Jones, G. Treatment with 4Jointz reduces knee pain over 12 weeks of treatment in patients with clinical knee osteoarthritis: A randomised controlled trial. *Osteoarthr. Cartil.* **2012**, *20*, 1209–1216. [CrossRef] [PubMed]
111. Grube, B.; Grünwald, J.; Krug, L.; Staiger, C. Efficacy of a comfrey root (*Symphyti offic. radix*) extract ointment in the treatment of patients with painful osteoarthritis of the knee: Results of a double-blind, randomised, bicenter, placebo-controlled trial. *Phytomedicine* **2007**, *14*, 2–10. [CrossRef] [PubMed]
112. Gracza, L.; Koch, H.; Loffler, E. Biochemical-pharmacologic studies of medicinal plants. 1. Isolation of rosmarinic acid from *Symphytum officinale* L. and its anti-inflammatory activity in an in vitro model. *Arch. Pharm.* **1985**, *318*, 1090–1095. [CrossRef]

113. Gracza, L. Prüfung der membranabdichtenden Wirkung eines Phytopharmakons und dessen Wirkstoffe. *Z. Phytother.* **1987**, *8*, 78–81.
114. Huang, S.-H.; Lee, C.-H.; Wang, H.-M.; Chang, Y.-W.; Lin, C.-Y.; Chen, C.-Y.; Chen, Y.-H. 6-Dehydrogingerdione restrains lipopolysaccharide-induced inflammatory responses in RAW 264.7 macrophages. *J. Agric. Food Chem.* **2014**, *62*, 9171–9179. [CrossRef] [PubMed]
115. Van Breemen, R.B.; Tao, Y.; Li, W. Cyclooxygenase-2 inhibitors in ginger (*Zingiber officinale*). *Fitoterapia* **2011**, *82*, 38–43. [CrossRef] [PubMed]
116. Grzanna, R.; Lindmark, L.; Frondoza, C.G. Ginger—An herbal medicinal product with broad anti-inflammatory actions. *J. Med. Food* **2005**, *8*, 125–132. [CrossRef] [PubMed]
117. Ueda, H.; Ippoushi, K.; Takeuchi, A. Repeated oral administration of a squeezed ginger (*Zingiber officinale*) extract augmented the serum corticosterone level and had anti-inflammatory properties. *Biosci. Biotechnol. Biochem.* **2010**, *74*, 2248–2252. [CrossRef] [PubMed]
118. Naderi, Z.; Mozaffari-Khosravi, H.; Dehghan, A.; Nadjarzadeh, A.; Huseini, H.F. Effect of ginger powder supplementation on nitric oxide and C-reactive protein in elderly knee osteoarthritis patients: A 12-week double-blind randomized placebo-controlled clinical trial. *J. Tradit. Complement. Med.* **2016**, *6*, 199–203. [CrossRef]
119. Altman, R.D.; Marcussen, K.C. Effects of a ginger extract on knee pain in patients with osteoarthritis. *Arthritis Rheum.* **2001**, *44*, 2531–2538. [CrossRef]
120. Alipour, Z.; Asadizaker, M.; Fayazi, S.; Yegane, N.; Kochak, M.; Haghighi Zadeh, M.H. The Effect of Ginger on Pain and Satisfaction of Patients with Knee Osteoarthritis. *Jundishapur J. Chronic Dis. Care* **2016**, *6*, e34798. [CrossRef]
121. Haghighi, M.; Khalvat, A.; Toliat, T.; Jallaei, S. Comparing the effects of ginger extract and ibuprofen in patients with osteoporosis. *Arch. Iran. Med.* **2005**, *8*, 267–271.
122. Drozdov, V.N.; Kim, V.A.; Tkachenko, E.V.; Varvanina, G.G. Influence of a specific ginger combination on gastropathy conditions in patients with osteoarthritis of the knee or hip. *J. Altern. Complement. Med.* **2012**, *18*, 583–588. [CrossRef] [PubMed]
123. Bliddal, H.; Rosetzsky, A.; Schlichting, P.; Weidner, M.S.; Andersen, L.A.; Ibfelt, H.H.; Christensen, K.; Jensen, O.N.; Barslev, J. A randomized, placebo-controlled, cross-over study of ginger extracts and ibuprofen in osteoarthritis. *Osteoarthr. Cartil.* **2000**, *8*, 9–12. [CrossRef] [PubMed]
124. Lee, H.Y.; Park, S.H.; Lee, M.; Kim, H.-J.; Ryu, S.Y.; Kim, N.D.; Hwang, B.Y.; Hong, J.T.; Han, S.-B.; Kim, Y. 1-Dehydro-[10]-gingerdione from ginger inhibits IKKβ activity for NF-κB activation and suppresses NF-κB-regulated expression of inflammatory genes. *Br. J. Pharmacol.* **2012**, *167*, 128–140. [CrossRef] [PubMed]
125. Singh, N.; Bhalla, M.; de Jager, P.; Gilca, M. An overview on Ashwagandha: A Rasayana (Rejuvenator) of Ayurveda. *Afr. J. Tradit. Complement. Altern. Med.* **2011**, *8*, 208–213. [CrossRef] [PubMed]
126. Singh, D.; Aggarwal, A.; Maurya, R.; Naik, S. Withania somnifera inhibits NF-κB and AP-1 transcription factors in human peripheral blood and synovial fluid mononuclear cells. *Phytother. Res.* **2007**, *21*, 905–913. [CrossRef] [PubMed]
127. Ganesan, K.; Sehgal, P.K.; Mandal, A.B.; Sayeed, S. Protective effect of Withania somnifera and Cardiospermum halicacabum extracts against collagenolytic degradation of collagen. *Appl. Biochem. Biotechnol.* **2011**, *165*, 1075–1091. [CrossRef] [PubMed]
128. Rasool, M.; Varalakshmi, P. Protective effect of Withania somnifera root powder in relation to lipid peroxidation, antioxidant status, glycoproteins and bone collagen on adjuvant-induced arthritis in rats. *Fundam. Clin. Pharmacol.* **2007**, *21*, 157–164. [CrossRef] [PubMed]
129. Ramakanth, G.S.H.; Uday Kumar, C.; Kishan, P.V.; Usharani, P. A randomized, double blind placebo controlled study of efficacy and tolerability of Withaina somnifera extracts in knee joint pain. *J. Ayurveda Integr. Med.* **2016**, *7*, 151–157. [CrossRef] [PubMed]
130. Sabina, E.P.; Chandal, S.; Rasool, M.K. Inhibition of monosodium urate crystal-induced inflammation by withaferin A. *J. Pharm. Pharm. Sci.* **2008**, *11*, 46–55. [PubMed]
131. Grover, A.; Shandilya, A.; Punetha, A.; Bisaria, V.S.; Sundar, D. Inhibition of the NEMO/IKKβ association complex formation, a novel mechanism associated with the NF-κB activation suppression by Withania somnifera's key metabolite withaferin A. *BMC Genom.* **2010**, *11* (Suppl. 4), S25. [CrossRef] [PubMed]

132. Heyninck, K.; Lahtela-Kakkonen, M.; van der Veken, P.; Haegeman, G.; Vanden Berghe, W. Withaferin A inhibits NF-κB activation by targeting cysteine 179 in IKKβ. *Biochem. Pharmacol.* **2014**, *91*, 501–509. [CrossRef] [PubMed]
133. Bee, T.A.; Liew, A.; Hons, P. Dietary Supplements Used in Osteoarthritis. *Proc. Singap. Healthc.* **2010**, *19*, 237–247. [CrossRef]
134. Posadzki, P.; Watson, L.; Ernst, E. Contamination and adulteration of herbal medicinal products (HMPs): An overview of systematic reviews. *Eur. J. Clin. Pharmacol.* **2013**, *69*, 295–307. [CrossRef] [PubMed]
135. Ernst, E. Risks of herbal medicinal products. *Pharmacoepidemiol. Drug Saf.* **2004**, *13*, 767–771. [CrossRef] [PubMed]
136. Posadzki, P.; Watson, L.; Ernst, E. Herb-drug interactions: An overview of systematic reviews. *Br. J. Clin. Pharmacol.* **2013**, *75*, 603–618. [CrossRef] [PubMed]
137. Bhattaram, V.A.; Graefe, U.; Kohlert, C.; Veit, M.; Derendorf, H. Pharmacokinetics and bioavailability of herbal medicinal products. *Phytomedicine* **2002**, *9* (Suppl. 3), 1–33. [CrossRef] [PubMed]

10

Protective Effect of Chokeberry (*Aronia melanocarpa* L.) Extract against Cadmium Impact on the Biomechanical Properties of the Femur: A Study in a Rat Model of Low and Moderate Lifetime Women Exposure to This Heavy Metal

Małgorzata M. Brzóska *, Alicja Roszczenko, Joanna Rogalska, Małgorzata Gałażyn-Sidorczuk and Magdalena Mężyńska

Department of Toxicology, Medical University of Bialystok, Adama Mickiewicza 2C street, 15-222 Bialystok, Poland; alicja.roszczenko@umb.edu.pl (A.R.); joanna.rogalska@umb.edu.pl (J.R.); malgorzata.galazyn-sidorczuk@umb.edu.pl (M.G.-S.); mmezynska1@student.umb.edu.pl (M.M.)

* Correspondence: malgorzata.brzoska@umb.edu.pl

Abstract: The hypothesis that the consumption of *Aronia melanocarpa* berries (chokeberries) extract, recently reported by us to improve bone metabolism in female rats at low-level and moderate chronic exposure to cadmium (1 and 5 mg Cd/kg diet for up to 24 months), may increase the bone resistance to fracture was investigated. Biomechanical properties of the neck (bending test with vertical head loading) and diaphysis (three-point bending test) of the femur of rats administered 0.1% aqueous chokeberry extract (65.74% of polyphenols) or/and Cd in the diet (1 and 5 mg Cd/kg) for 3, 10, 17, and 24 months were evaluated. Moreover, procollagen I was assayed in the bone tissue. The low-level and moderate exposure to Cd decreased the procollagen I concentration in the bone tissue and weakened the biomechanical properties of the femoral neck and diaphysis. Chokeberry extract administration under the exposure to Cd improved the bone collagen biosynthesis and femur biomechanical properties. The results allow for the conclusion that the consumption of chokeberry products under exposure to Cd may improve the bone biomechanical properties and protect from fracture. This study provides support for *Aronia melanocarpa* berries being a promising natural agent for skeletal protection under low-level and moderate chronic exposure to Cd.

Keywords: *Aronia melanocarpa* berries; bone biomechanical properties; cadmium; chokeberries; female rats; polyphenols; procollagen; protection

1. Introduction

The growing occurrence of osteoporosis with bone fracture in inhabitants of industrialized countries, which has generated an increasing amount of attention in recent years, has been focused on environmental risk factors for bone damage [1–3] and numerous efforts have been undertaken to find effective ways of protecting bone [4–6]. Among the factors that may be useful in this protection, a subject of special interest is dietary products that are rich in biologically active substances, characterized by a well-defined beneficial impact on bone metabolism, including polyphenolic compounds that occur in green tea and some fruit and vegetables [4–7].

More numerous epidemiological data provide evidence that important environmental risk factors for the increasing incidence of osteoporosis are toxic heavy metals, including cadmium (Cd) [1–3,8–10]. Due to the wide distribution of this metal in the environment and food pollution, as well as its presence in tobacco smoke, the whole population is exposed to this metal during their lifetime [8–12].

Bone damage is one of the main unfavourable health effects of long-term exposure to this xenobiotic in both human [1,8–12] and experimental animals [13–19]. We have reported, for a rat model with environmental human exposure to Cd, that this metal disturbs bone metabolism and weakens the biomechanical properties of long bones and lumbar spine vertebral bodies, which may even result in femoral neck and vertebral fractures [13–18]. In recent years, numerous epidemiological data have shown that even low-level lifetime exposure to this heavy metal may decrease the bone mineral density (BMD) and contribute to osteoporosis with an increased risk of bone fracture in the general population [1,8–10]. Moreover, the forecasts indicate that the exposure of the general population to this xenobiotic will increase in the future decades [11]. Thus, it seems very important to recognize effective ways of preventing these health effects due to exposure to Cd, including its impact on the skeleton.

The attention of researchers regarding effective agents that may play a role in protecting against the effects of Cd action has been focused on natural products, including those rich in polyphenolic compounds [20–22]. Due to the multidirectional favourable action of polyphenols (antioxidative, anti-inflammatory, anticoagulative, antiatherogenic, antidiabetic, antibacterial, and anticancer), products abundant in these compounds are recommended to be used as functional food in the case of cardiovascular diseases, diabetes, neurodegenerative disorders, urinary tract infection, non-alcoholic fatty liver disease, and chemotherapy [20,22,23]. Moreover, polyphenols are also known for their beneficial impact on the skeleton [4,6,7,24].

Available data, including our own findings, show that some plant products rich in polyphenolic compounds, including the berries of *Aronia melanocarpa* (chokeberries; [Michx.] Elliott, Rosaceae), possess the potential to protect from various unfavourable effects that result from the exposure to Cd [21,22,25–27]. Recently, using a rat model of lifetime low-level and moderate female exposure to Cd (1 and 5 mg Cd/kg diet), we have revealed that the consumption of an extract from the berries of *A. melanocarpa* (AE) protected against these heavy metal-induced disturbances in the bone turnover and bone mineral status (findings are summarized as Tables S1 and S2) [26,27]. Because the mineral status of the bone tissue determines its biomechanical properties and susceptibility to fracture [28], taking into account our recent findings [25–27], we have hypothesized that the consumption of AE under Cd exposure may also improve the bone biomechanical properties and, in this way, decrease the bone susceptibility to fracture. The aim of the present study was to investigate this hypothesis. For this purpose, the impact of AE administration under chronic low-level and moderate exposure to Cd on the biomechanical properties of the femoral neck and femoral diaphysis was estimated for the animals in which we have revealed the protective impact of the extract against the body burden of Cd and disorders in the bone tissue metabolism [25–27]. Moreover, because the bone biomechanical properties are determined not only by the bone mineral status, but also by the bone matrix composed mainly of collagen [29,30], the concentration of procollagen I (PC I) in the bone tissue, as a marker of collagen biosynthesis, was assayed.

2. Materials and Methods

2.1. Animals

One hundred and ninety-two young (aged three to four week) female Wistar rats [Crl: WI (Han)] purchased from the certified Laboratory Animal House (Brwinów, Poland) were used. The animals were housed in controlled conventional conditions (temperature 22 ± 2 °C, relative humidity 50 ± 10%, 12-h light/dark cycle) and had free access to drinking water and feed (Labofeed B diet through the first three months and then a Labofeed H diet; Label Food 'Morawski', Kcynia, Poland) [25,26].

2.2. Cd Diets

The diets containing 1 and 5 mg Cd/kg were prepared by the addition, at the stage of production, of appropriate amounts of $CdCl_2 \times H_2O$ (POCh, Gliwice, Poland) into the ingredients of the standard feed (Labofeed B and Labofeed H diets). The mean Cd concentration determined by us (by atomic absorption spectrometry method) in the diets reached 1.09 ± 0.11 mg/kg and 4.92 ± 0.78 mg/kg (mean ± SE), respectively, whereas its mean concentration in the standard Labofeed diets was 0.0584 ± 0.0046 mg/kg.

2.3. *A. melanocarpa* Extract

Powdered aronia extract was received from Adamed Consumer Healthcare (Tuszyn, Poland). According to the producer, the extract contained 65.74% of polyphenols (including 18.65% of anthocyanins). Although the polyphenols content in the powdered *A. melanocarpa* extract was certified and is widely reported [22,23,31,32], the phytochemical profile of the extract was evaluated and the concentrations of total polyphenols, phenolic acids (including chlorogenic acid), flavonoids, proanthocyanidins, and anthocyanins (including cyanidin 3-*O*-β-galactoside, cyanidin 3-*O*-α-arabinoside, and cyanidin 3-*O*-β-glucoside) were quantified by us [26] (Table S3). According to the producer's declaration and literature data [22,31], the extract also contained other components such as pectins, sugar, sugar alcohols (sorbitol, parasorboside), triterpenes, carotenoids, and phytosterols, as well as minerals and vitamins.

2.4. *Study Design*

The study was approved by the Local Ethics Committee for Animal Experiments in Bialystok (Poland) and was performed following the ethical principles, institutional guidelines, and international Guide for the Use of Animals in Biomedical Research.

The rats were allowed to adjust to the experimental facility for five days before the study was started and were randomly divided into six groups, each containing 32 animals. One group received 0.1% aqueous solution of aronia extract alone as the only drinking fluid (AE group), two groups were intoxicated with Cd alone via the diets containing 1 and 5 mg Cd/kg (Cd_1 group and Cd_5 group), and the next two groups received the AE during the whole course of the exposure to Cd (Cd_1 + AE group and Cd_5 + AE group) for 3, 10, 17, and 24 months. The Cd_1 group and Cd_5 group, unlike the Cd_1 + AE group and Cd_5 + AE group, did not receive the AE. The last group, maintained on redistilled water (containing < 0.05 μg Cd/L and not completely deprived of bioelements necessary for the bone health) and standard Labofeed diet, served as a control.

The daily intake of Cd throughout the 24-month exposure to the 1 and 5 mg Cd/kg diets, irrespective of whether this xenobiotic was administered alone or in conjunction with the AE, reached 37.50–84.88 μg/kg b.w. and 196.69–404.76 μg/kg b.w., respectively. Cd intake in the control group and AE group was negligible compared to its intake in the Cd_1, Cd_1 + AE, Cd_5, and Cd_5 + AE groups (Table S4) [25,26].

The 0.1% AE was prepared daily by dissolving 1 g of the powdered aronia extract in 1 L of redistilled water. The total polyphenols concentration in the 0.1% aqueous AE reached 0.612 ± 0.003 mg/mL (mean ± SE) and was stable for 24 h after this solution preparation, while the Cd concentration was <0.05 μg/L [26]. The daily intake of polyphenolic compounds during the whole experiment, irrespective of the manner of their administration, reached 41.5–104.6 mg/kg b.w. and did not differ, regardless of whether the AE was administered alone or under the treatment with Cd (Table S5) [26].

At the end of the 3rd, 10th, 17th, and 24th month of the experiment, eight rats of each group (except for seven animals in the AE group, and the groups treated with 1 and 5 mg Cd/kg diet alone after 24 months), after overnight starvation, were subjected to anaesthesia with Morbital (pentobarbital sodium and pentobarbital 5:1, 30 mg/kg b.w., *i.p.*). The whole blood was taken by cardiac puncture with and without anticoagulant (heparin), and various organs and tissues, including the right femur used in the present study, were dissected.

The femur was immediately cleaned of all adherent soft tissues and weighed with an automatic balance (OHAUS, Switzerland, accuracy to 0.0001 g). Moreover, the bone length and the anterior–posterior (A–P) and medial–lateral (M–L) diameters at the midpoint of the diaphysis were measured with an electronic calliper (±0.02 mm). All the measurements were performed by the same investigator. The precision of these measurements (determined by three measurements of three bones), expressed as a coefficient of variation (CV) for the femur length and diameter, was <0.45% and 0.5%, respectively. The femur of each rat was stored in physiological saline (0.9% sodium chloride) at −20 °C until biomechanical testing was performed. After biomechanical testing, the bone slices collected from the distal epiphysis and diaphysis of the femur were subjected to a PC I measurement.

The experimental model has been described in detail in our previous reports [25–27].

2.5. Bone Biomechanical Testing

The femur was subjected to the mechanical study performed using a testing machine (Zwick 2.5; Zwick GmbH & Co. KG, Ulm, Germany) equipped with a load cell (range of forces up to 2.5 N) and a computer for data acquisition and storage (TestXpert II V3.31 software; Zwick GmbH & Co. KG, Ulm, Germany). A three-point bending test (Section 2.5.1) was performed to estimate the biomechanical properties of the femoral diaphysis (Figure 1A) [15]. Next, the proximal end of the broken femur was used for the measurement of the biomechanical properties of the femoral neck in a bending test (Section 2.5.1; Figure 1B) [15]. All of the tests were performed by the same operator. According to the producer, the measurement error of the method is 0.12% of the value recorded.

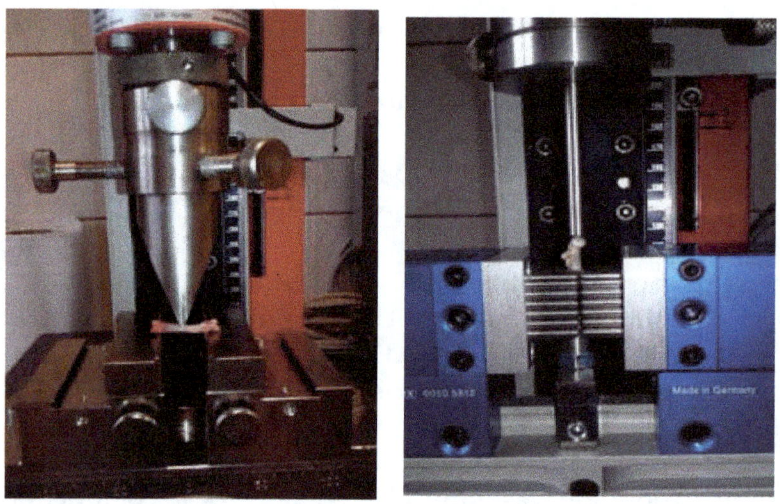

(A) (B)

Figure 1. Representation of the biomechanical testing of the femur (the photos originate from our private collection). (**A**) Three-point bending test of the femoral diaphysis; (**B**) Fracture test of the femoral neck.

The load-deformation curves were recorded during the testing (Sections 2.5.1 and 2.5.2). The yield load and fracture load were determined from the load-deformation curve and computer readings. The yield load is defined as the force causing the first bone damage visible in the load-deformation curve (the force at which the load-deformation curve broke from linearity), whereas the fracture load is the force causing bone fracture. These two forces (yield load and fracture load) describe the bone strength. The yield load (yield strength) reflects the maximum load-bearing capacity under elastic conditions, whereas the fracture load (fracture strength) is the force necessary to cause the bone fracture. Moreover, the bone stiffness was automatically calculated from the linear portion of the load-deformation curve as the ratio of the yield load and the bone deformation at the yield point. The area under the load-deformation curve, reflecting the total energy absorbed by the bone during the test, was measured as work to the bone fracture.

2.5.1. Three Point Bending Test of the Femoral Diaphysis

The femur placed horizontally on two rounded supporting bars, located at a distance of 18 mm, was loaded at the midpoint of the diaphysis in the A–P plane by lowering the third bar (stainless steel pin) at a rate of 2 mm/min, until the bone fracture (Figure 1A).

After finishing the three-point bending test, the vertical (A–P orientation) and horizontal (M–L) internal and external heights at the point of diaphysis fracture were measured. Based on the internal and external heights, geometric properties such as the wall thickness (WT), cross-sectional properties of the M–L axis like cross-sectional area (CSA), and cross-sectional moment of inertia (CSMI) at the point of diaphysis fracture were calculated [15].

The yield load, fracture load, and stiffness describe the "structural" properties of the femur as a whole anatomical unit. To better estimate the biomechanical properties of the femur, the "material" (intrinsic; independent of the tissue size) properties of the bone tissue at the femoral diaphysis were also evaluated. For this purpose, the structural properties of the femoral diaphysis, such as the yield load, fracture load, and stiffness, were normalized for their "geometric" properties, giving the yield stress, fracture stress, and elastic modulus (Young modulus of elasticity), respectively [15]. The yield stress and fracture stress reflect the strength of the bone tissue at the femoral diaphysis, and the values of these parameters were automatically calculated based on the recorded forces and the vertical and horizontal internal and external heights at the point of diaphysis fracture in the three-point bending test [15].

2.5.2. Fracture Test of the Femoral Neck

The proximal end of the broken femur was used for the measurement of the biomechanical properties of the femoral neck (Figure 1B) [15]. The proximal part of the femur was immobilized with special equipment of the Zwick 2.5 testing machine. Next, the bone head was vertically loaded at a displacement rate of 6 mm/min, until the neck fracture [15].

2.6. Determination of PC I

After the femur biomechanical testing, slices of the bone tissue collected from the femoral distal epiphysis (trabecular bone region) and diaphysis (cortical bone region) were separated, with the aim of determining the PC I concentration. The bone tissue was crumbled and washed in ice-cold physiological saline (0.9% sodium chloride), to eliminate the remove-available bone marrow. Next, known weight bone slices were homogenized in cold potassium phosphate buffer (50 mM, pH = 7.4) at 4 °C using a high-performance homogenizer (Ultra-Turrax T25; IKA®, Staufen, Germany) equipped with a stainless-steel dispersing element (S25N-8G; IKA®) to receive an appearing homogenous liquid. The prepared 10% homogenates were centrifuged (MPW-350R centrifugator, Medical Instruments, Warsaw, Poland) at 700× *g* for 20 min at 4 °C, and the aliquots were separated.

The concentration of PC I in the aliquots of the bone tissue was determined with the use of an Enzyme-linked Immunosorbent Assay Kit by Uscn Life Science Inc. (Wuhan, China). The precision of the measurement, expressed as the intra- and inter-assay CV, was <4.8% and 5.2%, respectively.

In order to adjust the bone tissue PC I for the protein concentration, the total protein was assayed in the bone aliquots with the use of a BioMaxima kit (Lublin, Poland).

2.7. Statistical Analysis

A one-way analysis of variance (Anova) was used to determine if there were statistically significant ($p < 0.05$) differences among the six experimental groups and then the Duncan's multiple range post hoc test was conducted for comparisons between individual groups and to determine which two means differed statistically significantly ($p < 0.05$). To discern whether the possible beneficial impact of the AE resulted from an independent action of the extract ingredients and/or their interaction with Cd, a two-way analysis of variance (Anova/Manova, test F) was performed. F values having $p < 0.05$ were considered statistically significant. With the aim of investigating the dependence between the impact of the AE consumption on the biomechanical properties and mineral status of the femur, Spearman rank correlation analysis between the variables describing the bone vulnerability to fracture in the females receiving the extract under the exposure to Cd and previously determined in these animals BMD of the femur [26], was conducted. Correlations were considered statistically significant at $p < 0.05$. All of the statistical calculations were performed using the Statistica package (StatSoft, Tulsa, OK, USA).

3. Results

3.1. Effect of AE on the Femur Weight in Rats Exposed to Cd

The mean absolute and relative weight of the femur in the control rats ranged from 0.6098 ± 0.014 g and 0.2006 ± 0.005 g/100 g b.w., respectively, after three months, up to 0.7703 ± 0.013 g and 0.1306 ± 0.002 g/100 g b.w., respectively, after 24 months of the experiment. The administration of the AE and Cd alone and together had no impact on the absolute and relative femur weight (Table S6).

3.2. Effect of AE on the Geometric Properties of the Femur in Rats Exposed to Cd

The femur length in the control rats ranged from 31.30 ± 0.42 mm after three months to 32.69 ± 0.29 mm after 24 months. The mid-diaphyseal femoral geometric properties such as the M–L and A–P within these animals reached 4.130 ± 0.057 mm and 2.791 ± 0.066 mm, respectively, after three months, and 4.618 ± 0.078 mm and 3.370 ± 0.170 mm, respectively, after 24 months. The administration of the AE and/or Cd for up to 24 months had no impact on the femur length and diameter at the mid-diaphysis (Table S7).

The administration of AE during the whole experiment had no impact on the geometric properties of the femoral diaphysis at the point of its fracture in the three-point bending test (WT, CSA, and CSMI; Table 1). The WT and CSA at the point of diaphysis fracture in the three-point bending test were lower in the animals exposed to the 1 and 5 mg Cd/kg diet for three months (by 14.6% and 15.6%, and 17.7% and 13.2%, respectively), whereas the CSMI was unaffected (Table 1). However, after the longer treatment with Cd, the WT and CSA at the point of diaphysis fracture did not differ compared to the control group, except for the increase (by 12.9%) in the CSA in the Cd_1 group (Table 1).

Table 1. Effect of the extract from the berries of *Aronia melanocarpa* (AE) on the geometric properties of the femur at the point of diaphysis fracture in the three-point bending test in rats exposed to cadmium (Cd).

Group	Experiment Duration			
	3 Months	10 Months	17 Months	24 Months
	WT (mm)			
Control	0.718 ± 0.047	0.691 ± 0.010	0.786 ± 0.036	0.799 ± 0.018
AE	0.636 ± 0.021	0.693 ± 0.017	0.860 ± 0.034	0.798 ± 0.019
Cd_1	0.613 ± 0.019 *	0.678 ± 0.018	0.848 ± 0.021	0.899 ± 0.038
Cd_1 + AE	0.636 ± 0.032 *	0.744 ± 0.023 †	0.756 ± 0.158	0.826 ± 0.051
Cd_5	0.591 ± 0.020 **	0.721 ± 0.020	0.753 ± 0.023	0.819 ± 0.043
Cd_5 + AE	0.633 ± 0.015	0.651 ± 0.020 †,‡‡	0.821 ± 0.054	0.869 ± 0.028
	CSA (mm^2)			
Control	7.610 ± 0.386	7.650 ± 0.083	9.114 ± 0.428	9.571 ± 0.247
AE	6.937 ± 0.365	7.642 ± 0.299	10.011 ± 0.478	9.082 ± 0.214
Cd_1	6.419 ± 0.274 *	7.871 ± 0.235	9.788 ± 0.246	10.810 ± 0.275 *
Cd_1 + AE	6.902 ± 0.335	8.362 ± 0.440	8.999 ± 0.250	9.926 ± 0.407
Cd_5	6.602 ± 0.221 *	8.122 ± 0.286	8.485 ± 0.449	9.616 ± 0.457 ‡
Cd_5 + AE	6.775 ± 0.278	7.277 ± 0.396 ‡	9.178 ± 0.584	10.039 ± 0.433
	CSMI			
Control	3.681 ± 0.208	4.342 ± 0.274	6.338 ± 0.382	8.615 ± 1.682
AE	4.080 ± 0.414	4.980 ± 0.472	7.660 ± 0.612	7.442 ± 0.175
Cd_1	3.606 ± 0.168	4.882 ± 0.200	6.963 ± 0.609	9.850 ± 0.524
Cd_1 + AE	3.778 ± 0.205	5.201 ± 0.381	7.061 ± 0.442	9.271 ± 0.200
Cd_5	4.395 ± 0.390	4.793 ± 0.188	5.239 ± 0.516 ‡	8.943 ± 0.726
Cd_5 + AE	3.721 ± 0.185	4.772 ± 0.356	5.801 ± 0.613	7.762 ± 0.670

Data are represented as mean ± SE for eight rats (except for seven animals in the AE, Cd_1, and Cd_5 groups after 24 months). Statistically significant differences (Anova, Duncan's multiple range test) compared to the control group (* $p < 0.05$, ** $p < 0.01$), respective group receiving Cd alone († $p < 0.05$), and respective group receiving 1 mg Cd/kg diet alone or with the AE (‡ $p < 0.05$, ‡‡ $p < 0.01$) are marked. WT, cortical width; CSA, cross-sectional area; CSMI, cross-sectional moment of inertia.

3.3. *Effect of AE on the Biomechanical Properties of the Femoral Neck in Rats Exposed to Cd*

The administration of the AE alone for three months increased the yield and fracture strength of the femoral neck (Figure 2), as well as the work to the neck fracture (Figure 3), but had no impact on its stiffness (Figure 3). After a longer administration of the extract, all evaluated biomechanical properties of the femoral neck were unchanged compared to the control, except for an increase in the work to the neck fracture after 17 months (Figures 2 and 3).

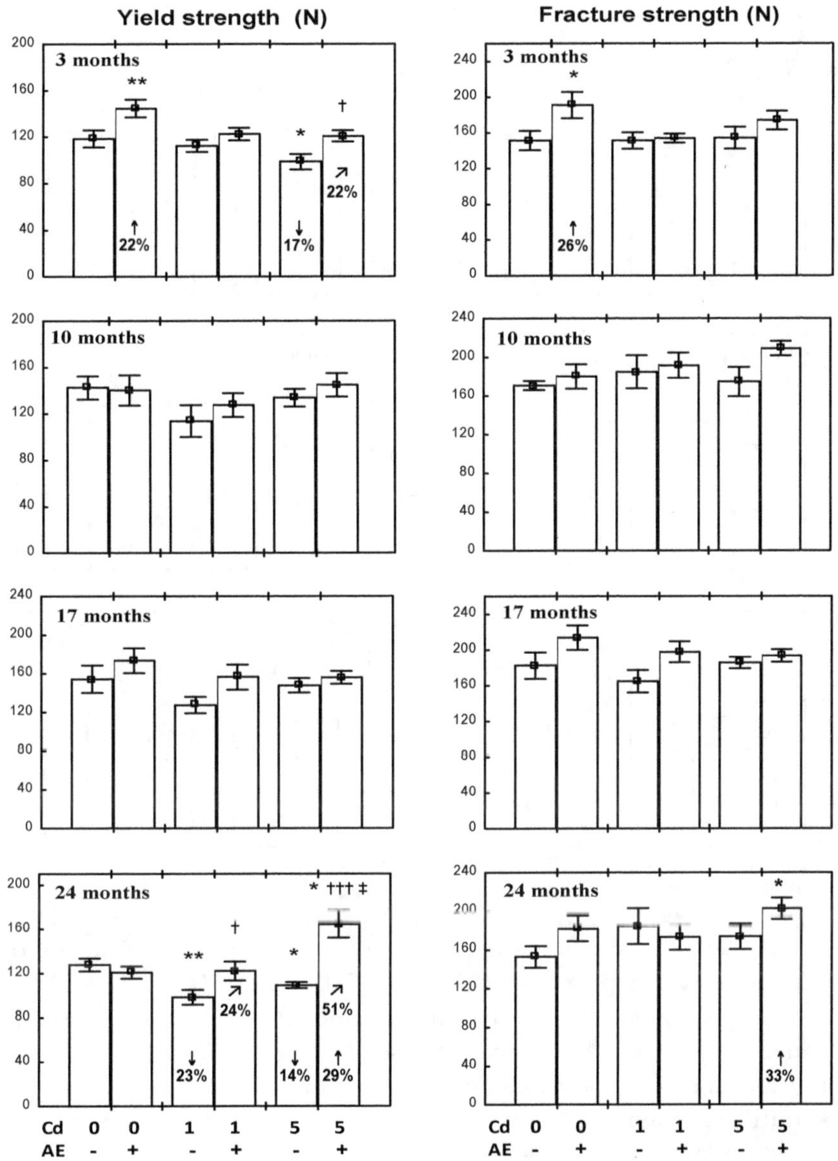

Figure 2. Effect of an extract from the berries of *Aronia melanocarpa* (AE) on the yield and fracture strength of the femoral neck in rats exposed to cadmium (Cd). The rats received 0.1% aqueous AE or not ("+" and "−", respectively) and Cd in diet at the concentration of 0, 1, and 5 mg/kg. Data are represented as mean ± SE for eight rats, except for seven animals in the AE group, and the groups treated with the 1 and 5 mg Cd/kg diet alone after 24 months. Statistically significant differences (Anova, Duncan's multiple range test): * $p < 0.05$, ** $p < 0.01$ vs. control group; † $p < 0.05$, ††† $p < 0.001$ vs. respective group receiving Cd alone; ‡ $p < 0.05$ vs. respective group receiving the 1 mg Cd/kg diet. Numerical values in bars indicate percentage change compared to the control group (↓, decrease; ↑, increase) or the respective group receiving Cd alone (↗, increase).

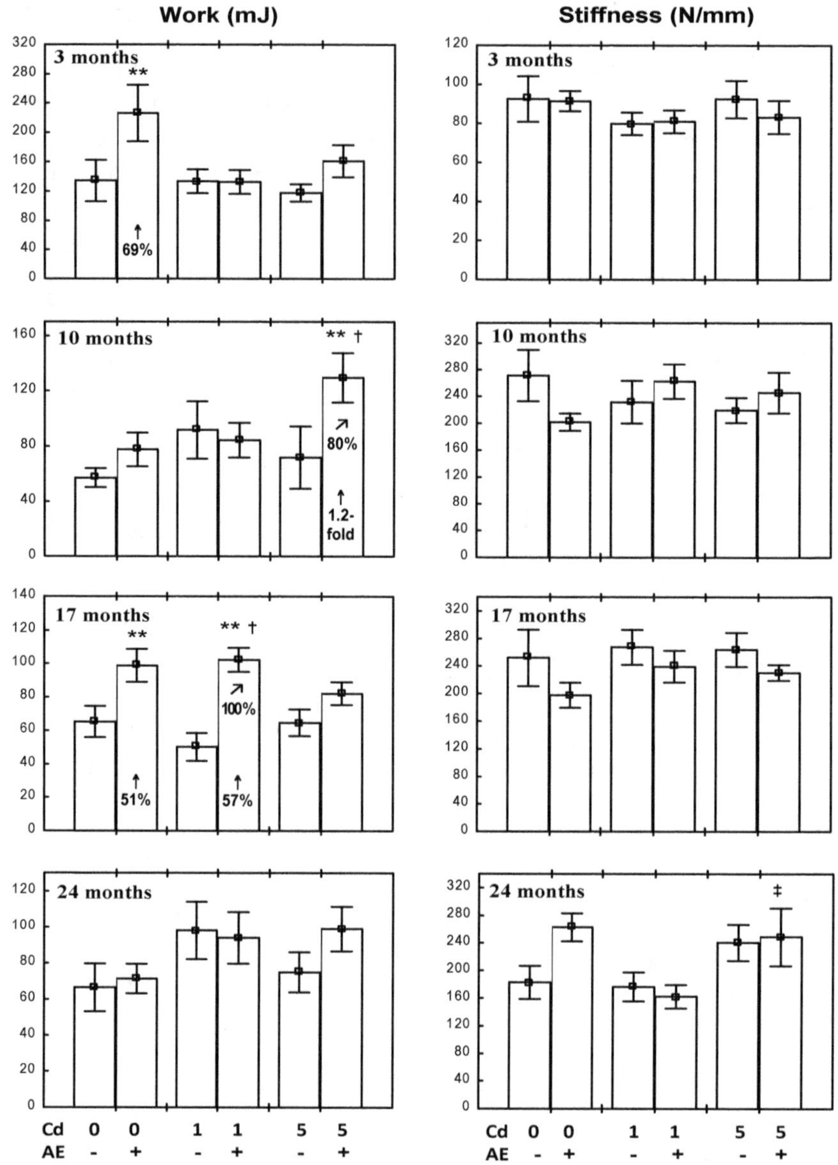

Figure 3. Effect of an extract from the berries of *Aronia melanocarpa* (AE) on the femoral neck stiffness and work to its fracture in rats exposed to cadmium (Cd). The rats received 0.1% aqueous AE or not ("+" and "−", respectively) and Cd in diet at the concentration of 0, 1, and 5 mg/kg. Data are represented as mean ± SE for eight rats, except for seven animals in the AE group, and the groups treated with the 1 and 5 mg Cd/kg diet alone after 24 months. Statistically significant differences (Anova, Duncan's multiple range test): ** $p < 0.01$ vs. control group; † $p < 0.05$ vs. respective group receiving Cd alone; ‡ $p < 0.05$ vs. respective group receiving the 1 mg Cd/kg diet. Numerical values in bars indicate percentage change or a factor of change compared to the control group (↑, increase) or the respective group receiving Cd alone (↗, increase).

The exposure to the 1 mg Cd/kg diet for 3, 10, and 17 months had no impact on the biomechanical properties of the femoral neck; however, after 24 months, the yield strength was decreased (Figures 2 and 3). In the animals treated with the 5 mg Cd/kg diet, the only change in the evaluated biomechanical parameters was a decrease in the yield strength after three and 24 months (Figures 2 and 3).

In the animals receiving the AE under the exposure to the 1 mg Cd/kg diet for 17 months, the work to the neck fracture was higher compared to the control group and the group treated with Cd alone (Figure 3). Moreover, the AE completely prevented the 24-month exposure to Cd-induced decrease in the yield strength (Figure 2). The Anova/Manova analysis revealed that the beneficial impact of the AE consumption under the low treatment with Cd on the yield strength of the femoral neck was an effect of the independent action of this extract's ingredients ($F = 4.309$, $p < 0.05$) and their interaction with this heavy metal ($F = 5.166$, $p < 0.05$). The AE administration to the animals treated with 5 mg Cd/kg diet completely prevented the three- and 24-month exposure-induced decrease in the yield strength of the femoral neck (Figure 2), and this effect resulted from the independent action of the extract ($F = 10.574$, $p < 0.001$) after three months and from its interaction with Cd ($F = 17.184$, $p < 0.001$) after 24 months. Moreover, the yield strength and fracture strength of the femoral neck in the Cd_5 + AE group after 24 months were higher than in the control group (Figure 2). The extract administration under the 10-month exposure to the 5 mg Cd/kg diet increased the work to the neck fracture compared to the control group and the Cd_5 group (Figure 3), as a result of its independent action ($F = 4.362$, $p < 0.05$).

3.4. *Effect of AE on the Biomechanical Properties of the Femoral Diaphysis in Rats Exposed to Cd*

The administration of the AE alone had no impact on the "structural" biomechanical properties (yield strength, fracture strength, stiffness, and work to fracture) of the femoral diaphysis, apart from an increase in the fracture strength after 24 months and a decrease in the stiffness after 10 months, as well as a decrease in the work to fracture after 10 months and its increase after 17 and 24 months (Figures 4 and 5). The only "material" biomechanical property influenced by the consumption of the AE alone was a decrease in the Young modulus of elasticity after 10 months (Figure 6).

The exposure to Cd affected both the "structural" and "material" biomechanical properties of the femoral diaphysis (Figures 4–6). In the rats treated with 1 mg Cd/kg diet, the yield strength, yield stress, and stiffness were decreased after 17 and 24 months (Figures 4–6). Moreover, after 17 months, the fracture strength and fracture stress were decreased, while after 24 months, the work to the diaphysis fracture was increased (Figures 4–6). At the higher exposure to Cd, the yield strength was decreased after 17 and 24 months and the fracture strength and stiffness decreased after 17 months, whereas the work to fracture was increased after 10 and 24 months (Figures 4 and 5). Moreover, the treatment with the 5 mg Cd/kg diet increased the fracture stress after 17 months and decreased the yield stress after 24 months (Figure 6).

The administration of the AE during the exposure to the 1 mg Cd/kg diet completely prevented this heavy metal-induced decrease in the femoral diaphysis yield strength (Figure 4), stiffness (Figure 5), yield stress, and fracture stress (Figure 6). Moreover, the stiffness and fracture strength in the Cd_1 + AE group after 24 months were increased compared to the control group and Cd_1 group (Figures 4 and 5). The Anova/Manova analysis revealed that the impact of the AE consumption under the low-level exposure to Cd on the fracture strength of the femoral diaphysis was an effect of the independent action of this extract's ingredients ($F = 8.206$, $p < 0.01$) and their interaction with this toxic metal ($F = 8.361$, $p < 0.01$). Apart from that, the administration of the AE under the 10-month treatment with the 1 mg Cd/kg diet resulted in a decrease in the stiffness of the femoral diaphysis and work to its fracture, and this impact was caused by the interactive action of the extract's ingredients and Cd ($F = 6.194$, $p < 0.05$ and $F = 7.507$, $p < 0.05$, respectively). The administration of the AE under the 17-month exposure to the 1 mg Cd/kg diet increased the work to the femoral diaphysis fracture compared to the control group and the Cd_1 group, whereas the extract consumption for 24 months had no impact on the Cd-increased value of this parameter. The consumption of the AE under the higher Cd treatment entirely prevented this heavy metal-caused decrease in the yield strength and fracture strength (Figure 4). The beneficial impact on the yield strength resulted from the independent action of the AE after 17 months ($F = 6.643$, $p < 0.05$) and its interaction with Cd after 24 months ($F = 11.43$, $p < 0.01$). The 24-month administration of the extract increased the femoral diaphysis fracture strength (Figure 4) and its stiffness compared to the control group and Cd_5 group (Figure 5), and the diaphysis fracture stress compared to the control group (Figure 6). According to the results of the Anova/Manova analysis, the favourable impact of the AE administration for 24 months on the fracture strength was an effect of its independent action ($F = 9.720$, $p < 0.01$), whereas the influence on the femoral diaphysis stiffness and yield stress of the bone tissue at the femoral diaphysis resulted from the AE–Cd interaction (F = 5.977, $p < 0.05$ and F = 6.883, $p < 0.05$, respectively). Moreover, this extract administration under the 10-month exposure to the 5 mg Cd/kg diet resulted in a decrease in the work to the diaphysis fracture compared to the control group and Cd_5 group, increased the value of this biomechanical parameter compared to the control group after 17 months, and completely prevented its increase after 24 months (Figure 5). The Anova/Manova analysis revealed that the impact of the AE administration on the work to the diaphysis fracture after 10 months was an effect of both its independent (F = 14.03, $p < 0.01$) and interactive action with Cd (F = 53.20, $p < 0.001$), whereas after 17 months, this was only a result of the AE–Cd interaction (F = 18.75, $p < 0.01$). Apart from that, the 10-month consumption of the AE under the exposure to the 5 mg Cd/kg diet decreased the stiffness of the femoral diaphysis (Figure 5) as a result of the interaction with Cd (F = 8.219, $p < 0.01$).

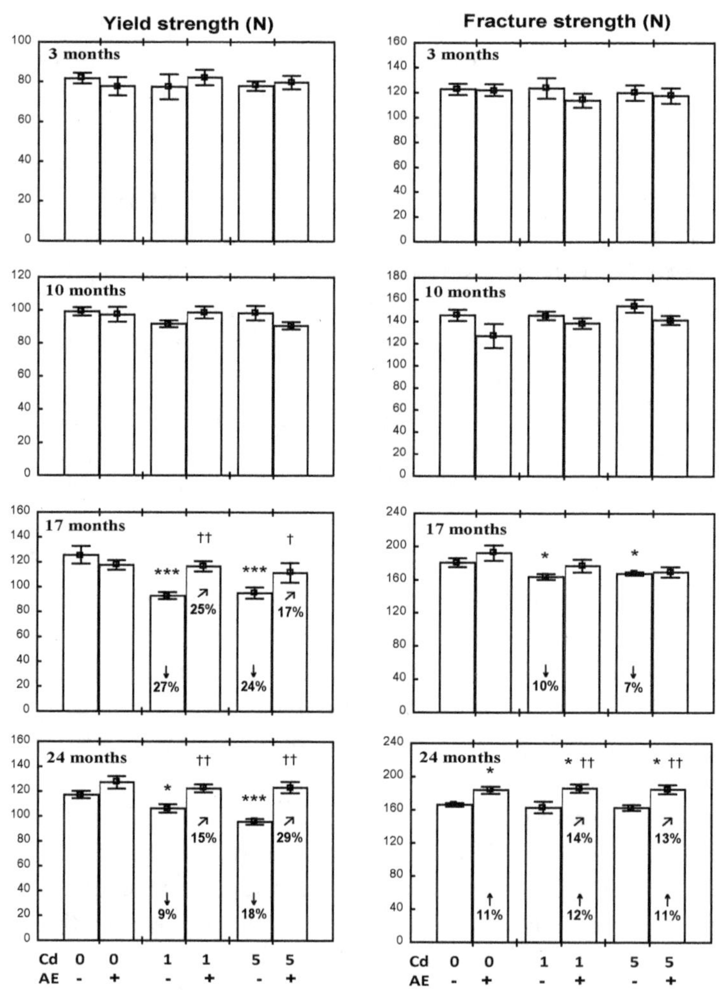

Figure 4. Effect of an extract from the berries of *Aronia melanocarpa* (AE) on the yield and fracture strength of the femoral diaphysis in rats exposed to cadmium (Cd). The rats received 0.1% aqueous AE or not ("+" and "−", respectively) and Cd in diet at the concentration of 0, 1, and 5 mg/kg. Data are represented as mean ± SE for eight rats, except for seven animals in the AE group, and the groups treated with the 1 and 5 mg Cd/kg diet alone after 24 months. Statistically significant differences (Anova, Duncan's multiple range test): * $p < 0.05$, *** $p < 0.001$ vs. control group; † $p < 0.05$, †† $p < 0.01$ vs. respective group receiving Cd alone. Numerical values in bars indicate percentage change compared to the control group (↑, increase; ↓, decrease) or the respective group receiving Cd alone (↗, increase).

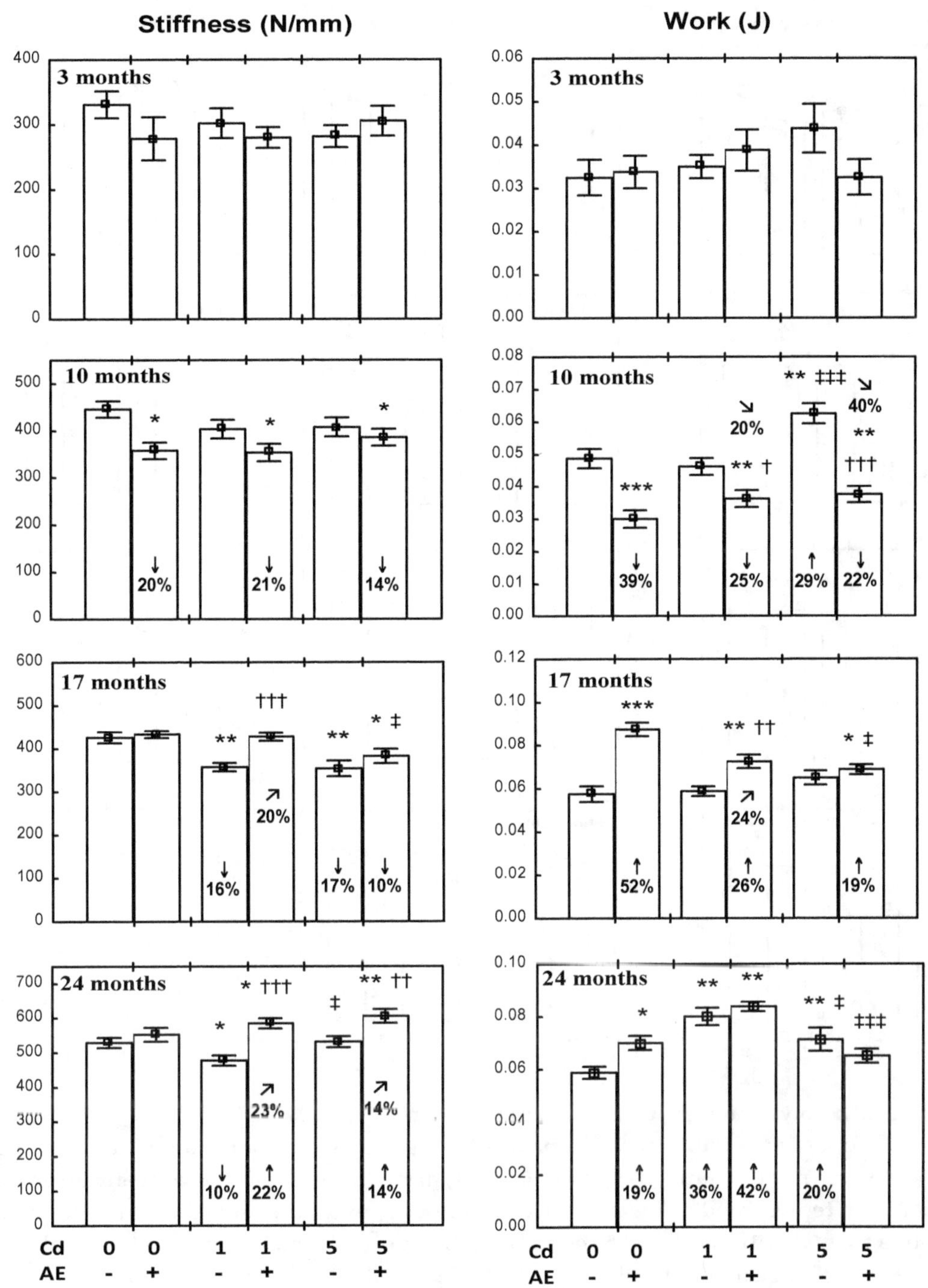

Figure 5. Effect of a polyphenol-rich extract from the berries of *Aronia melanocarpa* (AE) on the femoral diaphysis stiffness and work to its fracture in rats exposed to cadmium (Cd). The rats received 0.1% aqueous AE or not ("+" and "−", respectively) and Cd in diet at the concentration of 0, 1, and 5 mg/kg. Data are represented as mean ± SE for eight rats, except for seven animals in the AE group, and the groups treated with the 1 and 5 mg Cd/kg diet alone after 24 months. Statistically significant differences (Anova, Duncan's multiple range test): * $p < 0.05$, ** $p < 0.01$, *** $p < 0.001$ vs. control group; † $p < 0.05$, †† $p < 0.01$, ††† $p < 0.001$ vs. respective group receiving Cd alone; ‡ $p < 0.05$, ‡‡‡ $p < 0.001$ vs. respective group receiving the 1 mg Cd/kg diet. Numerical values in bars or above the bars indicate percentage change compared to the control group (↑, increase; ↓, decrease) or the respective group receiving Cd alone (↗, increase; ↘, decrease).

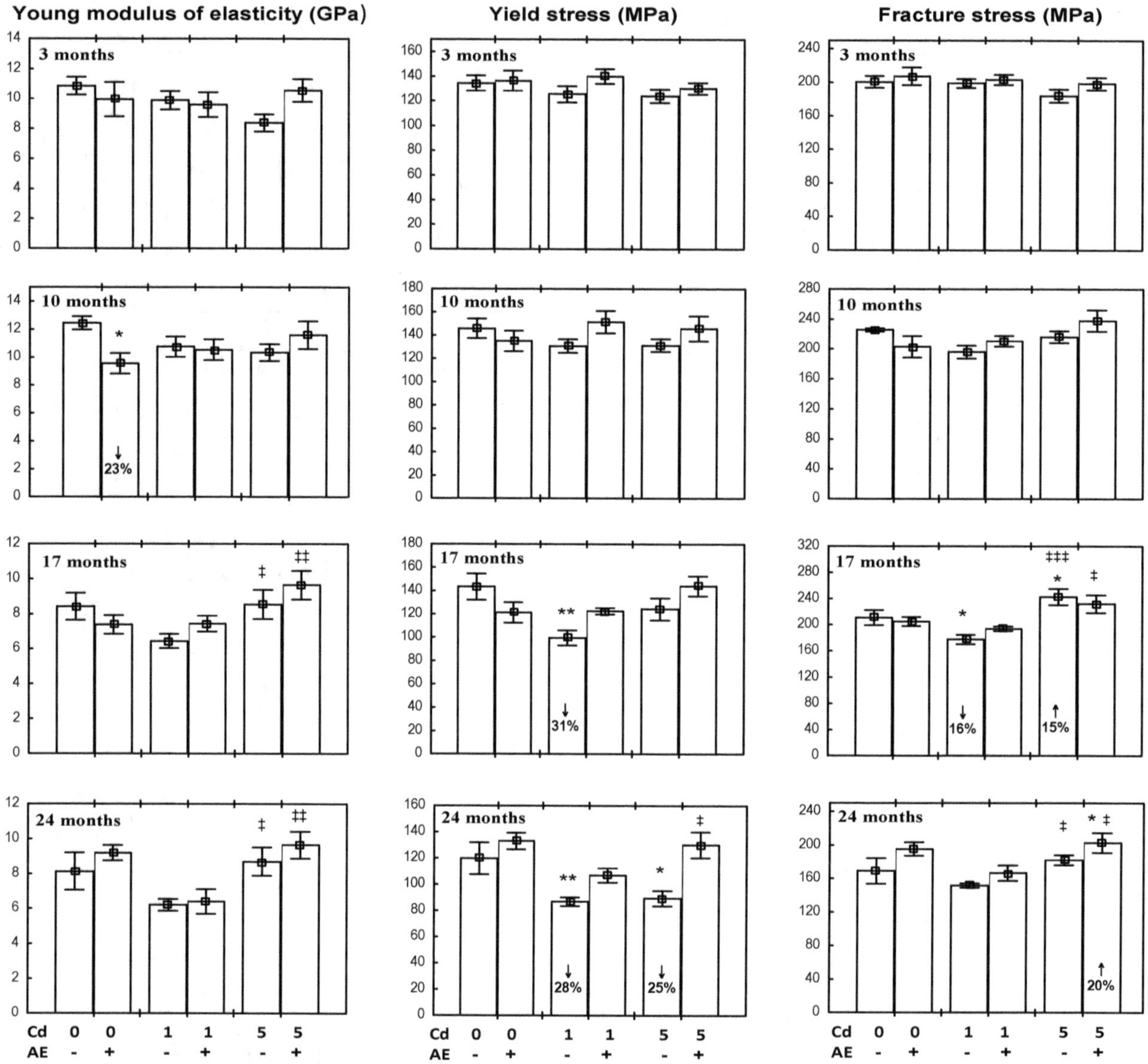

Figure 6. Effect of a polyphenol-rich extract from the berries of *Aronia melanocarpa* (AE) on the "material" biomechanical properties of the femoral diaphysis in rats exposed to cadmium (Cd). The rats received 0.1% aqueous AE or not ("+" and "−", respectively) and Cd in diet at the concentration of 0, 1, and 5 mg/kg. Data are represented as mean ± SE for eight rats, except for seven animals in the AE group, and the groups treated with the 1 and 5 mg Cd/kg diet alone after 24 months. Statistically significant differences (Anova, Duncan's multiple range test): * $p < 0.05$, ** $p < 0.01$ vs. control group; ‡ $p < 0.05$, ‡‡ $p < 0.01$, ‡‡‡ $p < 0.001$ vs. respective group receiving the 1 mg Cd/kg diet. Numerical values in bars indicate percentage change compared to the control group (↑, increase; ↓, decrease).

3.5. Effect of AE on PC I Concentration in the Bone Tissue in Rats Exposed to Cd

The administration of the AE alone for up to 24 months had no impact on the PC I concentration in the bone tissue at the distal epiphysis and diaphysis of the femur (Figure 7).

The exposure to the 1 mg Cd/kg diet for 10, 17, and 24 months resulted in a decrease in the bone tissue concentration of PC I, except for a lack of change in this parameter concentration at the distal femoral diaphysis after 24 months (Figure 7). At the higher exposure to Cd, the concentration of PC I in the bone tissue at the femoral epiphysis was decreased through the whole experiment, while the value of this parameter in the bone tissue at the femoral diaphysis was decreased after the 10th month (Figure 7).

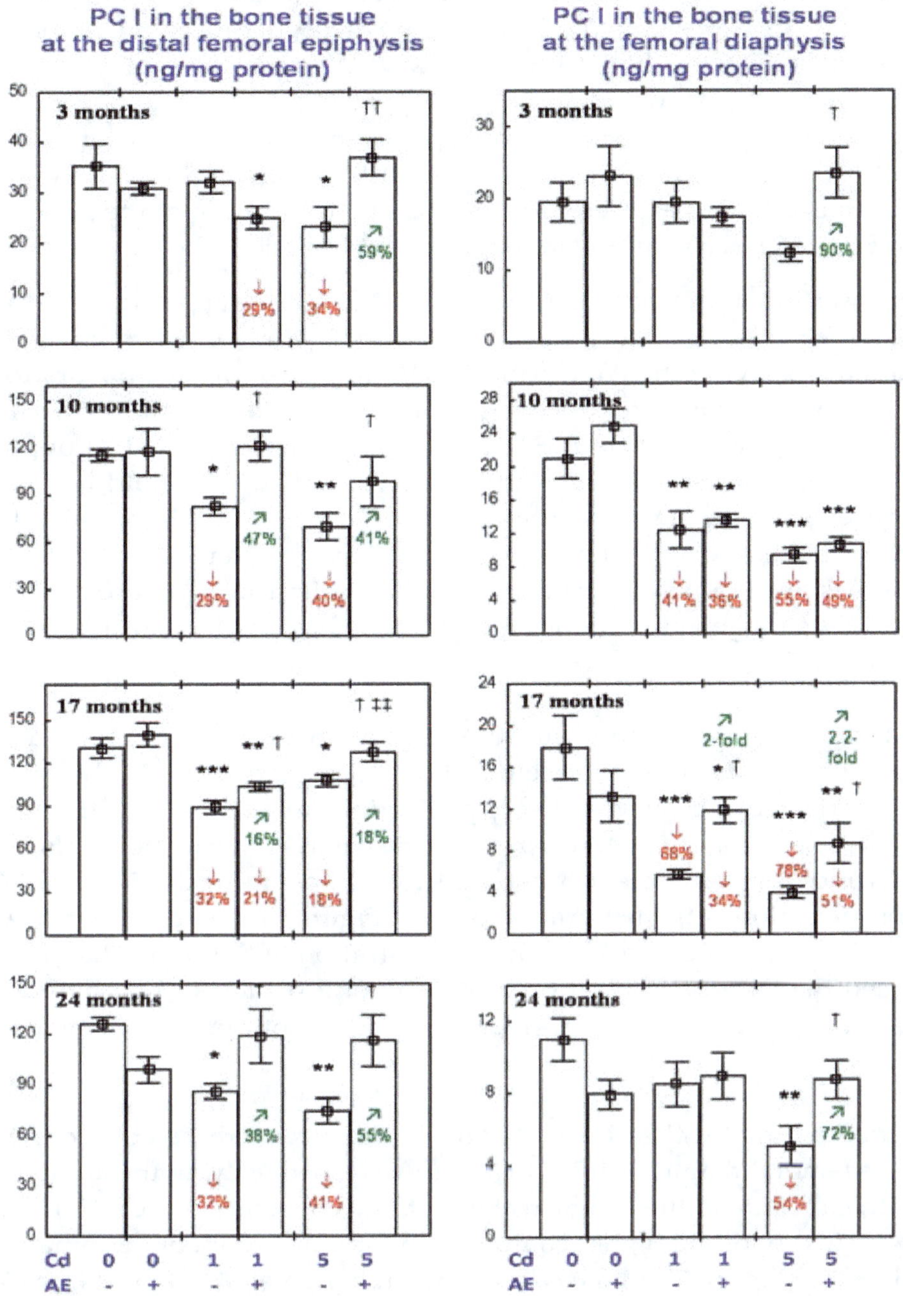

Figure 7. Effect of a polyphenol-rich extract from the berries of *Aronia melanocarpa* (AE) on procollagen I concentration in the bone tissue of rats exposed to cadmium (Cd). The rats received 0.1% aqueous AE or not ("+" and "−", respectively) and Cd in diet at the concentration of 0, 1, and 5 mg/kg. Data are represented as mean ± SE for eight rats, except for seven animals in the AE group, and the groups treated with the 1 and 5 mg Cd/kg diet alone after 24 months. Statistically significant differences (Anova, Duncan's multiple range test): * $p < 0.05$, ** $p < 0.01$, *** $p < 0.001$ vs. control group; † $p < 0.05$, †† $p < 0.01$ vs. respective group receiving Cd alone; ‡‡ $p < 0.01$ vs. respective group receiving the 1 mg Cd/kg diet. Numerical values in bars or above the bars indicate percentage change or a factor of change compared to the control group (↓, decrease) or the respective group receiving Cd alone (↗, increase).

The administration of the AE to the animals fed with the diets containing 1 and 5 mg Cd/kg completely prevented the above-described decrease in the concentration of PC I in the bone tissue at the distal femoral epiphysis, except for a partial protection after 17 months of the exposure to the 1 mg

Cd/kg diet (Figure 7). The effect of the AE on the PC I concentration in the bone tissue at the distal femoral epiphysis in the rats exposed to the 1 mg Cd/kg diet was caused by an independent action of the extract ($F = 4.621$, $p < 0.05$) after 10 months, whereas the impact after 24 months resulted from the interaction of ingredients of the AE with Cd ($F = 10.13$, $p < 0.01$). Moreover, the tendency of the AE and Cd to interactively impact the PC I concentration after 10 months ($F = 3.832$, $p = 0.06$) and the extract alone after 17 months ($F = 3.680$, $p = 0.06$) was noted. The AE consumption under the three-month treatment with the 1 mg Cd/kg diet decreased the PC I concentration in the bone tissue at the distal femoral epiphysis (Figure 7) as a result of an independent impact of the extract ($F = 4.246$, $p < 0.05$).

The PC I concentration in the bone tissue at the distal femoral epiphysis of the rats exposed to the 1 mg Cd/kg diet for 10–24 months was, on average, 29–32% lower than in the control group, whereas in the animals receiving the AE during the 10- and 24-month exposure to the 1 mg Cd/kg diet, the concentration of this biomarker of collagen biosynthesis did not differ when compared to the control group (and was higher by 47% and 38%, respectively, than in the Cd_1 group). After 17 months, the value of this parameter was 21% lower than in the control animals (and was 16% higher than in the Cd_1 group; Figure 7). The exposure to the 5 mg Cd/kg diet for 3–24 months decreased the PC I concentration in the bone tissue at the femoral epiphysis by an average of 18–41% compared to the control group, whereas in the animals receiving the AE under the exposure to Cd, the value of this parameter was within the range of the control group and was an average of 18–59% higher compared to the Cd_5 group (Figure 7).

The administration of the AE under the 10-month exposure to the 1 and 5 mg Cd/kg diet had no impact on the PC I concentration at the femoral diaphysis; however, in the case of the 17-month co-administration, partial, but clearly evident, protection, resulting from the AE ingredients–Cd interaction ($F = 6.771$, $p < 0.05$ and $F = 4.513$, $p < 0.05$, respectively), was noted (Figure 7). The extract consumption for 24 months completely prevented the exposure to the 5 mg Cd/kg diet-induced decrease in PC I concentration at the femoral diaphysis (Figure 7) as a result of the AE–Cd interaction ($F = 9.926$, $p < 0.01$). Moreover, the three-month administration of the AE to the rats fed with the 5 mg Cd/kg diet increased the PC I concentration at the femoral diaphysis compared to the Cd_5 group (Figure 7) and the effect resulted from an independent action of the extract's ingredients ($F = 5.603$, $p < 0.05$).

The exposure to the 1 mg Cd/kg diet for 10 and 17 months decreased the concentration of PC I in the bone tissue at the femoral diaphysis by 41% and 68%, respectively. In the animals receiving the AE during the 17-month exposure to the 1 mg Cd/kg diet, the concentration of PC I in the bone tissue at the femoral diaphysis was two-fold higher compared to the Cd_1 group, but it remained lower (by 34%) than in the control group (Figure 7). In the case of the higher level of Cd exposure (5 mg Cd/kg diet), the PC I concentration in the bone tissue at the femoral diaphysis after 17 and 24 months was 78% and 54% lower, respectively, compared to the control group, whereas in the case of the co-administration of Cd and the AE, the concentration was 2.2-fold and 72% higher, respectively, than in the Cd_5 group. Moreover, after 17 months, the concentration of PC I remained 51% lower than in the control group, while after 24 months, it did not differ compared to the proper values of the control animals.

3.6. Dependence Between the Femur BMD and Its Biomechanical Properties in Rats Exposed to Cd

In the animals receiving the AE under the exposure to Cd, positive correlations were noted between the femur BMD and the yield strength ($r = 0.525$, $p < 0.001$), fracture strength ($r = 0.499$, $p < 0.001$), stiffness ($r = 0.459$, $p < 0.001$), and work to the femoral diaphysis fracture ($r = 0.445$, $p < 0.001$). Moreover, the femur BMD negatively correlated ($r = -0.246$, $p < 0.05$) with the Young modulus of elasticity of the bone tissue at the femoral diaphysis. A positive correlation was also noted between the femur BMD and the stiffness of the femoral neck ($r = 0.260$, $p < 0.05$).

4. Discussion

The present study is the first that investigated and revealed the protective impact of AE consumption under low-level and moderate chronic exposure to Cd on the bone biomechanical properties and collagen biosynthesis in the bone tissue. Although this study was focused mainly on the possibility of the protective influence of the AE on the femur biomechanical properties under chronic exposure to Cd, it has also provided important data on the effect of low-level chronic exposure to Cd on bone vulnerability to fracture.

The study not only confirmed the previously reported results by us [15–18] relating to the unfavourable impact of low exposure to this heavy metal on the bone biomechanical properties, but it also provided evidence that the biomechanical properties of the femur may be weakened at a lower exposure than was previously shown and a very low Cd concentration in the blood and urine (0.185–0.324 μg/L and 0.107–0.285 μg/g creatinine, respectively; such concentrations were reached after 17–24 months of the exposure to the 1 mg Cd/kg diet [25]), comparable to the metal concentrations commonly noted in the general population. Weakening of the bone biomechanical properties at such a low Cd concentration in the blood and urine has been reported in the present paper for the first time. The impact of Cd on the biomechanical properties of the femoral neck and diaphysis evaluated in the current study was relatively subtle, but clearly evident taking into account the fact that the unfavourable effect occurred at low-level exposure, resulting in a blood and urinary Cd concentration comparable to this metal's concentration noted in the general population. The effect of Cd on the femur biomechanical properties in the female rats was less serious than that previously reported by us [15–18], but the investigated levels of exposure were also lower. The decrease in the yield and fracture strength of the femoral diaphysis after 17 months and in the yield strength of the femoral neck after 24 months provide evidence of decreased bone resistance to fracture, resulting in an enhancement in the risk of fracture due to long-term low-level exposure to this heavy metal. However, it should be clearly underlined that the changes in the biomechanical properties of the femur observed in the present study show that long-term, even very low-level, intoxication with this toxic metal has an unfavourable impact on the skeleton. At both levels of exposure, the impact of Cd on the strength of the femur was clearly evident after only 17 months of intoxication. As was reported in detail in our previous papers, the weakening of the biomechanical properties of the femur due to the treatment with Cd results from the unfavourable impact of this heavy metal on the mineral status and organic matrix (formed mainly by collagen) of the bone [15–18,33,34]. The proper amount and structure of collagen fibers play an important role in bone formation and strength [29,30,35]. The results of the present study show that the low exposure to Cd (1 mg Cd/kg diet) inhibited collagen biosynthesis in the bone tissue after 10 months. Because the impact of Cd on the "structural" and "material" biomechanical properties of the femoral diaphysis and the femoral neck susceptibility to fracture was previously reported by us [15–18,33], and the mechanisms leading to an increase in the bone susceptibility to fracture are known and reported, they are not discussed in the present paper. However, the very important finding of the present study regarding the impact of Cd on the femur susceptibility to fracture reveals that this heavy metal may weaken the biomechanical properties of the femoral neck and diaphysis at an exposure lower than has been revealed until now [16,18].

The biomechanical tests performed conclusively revealed that the consumption of the chokeberry extract under long-term low and moderate exposure to Cd improved the femur resistance to fracture. The protective impact of the AE may be explained by the recently reported results by us relating to the beneficial influence of the extract on bone turnover, reflected in an improvement in the femur BMD (Tables S1 and S2) [26] and revealed in the present study's protection from the Cd-induced inhibition of collagen biosynthesis. The possible mechanism of the extract's impact on the bone mineral status has been previously reported by us [26] and it consists of an inhibition of Cd-induced bone resorption and the stimulation of the processes of bone formation. It was also revealed by us that the mechanism of osteoprotective action of the AE extract is mediated by its antioxidative properties, as well as the improvement of the oxidative/antioxidative balance in the bone tissue and protection from oxidative stress and oxidative damage to macromolecules in the bone tissue [27].

The results of the Anova/Manova analysis allow us to recognize that the beneficial impact of the AE administration on the biomechanical properties of the femur resulted from both an independent action of the ingredients of the extract and their interaction with Cd, resulting in a lower body burden of this metal and its lower accumulation in the bone tissue [25–27]. As a result of the AE ingredients–Cd interaction, the direct and indirect damaging impact of this toxic metal on the skeleton has been weakened. The independent impact of the AE ingredients on the skeleton may be explained mainly by the action of polyphenolic compounds, being the most abundant active components of the aronia berries. Polyphenolic compounds are widely known from their osteoprotective impact related with the improvement of BMD, but the data mainly refers to green tea polyphenols [7,24,36]. In the available literature, apart from our recent reports [25–27], there is no data on the impact of the consumption of aronia berries and their products on bone metabolism and bone strength properties. However, our findings in the animals administered the AE alone for 3, 10, 17, and 24 months provide clear evidence for an independent influence of the extract's ingredients on the skeleton, including the impact on the bone turnover, bone mineral status, oxidative/antioxidative status of the bone tissue, and the bone biomechanical properties [22–24]. It seems possible that the main cause of the beneficial impact of the AE under exposure to Cd on the femur biomechanical properties is this extract-caused improvement of the bone mineral status [26]. The positive correlations noted in the current study between the femur BMD and biomechanical properties of the femoral diaphysis (yield and fracture strength, stiffness, work to fracture) in the animals administered with the AE under exposure to Cd confirm the validity of this reasoning. The bone mineral status is one of the main determinants of the bone vulnerability to fracture [28]. Thus, the improvement in the bone mineral status is also related to the improvement in the bone strength properties. Owing to the lack of any literature data on the impact of *A. melanocarpa* on the bone biomechanical properties and the bone susceptibility to fracture, a wider discussion of the results is impossible.

We are aware not only of the achievements, but also of the limitations, of our designed studies on the possible protective impact of AE on the skeleton. At this stage of our investigation, we are unable to explain the exact mechanisms of the beneficial impact of AE on the bone, including the bone susceptibility to fractures, nonetheless our experiment provided unquestionable evidence for this protection. Moreover, because our study was conducted on a female rat model of lifetime environmental exposure, the findings refer to the female skeleton and further study involving an evaluation of AE on the male skeleton is warranted.

5. Conclusions

In summary, the present study provides the first evidence that the consumption of AE under chronic exposure to Cd improves the biomechanical properties of the femur, increasing its resistance to fracture at the neck and diaphysis. Fracture is the most serious consequence of the damaging impact of any factor on bone, thus revealing the fact that chokeberry extract enhances the femur resistance to fracture under exposure to Cd is a very important and practically useful finding of our study. This finding, together with our previous results on the bone impact of AE in the experimental model of the lifetime women exposure to Cd [25–27], provide strong evidence, allowing us to recognize that the consumption of aronia berries and their products under chronic exposure to this heavy metal seems to be a promising natural strategy for preventing skeletal damage. However, the possible use of the *A. melanocarpa* berries as a prophylactic of bone diseases in humans needs further investigation. It seems necessary to analyse the relationship between the consumption of the aronia berries and the bone status in subjects chronically exposed to Cd, including both males and females.

Acknowledgments: This study was financially supported in part by the Grant (No. N N405 051140) from the National Science Centre (Poland) and Medical University of Bialystok (Poland). The study was conducted with the use of equipment by Medical University of Bialystok as part of the OP DEP 2007–2013, Priority Axis I.3, contract No. POPW.01.00-20-001/12.

Author Contributions: Małgorzata M. Brzóska designed the research, participated in the experiment, interpreted the data, and designed and wrote the paper; Alicja Roszczenko and Joanna Rogalska performed the experiment and statistical analysis, and participated in the manuscript preparation; Małgorzata Gałażyn-Sidorczuk performed the experiment and participated in the manuscript preparation; Magdalena Mężyńska participated in the experiment and manuscript preparation. All authors approved the final version of the manuscript.

Abbreviations

AE, extract from the berries of *Aronia melanocarpa*; A–P, anterior–posterior; BMD, bone mineral density; Cd, cadmium; CSA, cross-sectional area; CSMI, cross-sectional moment of inertia; CV, coefficient of variation; M–L, medial–lateral; PC I, procollagen I; WT, wall thickness.

References

1. Dahl, C.; Søgaard, A.J.; Tell, G.S.; Flaten, T.P.; Hongve, D.; Omsland, T.K.; Holvik, K.; Meyer, H.E.; Aamodt, G. Norwegian Epidemiologic Osteoporosis Study (NOREPOS) Core Research Group. Do cadmium, lead, and aluminum in drinking water increase the risk of hip fractures? A NOREPOS study. *Biol. Trace Elem. Res.* **2014**, *157*, 14–23. [CrossRef] [PubMed]
2. Søgaard, A.J.; Meyer, H.E.; Emaus, N.; Grimnes, G.; Gjesdal, C.G.; Forsmo, S.; Schei, B.; Tell, G.S. Cohort profile: Norwegian Epidemiologic Osteoporosis Studies (NOREPOS). *Scand. J. Public Health* **2014**, *42*, 804–813. [CrossRef] [PubMed]
3. Wong, A.K.O.; Beattie, K.A.; Bhargava, A.; Cheung, M.; Webber, C.E.; Chettle, D.R.; Papaioannou, A.; Adach, J.D. Bone lead (Pb) content at the tibia is associated with thinner distal tibia cortices and lower volumetric bone density in postmenopausal women. *Bone* **2015**, *79*, 58–64. [CrossRef] [PubMed]
4. Shen, C.L.; Yeh, J.K.; Cao, J.J.; Wang, J.S. Green tea and bone metabolism. *Nutr. Res.* **2009**, *29*, 437–456. [CrossRef] [PubMed]
5. Gunn, C.A.; Weber, J.L.; McGill, A.T.; Kruger, M.C. Increased intake of selected vegetables, herbs and fruit may reduce bone turnover in post-menopausal women. *Nutrients* **2015**, *7*, 2499–2517. [CrossRef] [PubMed]
6. Hardcastle, A.C.; Aucott, L.; Reid, D.M.; Macdonald, H.M. Associations between dietary flavonoid intakes and bone health in a Scottish population. *J. Bone Miner. Res.* **2011**, *26*, 941–947. [CrossRef] [PubMed]
7. Shen, C.L.; Chyu, M.C.; Wang, J.S. Tea and bone health: Steps forward in translational nutrition. *Am. J. Clin. Nutr.* **2013**, *98*, 1694S–1699S. [CrossRef] [PubMed]
8. Chen, X.; Wang, K.; Wang, Z.; Gan, C.; He, P.; Liang, Y.; Jin, T.; Zhu, G. Effects of lead and cadmium co-exposure on bone mineral density in a Chinese population. *Bone* **2014**, *63*, 76–80. [CrossRef] [PubMed]
9. Callan, A.C.; Devine, A.; Qi, L.; Ng, J.C.; Hinwood, A.L. Investigation of the relationship between low environmental exposure to metals and bone mineral density, bone resorption and renal function. *Int. J. Hyg. Environ. Health* **2015**, *218*, 444–451. [CrossRef] [PubMed]
10. Wallin, M.; Barregard, L.; Sallsten, G.; Lundh, T.; Karlsson, M.K.; Lorentzon, M.; Ohlsson, C.; Mellström, D. Low-level cadmium exposure is associated with decreased bone mineral density and increased risk of incident fractures in elderly men: The MrOS Sweden study. *J. Bone Miner. Res.* **2015**, *31*, 732–741. [CrossRef] [PubMed]
11. Nawrot, T.S.; Staessen, J.A.; Roels, H.A.; Munters, E.; Cuypers, A.; Richart, T.; Ruttens, A.; Smeets, K.; Clijsters, H.; Vangronsveld, J. Cadmium exposure in the population: From health risks to strategies of prevention. *Biometals* **2010**, *23*, 769–782. [CrossRef] [PubMed]
12. Satarug, S.; Vesey, D.A.; Gobe, G.C. Health risk assessment of dietary cadmium intake: Do current guidelines indicate how much is safe? *Environ. Health Perspect.* **2017**, *125*, 284–288. [CrossRef] [PubMed]
13. Brzóska, M.M.; Moniuszko-Jakoniuk, J. Low-level exposure to cadmium during the lifetime increases the risk of osteoporosis and fractures of the lumbar spine in the elderly: Studies on a rat model of human environmental exposure. *Toxicol. Sci.* **2004**, *82*, 468–477. [CrossRef] [PubMed]

14. Brzóska, M.M.; Moniuszko-Jakoniuk, J. Low-level lifetime exposure to cadmium decreases skeletal mineralization and enhances bone loss in aged rats. *Bone* **2004**, *35*, 1180–1191. [CrossRef] [PubMed]
15. Brzóska, M.M.; Majewska, K.; Moniuszko-Jakoniuk, J. Mechanical properties of femoral diaphysis and femoral neck of female rats chronically exposed to various levels of cadmium. *Calcif. Tissue Int.* **2005**, *76*, 287–298. [CrossRef] [PubMed]
16. Brzóska, M.M.; Majewska, K.; Moniuszko-Jakoniuk, J. Weakness in the mechanical properties of the femur of growing female rats exposed to cadmium. *Arch. Toxicol.* **2005**, *79*, 277–288. [CrossRef] [PubMed]
17. Brzóska, M.M.; Majewska, K.; Kupraszewicz, E. Effects of low, moderate and relatively high chronic exposure to cadmium on long bones susceptibility to fracture in male rats. *Environ. Toxicol. Pharmacol.* **2010**, *29*, 235–245. [CrossRef] [PubMed]
18. Brzóska, M.M. Low-level chronic exposure to cadmium enhances the risk of long bone fractures: A study on a female rat model of human lifetime exposure. *J. Appl. Toxicol.* **2011**, *32*, 34–44. [CrossRef] [PubMed]
19. Olgun, O. The effect of dietary cadmium supplementation on performance, egg quality, tibia biomechanical properties and eggshell and bone mineralisation in laying quails. *Animal* **2015**, *9*, 1298–1303. [CrossRef] [PubMed]
20. Brzóska, M.M.; Borowska, S.; Tomczyk, M. Antioxidants as a potential preventive and therapeutic strategy for cadmium. *Curr. Drug Targets* **2016**, *17*, 1350–1384. [CrossRef] [PubMed]
21. Kopeć, A.; Sikora, A.; Piątkowska, E.; Borczak, B.; Czech, T. Possible protective role of elderberry fruit lyophilizate against selected effects of cadmium and lead intoxication in Wistar rats. *Environ. Sci. Pollut. Res.* **2016**, *23*, 8837–8848. [CrossRef] [PubMed]
22. Borowska, S.; Brzóska, M.M. Chokeberries (*Aronia melanocarpa*) and their products as a possible means for the prevention and treatment of noncommunicable diseases and unfavorable health effects due to exposure to xenobiotics. *Compr. Rev. Food Sci. Food Saf.* **2016**, *15*, 982–1017. [CrossRef]
23. Denev, P.N.; Kratchanov, C.G.; Ciz, M.; Lojek, A.; Kratchanova, M.G. Bioavailability and antioxidant activity of black chokeberry (*Aronia melanocarpa*) polyphenols: In vitro and in vivo evidences and possible mechanisms of action: A review. *Compr. Rev. Food Sci. Food Saf.* **2012**, *11*, 471–489. [CrossRef]
24. Shen, C.L.; Wang, P.; Guerrieri, J.; Yeh, J.K.; Wang, J.S. Protective effect of green tea polyphenols on bone loss in middle-aged female rats. *Osteoporos. Int.* **2008**, *19*, 979–990. [CrossRef] [PubMed]
25. Brzóska, M.M.; Galazyn-Sidorczuk, M.; Jurczuk, M.; Tomczyk, M. Protective effect of *Aronia melanocarpa* polyphenols on cadmium accumulation in the body: A study in a rat model of human exposure to this metal. *Curr. Drug Targets* **2015**, *16*, 1470–1487. [CrossRef]
26. Brzóska, M.M.; Rogalska, J.; Galazyn-Sidorczuk, M.; Jurczuk, M.; Roszczenko, A.; Tomczyk, M. Protective effect of *Aronia melanocarpa* polyphenols against cadmium-induced disorders in bone metabolism: A study in a rat model of lifetime human exposure to this heavy metal. *Chem. Biol. Interact.* **2015**, *229*, 132–146. [CrossRef] [PubMed]
27. Brzóska, M.M.; Rogalska, J.; Roszczenko, A.; Galazyn-Sidorczuk, A.; Tomczyk, M. The mechanism of the osteoprotective action of a polyphenol-rich *Aronia melanocarpa* extract during chronic exposure to cadmium is mediated by the oxidative defense system. *Planta Med.* **2016**, *82*, 621–631. [CrossRef] [PubMed]
28. Follet, H.; Boivin, G.; Rumelhart, C.; Meunier, P.J. The degree of mineralization is a determinant of bone strength: A study on human calcanei. *Bone* **2004**, *34*, 783–789. [CrossRef] [PubMed]
29. Osterhoff, G.; Morgan, E.F.; Shefelbine, S.J.; Karim, L.; McNamarae, L.M.; Augat, P. Bone mechanical properties and changes with osteoporosis. *Inj. Int. J. Care Inj.* **2016**, *47*, S11–S20. [CrossRef]
30. Garnero, P. The role of collagen organization on the properties of bone. *Calcif. Tissue Int.* **2015**, *97*, 229–240. [CrossRef] [PubMed]
31. Kulling, S.E.; Rawel, H.M. Chokeberry (*Aronia melanocarpa*)—A review on the characteristic components and potential health effects. *Planta Med.* **2008**, *74*, 1625–1634. [CrossRef] [PubMed]
32. Kokotkiewicz, A.; Jaremicz, Z.; Łuczkiewicz, M. Aronia plants: A review of traditional use, biological activities, and perspectives for modern medicine. *J. Med. Food* **2010**, *13*, 255–269. [CrossRef] [PubMed]
33. Brzóska, M.M.; Galażyn-Sidorczuk, M.; Rogalska, J.; Roszczenko, A.; Jurczuk, M.; Majewska, K.; Moniuszko-Jakoniuk, J. Beneficial effect of zinc supplementation on biomechanical properties of femoral distal end and femoral diaphysis of male rats chronically exposed to cadmium. *Chem. Biol. Interact.* **2008**, *171*, 312–324. [CrossRef] [PubMed]

11

Dietary Protein and Physical Activity Interventions to Support Muscle Maintenance in End-Stage Renal Disease Patients on Hemodialysis

Floris K. Hendriks [1,2], Joey S.J. Smeets [1], Frank M. van der Sande [3], Jeroen P. Kooman [2,3] and Luc J.C. van Loon [1,*]

1 Department of Human Biology, NUTRIM School of Nutrition and Translational Research in Metabolism, Maastricht University Medical Centre+, P.O. Box 616, 6200 MD Maastricht, The Netherlands; f.hendriks@maastrichtuniversity.nl (F.K.H.); joey.smeets@maastrichtuniversity.nl (J.S.J.S.)
2 Department of Internal Medicine, NUTRIM School of Nutrition and Translational Research in Metabolism, Maastricht University Medical Centre+, P.O. Box 616, 6200 MD Maastricht, The Netherlands; jeroen.kooman@mumc.nl
3 Division of Nephrology, Department of Internal Medicine, Maastricht University Medical Centre+, P.O. Box 5800, 6202 AZ Maastricht, The Netherlands; f.vander.sande@mumc.nl
* Correspondence: L.vanLoon@maastrichtuniversity.nl

Abstract: End-stage renal disease patients have insufficient renal clearance capacity left to adequately excrete metabolic waste products. Hemodialysis (HD) is often employed to partially replace renal clearance in these patients. However, skeletal muscle mass and strength start to decline at an accelerated rate after initiation of chronic HD therapy. An essential anabolic stimulus to allow muscle maintenance is dietary protein ingestion. Chronic HD patients generally fail to achieve recommended protein intake levels, in particular on dialysis days. Besides a low protein intake on dialysis days, the protein equivalent of a meal is extracted from the circulation during HD. Apart from protein ingestion, physical activity is essential to allow muscle maintenance. Unfortunately, most chronic HD patients have a sedentary lifestyle. Yet, physical activity and nutritional interventions to support muscle maintenance are generally not implemented in routine patient care. To support muscle maintenance in chronic HD patients, quantity and timing of protein intake should be optimized, in particular throughout dialysis days. Furthermore, implementing physical activity either during or between HD sessions may improve the muscle protein synthetic response to protein ingestion. A well-orchestrated combination of physical activity and nutritional interventions will be instrumental to preserve muscle mass in chronic HD patients.

Keywords: muscle wasting; exercise; nutrition; kidney disease

---

1. Introduction

Chronic kidney disease (CKD) is currently a public health problem with a global prevalence of 10% and the cause of approximately 33 million disability-adjusted life-years worldwide [1,2]. Development and progression of CKD are associated with the age-related decline in renal function, especially in individuals with hypertension and diabetes mellitus [3–5]. Therefore, the rapid ageing of our population is expected to further increase prevalence of CKD and its progression to end-stage renal disease (ESRD) [6,7]. The glomerular filtration rate in ESRD patients is below 15 mL/min/1.73 m^2 and insufficient to adequately remove metabolic waste products and fluids from the body [8,9]. Due to the accumulation of metabolic waste products in their body, ESRD patients experience phenotypic changes that resemble the ageing process, with a progressive loss of skeletal muscle mass and strength [10].

To prevent lethal consequences of metabolic waste product accumulation in ESRD patients, hemodialysis (HD) can be used to partially replace renal solute removal [11]. Over the past decades, survival of patients undergoing HD has improved substantially [12,13]. However, prevention of the adverse effects of HD on body composition has made less progression. After initiation of chronic hemodialysis (CHD) therapy, the age-related loss of skeletal muscle mass and strength accelerates and patients typically develop impairments in physical function [14–17]. Protein-energy wasting, a severe state of malnutrition, is observed in 28%–54% of CHD patients [18,19]. Loss of skeletal muscle mass and strength predisposes CHD patients to frailty and substantially reduces their quality of life [20]. Furthermore, the decline in skeletal muscle mass and strength is associated with higher hospitalization and mortality rates in CHD patients [20–22]. As the duration of CHD treatment is associated with its detrimental effects on body composition, the improved survival rate of CHD patients will generate new challenges for healthcare [14]. This emphasizes the need to understand and counteract skeletal muscle mass and strength loss in CHD patients.

2. Muscle Maintenance

Skeletal muscle mass is regulated through a dynamic balance between continuous synthesis and breakdown of muscle proteins. The muscle protein pool has shown to possess a turnover rate of 1%–2% per day, allowing skeletal muscle tissue to adapt to circumstances such as changes in physical activity pattern (e.g., muscle hypertrophy following resistance-type exercise training) [23]. Ingesting several protein-containing meals throughout the day results in a sinusoidal pattern of subsequent increases and decreases in skeletal muscle protein synthesis and breakdown rates [24]. Skeletal muscle protein synthesis rates are high during post-prandial periods and low during post-absorptive periods, whilst skeletal muscle protein breakdown rates follow a reverse pattern. Muscle maintenance is achieved when skeletal muscle protein synthesis rates equal skeletal muscle protein breakdown rates over a given period.

Protein ingestion is an essential requirement to maintain skeletal muscle mass. After consumption, dietary protein is absorbed as amino acids in the intestine, with a large fraction being subsequently released into the circulation [25]. The release of amino acids into the circulation following protein ingestion elevates plasma amino acid concentrations for a post-prandial period of up to 5 h [26]. These circulating plasma amino acids serve as precursors for de novo synthesis of muscle protein [27]. However, amino acids are more than simply building blocks for muscle protein synthesis, as they can function as signaling molecules. The post-prandial increase in plasma essential amino acid concentrations, and leucine in particular, stimulates anabolic signaling through several molecular pathways, such as the mammalian target of rapamycin complex 1 (mTORC1) pathway [28,29]. This post-prandial anabolic signaling increases skeletal muscle protein synthesis rates and inhibits proteolysis, allowing net muscle protein accretion [27].

Muscle loss can be attributed both to an increase in muscle protein breakdown as well as to a decline in muscle protein synthesis rates. Previous work has reported increased muscle proteolysis in CHD patients due to inflammation, metabolic acidosis, and the dialysis procedure itself [30–33]. Furthermore, it has been suggested that the muscle protein synthetic response to feeding is impaired in patients with CKD [34]. Whereas a maximal post-prandial muscle protein synthetic response has been reported after ingesting up to 20 g of a high-quality protein in healthy young adults, a lesser response has been observed in older individuals [27,35,36]. More recently, van Vliet et al. were unable to detect a measurable increase in skeletal muscle protein synthesis rates in CHD patients following ingestion of a meal containing 20 g protein [37]. The latter suggests that CHD patients suffer from a blunted muscle protein synthetic response to feeding, a phenomenon that has been coined anabolic resistance. In healthy elderly individuals, it has been shown that the anabolic resistance of skeletal muscle tissue can be overcome through ingesting a greater amount of protein (at least 30 g of a high-quality protein) [38] and/or performing a bout of resistance-type exercise prior to feeding [39]. When tailored specific to CHD patients, these anabolic strategies may prove essential to attenuate or even prevent the accelerated loss of skeletal muscle mass and strength in ESRD patients undergoing HD.

3. Dietary Protein Intake in ESRD Patients on HD

For healthy young adults, the recommended dietary protein intake to achieve a net balance between muscle protein synthesis and breakdown rates has been set at 0.8 g protein/kg body weight/day by the World Health Organization [40,41]. This level of protein intake may not be sufficient to support muscle maintenance in CHD patients. According to the National Kidney Foundation K/DOQI Clinical Practice Guidelines, these patients are recommended to ingest >1.2 g protein/kg body weight/day [42–45]. However, CHD patients generally do not meet this recommended level of protein intake. Previous studies in this population have observed a dietary protein intake of 0.9–1.0 g protein/kg body weight/day [46–51]. Especially on dialysis days, factors such as time constraints and reduced appetite make it difficult for patients to consume ample dietary protein [52]. As a result, dietary protein intake in CHD patients has been reported to be ~0.8 g protein/kg body weight on dialysis days compared to ~1.0 g protein/kg body weight on non-dialysis days [50].

In addition to low protein intake, another factor compromises plasma amino acid availability on dialysis days. During HD, both metabolic waste products as well as circulating amino acids are able to diffuse through the semipermeable dialysis membrane [11]. The diffusion into the dialysate results in a considerable extraction of circulating amino acids throughout HD [30,53–56]. We have recently shown that during a single HD session, ~12 g amino acids are extracted from the circulation in CHD patients who ingest their habitual diet during HD [57]. This amount equals the quantity of amino acids that is released into the circulation following ingestion of a typical meal (containing 20–25 g protein). Loss of circulating amino acids causes a significant decline of plasma amino acid concentrations throughout HD [55,57]. Moreover, Ikizler et al. showed that in fasting CHD patients, plasma amino acid concentrations remain low for at least 2 h after cessation of HD [30]. The HD-induced decline in plasma amino acid concentrations has been shown to cause substantial catabolism of skeletal muscle tissue in fasted CHD patients [58,59]. The continuous extraction of amino acids throughout HD stimulates skeletal muscle tissue to release amino acids into the circulation [60,61]. This homeostatic process attenuates the decline in plasma amino acid concentrations and may prevent subsequent detrimental effects on organs that are necessary to sustain life [62]. In addition, the decline in plasma amino acid concentrations reduces the availability of precursors for de novo synthesis of muscle proteins during and following HD. To allow a muscle protein synthetic response during this period, the extraction of circulating amino acids should be compensated for through amino acid and/or protein administration.

Provision of protein-rich nutrition during HD is often recommended to increase dietary protein intake on dialysis days [63–66]. Ingestion of 40–60 g protein has been shown to prevent the HD-induced decline in plasma amino acid concentrations in multiple studies [58,59,67,68]. Furthermore, Pupim et al. demonstrated that ingestion of 57 g protein resulted in a positive forearm amino acid balance throughout HD [58]. Thus, HD-associated skeletal muscle catabolism may be prevented through ingestion of sufficient protein during HD. Several studies have also observed long-term beneficial effects of protein supplementation during HD, such as an increase in lean body mass, improvement in physical function, and decrease in mortality [69–71]. However, data from our lab [57] and others [56,67] indicate that protein ingestion during HD is also accompanied by an increase in amino acid extraction, presumably due to a higher subsequent plasma-dialysate diffusion gradient (Figure 1). Due to this extraction following protein ingestion during HD, less amino acids become available to stimulate muscle protein synthesis rates and serve as precursors for de novo synthesis of muscle protein. Considering the anabolic resistance of skeletal muscle tissue that is also present in this population, CHD patients will need to ingest well above 20 g high-quality protein during HD to allow a post-prandial increase in skeletal muscle protein synthesis and an inhibition of proteolysis.

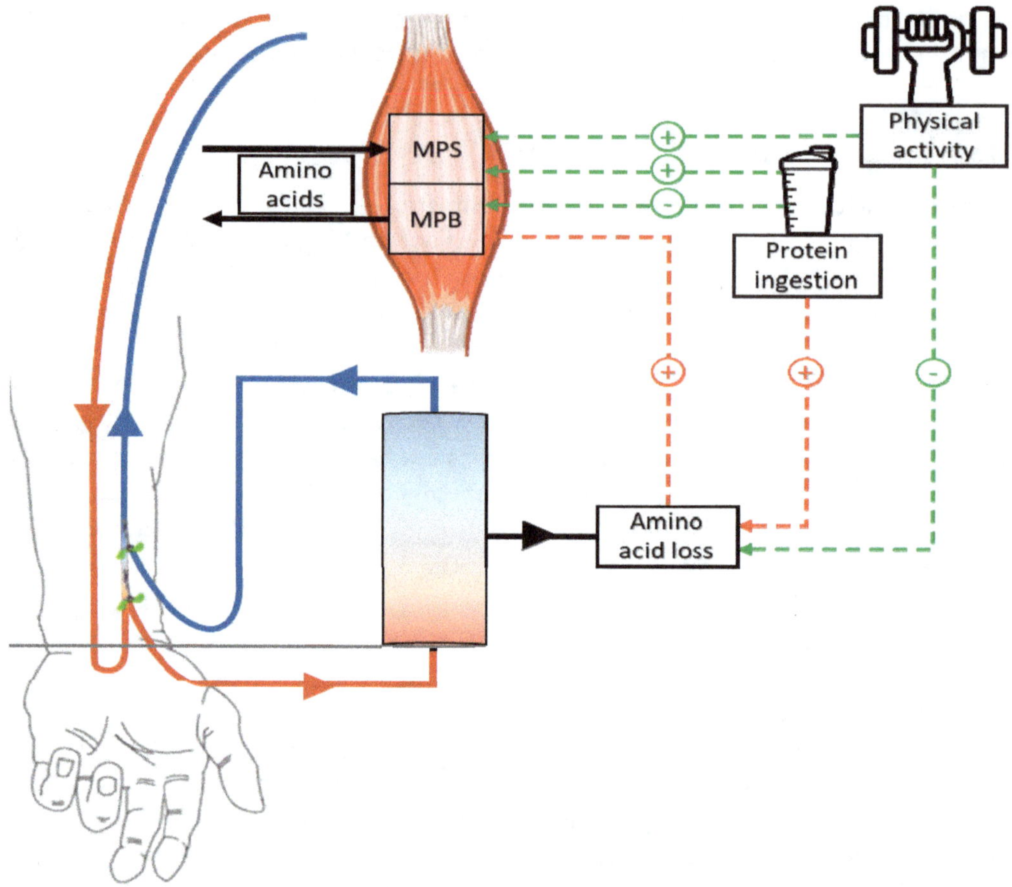

Figure 1. Conceptual overview of the effects of hemodialysis, protein ingestion, and physical activity on the muscle protein synthetic and proteolytic response. The extraction of amino acids during hemodialysis (HD) stimulates muscle protein breakdown (MPB) rates due to decreased plasma amino acid concentrations. Protein ingestion can maintain, or even increase, plasma amino acid concentrations throughout HD, which increases muscle protein synthesis (MPS) rates, while it may attenuate the HD-induced increase in MPB rates. However, elevated plasma amino acid concentrations also increase the amount of amino acids that are extracted during HD. Physical activity before or during HD may increase the use of plasma amino acids for de novo MPS, and thereby reduce the amount of amino acids that are extracted from the circulation during HD. Dashed lines in green represent processes that support muscle maintenance, whereas dashed lines in red represent processes that compromise muscle maintenance.

However, high quality (animal-derived) protein is rich in phosphorous [72]. In CHD patients, an increased dietary protein intake may lead to hyperphosphatemia or the need for phosphate binders. Furthermore, it has been suggested that an increased dietary protein intake in CHD patients provides more uremic toxin precursors and leads to higher uremic solute concentrations between HD sessions [73]. Recently, our laboratory has shown that the ingestion of branched-chain ketoacids, which contain no phosphorous or nitrogen, significantly stimulates skeletal muscle protein synthesis rates in healthy elderly individuals [74]. Ketoacid supplementation in CKD patients has been shown to reduce the generation of toxic metabolic waste products, while maintaining a good nutritional status [75]. However, it remains to be established whether ketoacid supplementation could support muscle maintenance in CHD patients.

4. Physical Activity in ESRD Patients on HD

Another key component for muscle maintenance is physical activity. Physical activity and exercise stimulate skeletal muscle protein synthesis rates, with post-absorptive muscle protein synthesis rates being elevated for up to 24 or even 48 h [76,77]. Furthermore, physical activity performed prior to food intake augments the post-prandial muscle protein synthetic response to feeding [78–81]. In contrast, a decline in physical activity reduces the muscle protein synthetic response to feeding [82–84]. In other words, whereas physical activity makes skeletal muscle tissue more sensitive to the anabolic properties of amino acids, muscle disuse leads to anabolic resistance of skeletal muscle tissue [85]. In support, daily exercise has been shown to increase skeletal muscle protein synthesis rates throughout the day [86], while a decline in physical activity has been shown to lower daily muscle protein synthesis rates [87]. Consequently, ample physical activity has been associated with a reduced age-related loss of muscle mass and strength [88,89], whereas a decline in the level of physical activity (e.g., during bed rest or limb immobilization) has been shown to induce a rapid decline in muscle mass and strength [90,91].

According to the Physical Activity Guidelines for Americans, patients with chronic diseases should follow the key physical activity guidelines for healthy adults to achieve substantial health benefits [92]. These guidelines recommend patients to perform at least 150–300 min per week of moderate-intensity aerobic exercise, 75–150 min of vigorous-intensity aerobic exercise per week, or an equivalent combination of both. In addition, muscle-strengthening activities that involve all major muscle groups should be performed at least twice per week. However, these guidelines do not contain specific recommendations for CHD patients. The Renal Association Clinical Practice Guideline on Hemodialysis recommends that all CHD patients without contraindication should perform at least 30 min of supervised moderate-intensity exercise during every dialysis session [93]. In addition, the guideline states that CHD patients should be encouraged to undertake physical activity on non-dialysis days. In line with this recommendation, it has recently been suggested that mortality rates are reduced in CHD patients who perform at least 4000 steps on non-dialysis days [94].

However, CHD patients typically adopt a sedentary lifestyle and spend less time being physically active than healthy adults [95,96]. In the United States, almost 50% of CHD patients perform exercise once or less than once per week [96]. A HD session represents a long (3–4 h) sedentary period, which often hinders CHD patients to engage in physical activity and, as such, dialysis treatments contribute to the lower physical activity levels [97,98]. Gomes et al. observed that CHD patients took 4362 ± 2084 and 7007 ± 3437 steps on dialysis and non-dialysis days, respectively, compared to 8792 ± 2870 steps taken by age-matched healthy controls [98]. The low habitual physical activity level in these patients is another key factor responsible for the accelerated loss of muscle mass and strength in CHD patients [17]. Interventions in CHD patients targeted to preserve or even increase muscle mass should not only provide nutritional support but also increase physical activity levels to maximize their impact.

5. Interventions to Support Muscle Maintenance in ESRD Patients on HD

Physical activity interventions for CHD patients may implement exercise during HD (intradialytic) or between HD sessions (interdialytic). A recent meta-analysis by Clarckson et al. reported no differences in the efficacy of intradialytic when compared with interdialytic exercise on improvements of physical function in CHD patients [99]. Due to exercise intolerance, CHD patients typically show low adherence and poor compliance to long-term unsupervised physical activity intervention programs [100]. HD sessions represent an opportunity to integrate supervised physical activity in the weekly routine of CHD patients. Intradialytic physical activity is considered safe and shows greater adherence rates than interdialytic physical activity [100–102]. Furthermore, supervision of intradialytic exercise sessions provides the opportunity to prescribe a patient-specific and progressive exercise program. Physical activity during HD has some limitations compared to interdialytic physical activity, such as constrains regarding exercise intensity and upper limb exercises. On the other hand, intradialytic physical activity provides distraction for CHD patients during their treatment and has been shown to improve their quality of life [101]. Therefore, we would advocate the implementation of an intradialytic exercise program in lifestyle interventions designed for (sedentary) CHD patients.

In addition to timing, the type of exercise is an important determinant of its potential to support muscle maintenance. Resistance-type exercise training is considered most potent to augment muscle mass and strength. In healthy adults, resistance-type exercise training has been shown to induce a robust increase in both skeletal muscle mass as well as strength [103–105]. Furthermore, resistance-type exercise also sensitizes skeletal muscle tissue to the anabolic properties of amino acids and, as such, increases the post-prandial muscle protein synthetic response to feeding [78,79,81]. In support, it has been reported that a single bout of resistance-type exercise performed prior to HD increases amino acid uptake by muscle tissue following intradialytic protein ingestion [106]. Intradialytic resistance-type exercise programs have shown to increase skeletal muscle strength, thereby improving physical function outcome measures such as the 6-min walk test [99,107–110]. In a systematic review of nine trials that assessed progressive resistance-type exercise training in ESRD patients on HD, Chan and Cheema concluded that resistance-type exercise training can effectively induce regional skeletal muscle hypertrophy [111]. However, due to inconsistent results of previous studies [69,112–118], it remains unclear whether resistance-type exercise can increase skeletal muscle mass on a whole-body level in CHD patients.

Protein ingestion during recovery from resistance-type exercise is required to achieve a positive net protein balance and, as such, to allow net muscle protein accretion [76]. Due to practical matters, the majority of studies that assessed the impact of resistance-type exercise training in CHD patients implemented their training sessions before or during HD [119]. As circulating amino acids are extracted during HD, recovery from those exercise sessions typically occurred during conditions of reduced amino acid availability. This may have attenuated the anabolic effects of the exercise training programs. Furthermore, the combination of amino acid extraction during HD and the anabolic resistance of skeletal muscle tissue in CHD patients likely increases the amount of protein that is required following intradialytic resistance-type exercise. We suggest that at least 30 g protein should be provided to CHD patients during recovery from resistance-type exercise performed immediately prior or during HD to allow a muscle protein synthetic response.

Besides protein ingestion during recovery from exercise, it has been advocated that every main meal (breakfast, lunch, and dinner) should contain 20 g high-quality protein to optimally stimulate muscle protein synthesis rates throughout the day [120,121]. We suggest that CHD patients should ingest well above 20 g high-quality protein per main meal to compensate for the blunted muscle protein synthetic response to feeding, recognizing that additional measures to prevent hyperphosphatemia might be necessary. In addition, ingesting a protein-rich snack prior to sleep, especially on training days, may further support muscle mass maintenance [24]. Though the impact of these nutritional strategies has not been assessed in CHD patients, they would likely be supplemental in the prevention of protein malnutrition in this population. Effectiveness of any nutritional intervention largely depends on long-term adherence and compliance. However, adherence to dietary interventions in CHD patients is often poor due to barriers such as dialysis time, motivation, and lack of social support [122]. Therefore, CHD patients should be advised on protein options that are easy to prepare, convenient to consume, and have an acceptable taste.

A well-orchestrated lifestyle intervention program combining exercise and nutritional interventions for CHD patients is required to attenuate or even prevent the loss of muscle mass, strength, and functional capacity in this population. For such a multimodal interventional approach to be effective, a (more) personalized supervision of CHD patients provided by a team of healthcare specialists with physical activity and nutritional expertise is required. A close collaboration between nephrologists, physical therapists, and dietitians in both research and clinical care will be essential to improve the health and well-being of the growing number of CHD patients.

6. Conclusions

The gradual loss of skeletal muscle mass in CHD patients accelerates after initiation of intermittent HD treatment. Muscle protein breakdown rates in CHD patients are increased, while muscle protein synthesis rates fail to match this increase due to insufficient protein ingestion, amino acid extraction during HD, and the prevalence of anabolic resistance. Protein intake of CHD patients should be increased on dialysis days to compensate for extraction of circulating amino acids during HD and to compensate for the blunted muscle protein synthetic response to feeding in these patients. Implementing structured physical activity in the daily routine of CHD patients represents a feasible strategy to increase the skeletal muscle protein synthetic response to protein ingestion and, as such, to alleviate anabolic resistance. More insight in the impact of protein ingestion and exercise in CHD patients on both dialysis as well as non-dialysis days is required to develop more effective nutritional and exercise intervention programs that can attenuate or even prevent muscle loss in CHD patients.

Author Contributions: Writing—original draft preparation, F.K.H. and L.J.C.v.L.; writing—review and editing, J.S.J.S., F.M.v.d.S., and J.P.K., All authors read and approved the final manuscript.

References

1. Mortality, G.B.D. Catrgory: Causes of Death. Global, regional, and national life expectancy, all-cause mortality, and cause-specific mortality for 249 causes of death, 1980–2015: A systematic analysis for the Global Burden of Disease Study 2015. *Lancet* **2016**, *388*, 1459–1544. [CrossRef]
2. Dalys, G.B.D.; Collaborators, H.; Murray, C.J.; Barber, R.M.; Foreman, K.J.; Abbasoglu Ozgoren, A.; Abd-Allah, F.; Abera, S.F.; Aboyans, V.; Abraham, J.P.; et al. Global, regional, and national disability-adjusted life years (DALYs) for 306 diseases and injuries and healthy life expectancy (HALE) for 188 countries, 1990-2013: Quantifying the epidemiological transition. *Lancet* **2015**, *386*, 2145–2191. [CrossRef]
3. Gansevoort, R.T.; Correa-Rotter, R.; Hemmelgarn, B.R.; Jafar, T.H.; Heerspink, H.J.L.; Mann, J.F.; Matsushita, K.; Wen, C.P. Chronic kidney disease and cardiovascular risk: Epidemiology, mechanisms, and prevention. *Lancet* **2013**, *382*, 339–352. [CrossRef]
4. Hill, N.R.; Fatoba, S.T.; Oke, J.L.; Hirst, J.A.; O'Callaghan, C.A.; Lasserson, D.S.; Hobbs, F.D. Global Prevalence of Chronic Kidney Disease-A Systematic Review and Meta-Analysis. *PLoS ONE* **2016**, *11*, e0158765. [CrossRef] [PubMed]
5. Webster, A.C.; Nagler, E.V.; Morton, R.L.; Masson, P. Chronic Kidney Disease. *Lancet* **2017**, *389*, 1238–1252. [CrossRef]
6. Van Oostrom, S.H.; Gijsen, R.; Stirbu, I.; Korevaar, J.C.; Schellevis, F.G.; Picavet, H.S.; Hoeymans, N. Time Trends in Prevalence of Chronic Diseases and Multimorbidity Not Only due to Aging: Data from General Practices and Health Surveys. *PLoS ONE* **2016**, *11*, e0160264. [CrossRef]
7. Tonelli, M.; Riella, M. Chronic kidney disease and the ageing population. *Nephron Clin. Pract.* **2014**, *128*, 319–322. [CrossRef]
8. Levey, A.S.; Eckardt, K.U.; Tsukamoto, Y.; Levin, A.; Coresh, J.; Rossert, J.; De Zeeuw, D.; Hostetter, T.H.; Lameire, N.; Eknoyan, G. Definition and classification of chronic kidney disease: A position statement from Kidney Disease: Improving Global Outcomes (KDIGO). *Kidney Int.* **2005**, *67*, 2089–2100. [CrossRef]
9. Agarwal, R. Defining end-stage renal disease in clinical trials: A framework for adjudication. *Nephrol. Dial. Transplant.* **2016**, *31*, 864–867. [CrossRef]
10. Kooman, J.P.; Kotanko, P.; Schols, A.M.; Shiels, P.G.; Stenvinkel, P. Chronic kidney disease and premature ageing. *Nat. Rev. Nephrol.* **2014**, *10*, 732–742. [CrossRef]
11. Himmelfarb, J.; Ikizler, T.A. Hemodialysis. *N. Engl. J. Med.* **2010**, *363*, 1833–1845. [CrossRef] [PubMed]
12. Fleming, G.M. Renal replacement therapy review. *Organogenesis* **2014**, *7*, 2–12. [CrossRef] [PubMed]
13. Marshall, M.R.; Polkinghorne, K.R.; Kerr, P.G.; Agar, J.W.; Hawley, C.M.; McDonald, S.P. Temporal Changes in Mortality Risk by Dialysis Modality in the Australian and New Zealand Dialysis Population. *Am. J. Kidney Dis.* **2015**, *66*, 489–498. [CrossRef] [PubMed]
14. Marcelli, D.; Brand, K.; Ponce, P.; Milkowski, A.; Marelli, C.; Ok, E.; Merello Godino, J.I.; Gurevich, K.; Jirka, T.; Rosenberger, J.; et al. Longitudinal Changes in Body Composition in Patients After Initiation of Hemodialysis Therapy: Results from an International Cohort. *J. Ren. Nutr.* **2016**, *26*, 72–80. [CrossRef] [PubMed]

15. Spiegel, B.M.; Melmed, G.; Robbins, S.; Esrailian, E. Biomarkers and health-related quality of life in end-stage renal disease: A systematic review. *Clin. J. Am. Soc. Nephrol.* **2008**, *3*, 1759–1768. [CrossRef]
16. Kurella Tamura, M.; Covinsky, K.E.; Chertow, G.M.; Yaffe, K.; Landefeld, C.S.; McCulloch, C.E. Functional status of elderly adults before and after initiation of dialysis. *N. Engl. J. Med.* **2009**, *361*, 1539–1547. [CrossRef]
17. Johansen, K.L.; Shubert, T.; Doyle, J.; Soher, B.; Sakkas, G.K.; Kent-Braun, J.A. Muscle atrophy in patients receiving hemodialysis: Effects on muscle strength, muscle quality, and physical function. *Kidney Int.* **2003**, *63*, 291–297. [CrossRef]
18. Carrero, J.J.; Thomas, F.; Nagy, K.; Arogundade, F.; Avesani, C.M.; Chan, M.; Chmielewski, M.; Cordeiro, A.C.; Espinosa-Cuevas, A.; Fiaccadori, E.; et al. Global Prevalence of Protein-Energy Wasting in Kidney Disease: A Meta-analysis of Contemporary Observational Studies From the International Society of Renal Nutrition and Metabolism. *J. Ren. Nutr.* **2018**, *28*, 380–392. [CrossRef]
19. Fouque, D.; Kalantar-Zadeh, K.; Kopple, J.; Cano, N.; Chauveau, P.; Cuppari, L.; Franch, H.; Guarnieri, G.; Ikizler, T.A.; Kaysen, G.; et al. A proposed nomenclature and diagnostic criteria for protein-energy wasting in acute and chronic kidney disease. *Kidney Int.* **2008**, *73*, 391–398. [CrossRef]
20. Broers, N.J.; Usvyat, L.A.; Kooman, J.P.; van der Sande, F.M.; Lacson, E., Jr.; Kotanko, P.; Maddux, F.W. Quality of Life in Dialysis Patients: A Retrospective Cohort Study. *Nephron* **2015**, *130*, 105–112. [CrossRef]
21. Isoyama, N.; Qureshi, A.R.; Avesani, C.M.; Lindholm, B.; Barany, P.; Heimburger, O.; Cederholm, T.; Stenvinkel, P.; Carrero, J.J. Comparative associations of muscle mass and muscle strength with mortality in dialysis patients. *Clin. J. Am. Soc. Nephrol.* **2014**, *9*, 1720–1728. [CrossRef] [PubMed]
22. Borges, M.C.; Vogt, B.P.; Martin, L.C.; Caramori, J.C. Malnutrition Inflammation Score cut-off predicting mortality in maintenance hemodialysis patients. *Clin. Nutr. ESPEN* **2017**, *17*, 63–67. [CrossRef] [PubMed]
23. Mamerow, M.M.; Mettler, J.A.; English, K.L.; Casperson, S.L.; Arentson-Lantz, E.; Sheffield-Moore, M.; Layman, D.K.; Paddon-Jones, D. Dietary protein distribution positively influences 24-h muscle protein synthesis in healthy adults. *J. Nutr.* **2014**, *144*, 876–880. [CrossRef] [PubMed]
24. Trommelen, J.; van Loon, L.J. Pre-Sleep Protein Ingestion to Improve the Skeletal Muscle Adaptive Response to Exercise Training. *Nutrients* **2016**, *8*, 763. [CrossRef] [PubMed]
25. Groen, B.B.; Horstman, A.M.; Hamer, H.M.; de Haan, M.; van Kranenburg, J.; Bierau, J.; Poeze, M.; Wodzig, W.K.; Rasmussen, B.B.; van Loon, L.J. Post-Prandial Protein Handling: You Are What You Just Ate. *PLoS ONE* **2015**, *10*, e0141582. [CrossRef] [PubMed]
26. Kouw, I.W.; Gorissen, S.H.; Burd, N.A.; Cermak, N.M.; Gijsen, A.P.; van Kranenburg, J.; van Loon, L.J. Postprandial Protein Handling Is Not Impaired in Type 2 Diabetes Patients When Compared with Normoglycemic Controls. *J. Clin. Endocrinol. Metab.* **2015**, *100*, 3103–3111. [CrossRef]
27. Wall, B.T.; Gorissen, S.H.; Pennings, B.; Koopman, R.; Groen, B.B.; Verdijk, L.B.; van Loon, L.J. Aging Is Accompanied by a Blunted Muscle Protein Synthetic Response to Protein Ingestion. *PLoS ONE* **2015**, *10*, e0140903. [CrossRef]
28. Bohe, J.; Low, A.; Wolfe, R.R.; Rennie, M.J. Human muscle protein synthesis is modulated by extracellular, not intramuscular amino acid availability: A dose-response study. *J. Physiol.* **2003**, *552*, 315–324. [CrossRef]
29. Rieu, I.; Balage, M.; Sornet, C.; Giraudet, C.; Pujos, E.; Grizard, J.; Mosoni, L.; Dardevet, D. Leucine supplementation improves muscle protein synthesis in elderly men independently of hyperaminoacidaemia. *J. Physiol.* **2006**, *575*, 305–315. [CrossRef]
30. Ikizler, T.A.; Pupim, L.B.; Brouillette, J.R.; Levenhagen, D.K.; Farmer, K.; Hakim, R.M.; Flakoll, P.J. Hemodialysis stimulates muscle and whole body protein loss and alters substrate oxidation. *Am. J. Physiol. Endocrinol. Metab.* **2002**, *282*, E107–E116. [CrossRef]
31. Wang, X.H.; Mitch, W.E. Mechanisms of muscle wasting in chronic kidney disease. *Nat. Rev. Nephrol.* **2014**, *10*, 504–516. [CrossRef] [PubMed]
32. Kooman, J.P.; Dekker, M.J.; Usvyat, L.A.; Kotanko, P.; van der Sande, F.M.; Schalkwijk, C.G.; Shiels, P.G.; Stenvinkel, P. Inflammation and premature aging in advanced chronic kidney disease. *Am. J. Physiol. Ren. Physiol.* **2017**, *313*, F938–F950. [CrossRef] [PubMed]
33. Lofberg, E.; Gutierrez, A.; Anderstam, B.; Wernerman, J.; Bergstrom, J.; Price, S.R.; Mitch, W.E.; Alvestrand, A. Effect of bicarbonate on muscle protein in patients receiving hemodialysis. *Am. J. Kidney Dis.* **2006**, *48*, 419–429. [CrossRef] [PubMed]
34. Garibotto, G. Muscle amino acid metabolism and the control of muscle protein turnover in patients with chronic renal failure. *Nutrition* **1999**, *15*, 145–155. [CrossRef]

35. Cuthbertson, D.; Smith, K.; Babraj, J.; Leese, G.; Waddell, T.; Atherton, P.; Wackerhage, H.; Taylor, P.M.; Rennie, M.J. Anabolic signaling deficits underlie amino acid resistance of wasting, aging muscle. *FASEB J.* **2005**, *19*, 422–424. [CrossRef]
36. Morton, R.W.; McGlory, C.; Phillips, S.M. Nutritional interventions to augment resistance training-induced skeletal muscle hypertrophy. *Front. Physiol.* **2015**, *6*, 245. [CrossRef]
37. Van Vliet, S.; Skinner, S.K.; Beals, J.W.; Pagni, B.A.; Fang, H.Y.; Ulanov, A.V.; Li, Z.; Paluska, S.A.; Mazzulla, M.; West, D.W.D.; et al. Dysregulated Handling of Dietary Protein and Muscle Protein Synthesis After Mixed-Meal Ingestion in Maintenance Hemodialysis Patients. *Kidney Int. Rep.* **2018**, *3*, 1403–1415. [CrossRef]
38. Pennings, B.; Groen, B.; de Lange, A.; Gijsen, A.P.; Zorenc, A.H.; Senden, J.M.; van Loon, L.J. Amino acid absorption and subsequent muscle protein accretion following graded intakes of whey protein in elderly men. *Am. J. Physiol. Endocrinol. Metab.* **2012**, *302*, E992–E999. [CrossRef]
39. Yang, Y.; Breen, L.; Burd, N.A.; Hector, A.J.; Churchward-Venne, T.A.; Josse, A.R.; Tarnopolsky, M.A.; Phillips, S.M. Resistance exercise enhances myofibrillar protein synthesis with graded intakes of whey protein in older men. *Br. J. Nutr.* **2012**, *108*, 1780–1788. [CrossRef]
40. World Health Organization; Food and Agriculture Organization of the United Nations; United Nations University. *Protein and Amino Acid Requirements in Human Nutrition*; World Health Organization: Geneva, Switzerland, 2007.
41. Rand, W.M.; Pellett, P.L.; Young, V.R. Meta-analysis of nitrogen balance studies for estimating protein requirements in healthy adults. *Am. J. Clin. Nutr.* **2003**, *77*, 109–127. [CrossRef] [PubMed]
42. Borah, M.F.; Schoenfeld, P.Y.; Gotch, F.A.; Sargent, J.A.; Wolfson, M.; Humphreys, M.H. Nitrogen balance during intermittent dialysis therapy of uremia. *Kidney Int.* **1978**, *14*, 491–500. [CrossRef] [PubMed]
43. Rao, M.; Sharma, M.; Juneja, R.; Jacob, S.; Jacob, C.K. Calculated nitrogen balance in hemodialysis patients: Influence of protein intake. *Kidney Int.* **2000**, *58*, 336–345. [CrossRef] [PubMed]
44. Kopple, J.D. National Kidney Foundation K/DOQI Clinical Practice Guidelines for Nutrition in Chronic Renal Failure. *Am. J. Kidney Dis.* **2001**, *37*, S66–S70. [CrossRef] [PubMed]
45. Fouque, D.; Vennegoor, M.; ter Wee, P.; Wanner, C.; Basci, A.; Canaud, B.; Haage, P.; Konner, K.; Kooman, J.; Martin-Malo, A.; et al. EBPG guideline on nutrition. *Nephrol. Dial. Transplant.* **2007**, *22* (Suppl. 2), ii45–ii87. [CrossRef]
46. Burrowes, J.D.; Larive, B.; Cockram, D.B.; Dwyer, J.; Kusek, J.W.; McLeroy, S.; Poole, D.; Rocco, M.V.; Hemodialysis Study, G. Effects of dietary intake, appetite, and eating habits on dialysis and non-dialysis treatment days in hemodialysis patients: Cross-sectional results from the HEMO study. *J. Ren. Nutr.* **2003**, *13*, 191–198. [CrossRef]
47. Kalantar-Zadeh, K.; Kopple, J.D.; Deepak, S.; Block, D.; Block, G. Food intake characteristics of hemodialysis patients as obtained by food frequency questionnaire. *J. Ren. Nutr.* **2002**, *12*, 17–31. [CrossRef]
48. Lorenzo, V.; de Bonis, E.; Rufino, M.; Hernandez, D.; Rebollo, S.G.; Rodriguez, A.P.; Torres, A. Caloric rather than protein deficiency predominates in stable chronic haemodialysis patients. *Nephrol. Dial. Transplant.* **1995**, *10*, 1885–1889.
49. Wolfson, M.; Strong, C.J.; Minturn, D.; Gray, D.K.; Kopple, J.D. Nutritional status and lymphocyte function in maintenance hemodialysis patients. *Am. J. Clin. Nutr.* **1984**, *39*, 547–555. [CrossRef]
50. Martins, A.M.; Dias Rodrigues, J.C.; de Oliveira Santin, F.G.; Barbosa Brito Fdos, S.; Bello Moreira, A.S.; Lourenco, R.A.; Avesani, C.M. Food intake assessment of elderly patients on hemodialysis. *J. Ren. Nutr.* **2015**, *25*, 321–326. [CrossRef]
51. Bossola, M.; Leo, A.; Viola, A.; Carlomagno, G.; Monteburini, T.; Cenerelli, S.; Santarelli, S.; Boggi, R.; Miggiano, G.; Vulpio, C.; et al. Dietary intake of macronutrients and fiber in Mediterranean patients on chronic hemodialysis. *J. Nephrol.* **2013**, *26*, 912–918. [CrossRef] [PubMed]
52. Clark-Cutaia, M.N.; Sevick, M.A.; Thurheimer-Cacciotti, J.; Hoffman, L.A.; Snetselaar, L.; Burke, L.E.; Zickmund, S.L. Perceived Barriers to Adherence to Hemodialysis Dietary Recommendations. *Clin. Nurs. Res.* **2018**. [CrossRef] [PubMed]
53. Alp Ikizler, T.; Flakoll, P.J.; Parker, R.A.; Hakim, R.M. Amino acid and albumin losses during hemodialysis. *Kidney Int.* **1994**, *46*, 830–837. [CrossRef] [PubMed]
54. Yokomatsu, A.; Fujikawa, T.; Toya, Y.; Shino-Kakimoto, M.; Itoh, Y.; Mitsuhashi, H.; Tamura, K.; Hirawa, N.; Yasuda, G.; Umemura, S. Loss of amino acids into dialysate during hemodialysis using hydrophilic and

nonhydrophilic polyester-polymer alloy and polyacrylonitrile membrane dialyzers. *Ther. Apher. Dial.* **2014**, *18*, 340–346. [CrossRef]

55. Navarro, J.F.; Marcen, R.; Teruel, J.L.; Martin del Rio, R.; Gamez, C.; Mora, C.; Ortuno, J. Effect of different membranes on amino-acid losses during haemodialysis. *Nephrol. Dial. Transplant.* **1998**, *13*, 113–117. [CrossRef]
56. Wolfson, M.; Jones, M.R.; Kopple, J.D. Amino acid losses during hemodialysis with infusion of amino acids and glucose. *Kidney Int.* **1982**, *21*, 500–506. [CrossRef]
57. Hendriks, F.K.; Smeets, J.S.J.; Broers, N.J.H.; Van Kranenburg, J.M.X.; Sande, F.M.; Kooman, J.P.; Van Loon, L.J.C. Amino acid loss during hemodialysis in end-stage renal disease patients. *Clin. Nutr.* **2018**, *37*, S96. [CrossRef]
58. Pupim, L.B.; Majchrzak, K.M.; Flakoll, P.J.; Ikizler, T.A. Intradialytic oral nutrition improves protein homeostasis in chronic hemodialysis patients with deranged nutritional status. *J. Am. Soc. Nephrol.* **2006**, *17*, 3149–3157. [CrossRef]
59. Pupim, L.B.; Flakoll, P.J.; Brouillette, J.R.; Levenhagen, D.K.; Hakim, R.M.; Ikizler, T.A. Intradialytic parenteral nutrition improves protein and energy homeostasis in chronic hemodialysis patients. *J. Clin. Investig.* **2002**, *110*, 483–492. [CrossRef]
60. Frontera, W.R.; Ochala, J. Skeletal muscle: A brief review of structure and function. *Calcif. Tissue Int.* **2015**, *96*, 183–195. [CrossRef]
61. Raj, D.S.; Adeniyi, O.; Dominic, E.A.; Boivin, M.A.; McClelland, S.; Tzamaloukas, A.H.; Morgan, N.; Gonzales, L.; Wolfe, R.; Ferrando, A. Amino acid repletion does not decrease muscle protein catabolism during hemodialysis. *Am. J. Physiol. Endocrinol. Metab.* **2007**, *292*, E1534–E1542. [CrossRef] [PubMed]
62. Lim, V.S.; Ikizler, T.A.; Raj, D.S.; Flanigan, M.J. Does hemodialysis increase protein breakdown? Dissociation between whole-body amino acid turnover and regional muscle kinetics. *J. Am. Soc. Nephrol.* **2005**, *16*, 862–868. [CrossRef] [PubMed]
63. Ikizler, T.A.; Cano, N.J.; Franch, H.; Fouque, D.; Himmelfarb, J.; Kalantar-Zadeh, K.; Kuhlmann, M.K.; Stenvinkel, P.; TerWee, P.; Teta, D.; et al. Prevention and treatment of protein energy wasting in chronic kidney disease patients: A consensus statement by the International Society of Renal Nutrition and Metabolism. *Kidney Int.* **2013**, *84*, 1096–1107. [CrossRef] [PubMed]
64. Kalantar-Zadeh, K.; Ikizler, T.A. Let them eat during dialysis: An overlooked opportunity to improve outcomes in maintenance hemodialysis patients. *J. Ren. Nutr.* **2013**, *23*, 157–163. [CrossRef]
65. Kistler, B.M.; Benner, D.; Burrowes, J.D.; Campbell, K.L.; Fouque, D.; Garibotto, G.; Kopple, J.D.; Kovesdy, C.P.; Rhee, C.M.; Steiber, A.; et al. Eating During Hemodialysis Treatment: A Consensus Statement from the International Society of Renal Nutrition and Metabolism. *J. Ren. Nutr.* **2018**, *28*, 4–12. [CrossRef] [PubMed]
66. Sabatino, A.; Regolisti, G.; Karupaiah, T.; Sahathevan, S.; Sadu Singh, B.K.; Khor, B.H.; Salhab, N.; Karavetian, M.; Cupisti, A.; Fiaccadori, E. Protein-energy wasting and nutritional supplementation in patients with end-stage renal disease on hemodialysis. *Clin. Nutr.* **2017**, *36*, 663–671. [CrossRef]
67. Veeneman, J.M.; Kingma, H.A.; Boer, T.S.; Stellaard, F.; De Jong, P.E.; Reijngoud, D.J.; Huisman, R.M. Protein intake during hemodialysis maintains a positive whole body protein balance in chronic hemodialysis patients. *Am. J. Physiol. Endocrinol. Metab.* **2003**, *284*, E954–E965. [CrossRef]
68. Sundell, M.B.; Cavanaugh, K.L.; Wu, P.; Shintani, A.; Hakim, R.M.; Ikizler, T.A. Oral protein supplementation alone improves anabolism in a dose-dependent manner in chronic hemodialysis patients. *J. Ren. Nutr.* **2009**, *19*, 412–421. [CrossRef]
69. Dong, J.; Sundell, M.B.; Pupim, L.B.; Wu, P.; Shintani, A.; Ikizler, T.A. The effect of resistance exercise to augment long-term benefits of intradialytic oral nutritional supplementation in chronic hemodialysis patients. *J. Ren. Nutr.* **2011**, *21*, 149–159. [CrossRef]
70. Weiner, D.E.; Tighiouart, H.; Ladik, V.; Meyer, K.B.; Zager, P.G.; Johnson, D.S. Oral intradialytic nutritional supplement use and mortality in hemodialysis patients. *Am. J. Kidney Dis.* **2014**, *63*, 276–285. [CrossRef]
71. Tomayko, E.J.; Kistler, B.M.; Fitschen, P.J.; Wilund, K.R. Intradialytic protein supplementation reduces inflammation and improves physical function in maintenance hemodialysis patients. *J. Ren. Nutr.* **2015**, *25*, 276–283. [CrossRef] [PubMed]
72. Kalantar-Zadeh, K.; Gutekunst, L.; Mehrotra, R.; Kovesdy, C.P.; Bross, R.; Shinaberger, C.S.; Noori, N.; Hirschberg, R.; Benner, D.; Nissenson, A.R.; et al. Understanding sources of dietary phosphorus in the

treatment of patients with chronic kidney disease. *Clin. J. Am. Soc. Nephrol.* **2010**, *5*, 519–530. [CrossRef] [PubMed]

73. Eloot, S.; Van Biesen, W.; Glorieux, G.; Neirynck, N.; Dhondt, A.; Vanholder, R. Does the adequacy parameter Kt/V (urea) reflect uremic toxin concentrations in hemodialysis patients? *PLoS ONE* **2013**, *8*, e76838. [CrossRef] [PubMed]
74. Fuchs, C.J.; Hermans, W.J.H.; Holwerda, A.M.; Smeets, J.S.J.; Senden, J.M.; van Kranenburg, J.; Gijsen, A.P.; Wodzig, W.K.H.W.; Schierbeek, H.; Verdijk, L.B.; et al. Branched-chain amino acid and branched-chain ketoacid ingestion increases muscle protein synthesis rates in vivo in older adults: A double-blind, randomized trial. *Am. J. Clin. Nutr.* **2019**, *110*, 862–872. [CrossRef] [PubMed]
75. Shah, A.P.; Kalantar-Zadeh, K.; Kopple, J.D. Is there a role for ketoacid supplements in the management of CKD? *Am. J. Kidney Dis.* **2015**, *65*, 659–673. [CrossRef] [PubMed]
76. Phillips, S.M.; Tipton, K.D.; Aarsland, A.; Wolf, S.E.; Wolfe, R.R. Mixed muscle protein synthesis and breakdown after resistance exercise in humans. *Am. J. Physiol.* **1997**, *273*, E99–E107. [CrossRef]
77. Biolo, G.; Maggi, S.P.; Williams, B.D.; Tipton, K.D.; Wolfe, R.R. Increased rates of muscle protein turnover and amino acid transport after resistance exercise in humans. *Am. J. Physiol.* **1995**, *268*, E514–E520. [CrossRef]
78. Burd, N.A.; West, D.W.; Moore, D.R.; Atherton, P.J.; Staples, A.W.; Prior, T.; Tang, J.E.; Rennie, M.J.; Baker, S.K.; Phillips, S.M. Enhanced amino acid sensitivity of myofibrillar protein synthesis persists for up to 24 h after resistance exercise in young men. *J. Nutr.* **2011**, *141*, 568–573. [CrossRef]
79. Trommelen, J.; Holwerda, A.M.; Kouw, I.W.; Langer, H.; Halson, S.L.; Rollo, I.; Verdijk, L.B.; LJ, V.A.N.L. Resistance Exercise Augments Postprandial Overnight Muscle Protein Synthesis Rates. *Med. Sci. Sports Exerc.* **2016**, *48*, 2517–2525. [CrossRef]
80. Pennings, B.; Koopman, R.; Beelen, M.; Senden, J.M.; Saris, W.H.; van Loon, L.J. Exercising before protein intake allows for greater use of dietary protein-derived amino acids for de novo muscle protein synthesis in both young and elderly men. *Am. J. Clin. Nutr.* **2011**, *93*, 322–331. [CrossRef]
81. Holwerda, A.M.; Kouw, I.W.; Trommelen, J.; Halson, S.L.; Wodzig, W.K.; Verdijk, L.B.; van Loon, L.J. Physical Activity Performed in the Evening Increases the Overnight Muscle Protein Synthetic Response to Presleep Protein Ingestion in Older Men. *J. Nutr.* **2016**, *146*, 1307–1314. [CrossRef] [PubMed]
82. Glover, E.I.; Phillips, S.M.; Oates, B.R.; Tang, J.E.; Tarnopolsky, M.A.; Selby, A.; Smith, K.; Rennie, M.J. Immobilization induces anabolic resistance in human myofibrillar protein synthesis with low and high dose amino acid infusion. *J. Physiol.* **2008**, *586*, 6049–6061. [CrossRef] [PubMed]
83. Wall, B.T.; Dirks, M.L.; Snijders, T.; van Dijk, J.W.; Fritsch, M.; Verdijk, L.B.; van Loon, L.J. Short-term muscle disuse lowers myofibrillar protein synthesis rates and induces anabolic resistance to protein ingestion. *Am. J. Physiol. Endocrinol. Metab.* **2016**, *310*, E137–E147. [CrossRef] [PubMed]
84. Breen, L.; Stokes, K.A.; Churchward-Venne, T.A.; Moore, D.R.; Baker, S.K.; Smith, K.; Atherton, P.J.; Phillips, S.M. Two weeks of reduced activity decreases leg lean mass and induces "anabolic resistance" of myofibrillar protein synthesis in healthy elderly. *J. Clin. Endocrinol. Metab.* **2013**, *98*, 2604–2612. [CrossRef] [PubMed]
85. Dideriksen, K.; Reitelseder, S.; Holm, L. Influence of amino acids, dietary protein, and physical activity on muscle mass development in humans. *Nutrients* **2013**, *5*, 852–876. [CrossRef] [PubMed]
86. Holwerda, A.M.; Paulussen, K.J.M.; Overkamp, M.; Smeets, J.S.J.; Gijsen, A.P.; Goessens, J.P.B.; Verdijk, L.B.; van Loon, L.J.C. Daily resistance-type exercise stimulates muscle protein synthesis in vivo in young men. *J. Appl. Physiol. (1985)* **2018**, *124*, 66–75. [CrossRef] [PubMed]
87. Shad, B.J.; Thompson, J.L.; Holwerda, A.M.; Stocks, B.; Elhassan, Y.S.; Philp, A.; LJC, V.A.N.L.; Wallis, G.A. One Week of Step Reduction Lowers Myofibrillar Protein Synthesis Rates in Young Men. *Med. Sci. Sports Exerc.* **2019**, *51*, 2125–2134. [CrossRef]
88. Peterson, M.J.; Giuliani, C.; Morey, M.C.; Pieper, C.F.; Evenson, K.R.; Mercer, V.; Cohen, H.J.; Visser, M.; Brach, J.S.; Kritchevsky, S.B.; et al. Physical activity as a preventative factor for frailty: The health, aging, and body composition study. *J. Gerontol. Ser. A Biol. Sci. Med. Sci.* **2009**, *64*, 61–68. [CrossRef]
89. Zampieri, S.; Pietrangelo, L.; Loefler, S.; Fruhmann, H.; Vogelauer, M.; Burggraf, S.; Pond, A.; Grim-Stieger, M.; Cvecka, J.; Sedliak, M.; et al. Lifelong physical exercise delays age-associated skeletal muscle decline. *J. Gerontol. Ser. A Biol. Sci. Med. Sci.* **2015**, *70*, 163–173. [CrossRef]

90. Dirks, M.L.; Wall, B.T.; van de Valk, B.; Holloway, T.M.; Holloway, G.P.; Chabowski, A.; Goossens, G.H.; van Loon, L.J. One Week of Bed Rest Leads to Substantial Muscle Atrophy and Induces Whole-Body Insulin Resistance in the Absence of Skeletal Muscle Lipid Accumulation. *Diabetes* **2016**, *65*, 2862–2875. [CrossRef]
91. Dirks, M.L.; Wall, B.T.; Nilwik, R.; Weerts, D.H.; Verdijk, L.B.; van Loon, L.J. Skeletal muscle disuse atrophy is not attenuated by dietary protein supplementation in healthy older men. *J. Nutr.* **2014**, *144*, 1196–1203. [CrossRef] [PubMed]
92. Piercy, K.L.; Troiano, R.P.; Ballard, R.M.; Carlson, S.A.; Fulton, J.E.; Galuska, D.A.; George, S.M.; Olson, R.D. The Physical Activity Guidelines for Americans. *JAMA* **2018**, *320*, 2020–2028. [CrossRef] [PubMed]
93. Ashby, D.; Borman, N.; Burton, J.; Corbett, R.; Davenport, A.; Farrington, K.; Flowers, K.; Fotheringham, J.; Andrea Fox, R.N.; Franklin, G.; et al. Renal Association Clinical Practice Guideline on Haemodialysis. *BMC Nephrol.* **2019**, *20*, 379. [CrossRef] [PubMed]
94. Matsuzawa, R.; Roshanravan, B.; Shimoda, T.; Mamorita, N.; Yoneki, K.; Harada, M.; Watanabe, T.; Yoshida, A.; Takeuchi, Y.; Matsunaga, A. Physical Activity Dose for Hemodialysis Patients: Where to Begin? Results from a Prospective Cohort Study. *J. Ren. Nutr.* **2018**, *28*, 45–53. [CrossRef]
95. Broers, N.J.H.; Martens, R.J.H.; Cornelis, T.; van der Sande, F.M.; Diederen, N.M.P.; Hermans, M.M.H.; Wirtz, J.; Stifft, F.; Konings, C.; Dejagere, T.; et al. Physical Activity in End-Stage Renal Disease Patients: The Effects of Starting Dialysis in the First 6 Months after the Transition Period. *Nephron* **2017**, *137*, 47–56. [CrossRef]
96. Tentori, F.; Elder, S.J.; Thumma, J.; Pisoni, R.L.; Bommer, J.; Fissell, R.B.; Fukuhara, S.; Jadoul, M.; Keen, M.L.; Saran, R.; et al. Physical exercise among participants in the Dialysis Outcomes and Practice Patterns Study (DOPPS): Correlates and associated outcomes. *Nephrol. Dial. Transpl.* **2010**, *25*, 3050–3062. [CrossRef]
97. Da Costa Rosa, C.S.; Nishimoto, D.Y.; Freitas Junior, I.F.; Ciolac, E.G.; Monteiro, H.L. Factors Associated with Levels of Physical Activity in Chronic Kidney Disease Patients Undergoing Hemodialysis: The Role of Dialysis Versus Nondialysis Day. *J. Phys. Act. Health* **2017**, *14*, 726–732. [CrossRef]
98. Gomes, E.P.; Reboredo, M.M.; Carvalho, E.V.; Teixeira, D.R.; Carvalho, L.F.; Filho, G.F.; de Oliveira, J.C.; Sanders-Pinheiro, H.; Chebli, J.M.; de Paula, R.B.; et al. Physical Activity in Hemodialysis Patients Measured by Triaxial Accelerometer. *Biomed. Res. Int.* **2015**, *2015*, 645645. [CrossRef] [PubMed]
99. Clarkson, M.J.; Bennett, P.N.; Fraser, S.F.; Warmington, S.A. Exercise interventions for improving objective physical function in patients with end-stage kidney disease on dialysis: A systematic review and meta-analysis. *Am. J. Physiol. Ren. Physiol.* **2019**, *316*, F856–F872. [CrossRef]
100. Koh, K.P.; Fassett, R.G.; Sharman, J.E.; Coombes, J.S.; Williams, A.D. Effect of intradialytic versus home-based aerobic exercise training on physical function and vascular parameters in hemodialysis patients: A randomized pilot study. *Am. J. Kidney Dis.* **2010**, *55*, 88–99. [CrossRef]
101. Salhab, N.; Karavetian, M.; Kooman, J.; Fiaccadori, E.; El Khoury, C.F. Effects of intradialytic aerobic exercise on hemodialysis patients: A systematic review and meta-analysis. *J. Nephrol.* **2019**. [CrossRef] [PubMed]
102. Anding, K.; Bar, T.; Trojniak-Hennig, J.; Kuchinke, S.; Krause, R.; Rost, J.M.; Halle, M. A structured exercise programme during haemodialysis for patients with chronic kidney disease: Clinical benefit and long-term adherence. *BMJ Open* **2015**, *5*, e008709. [CrossRef] [PubMed]
103. Campbell, W.W.; Crim, M.C.; Young, V.R.; Evans, W.J. Increased energy requirements and changes in body composition with resistance training in older adults. *Am. J. Clin. Nutr.* **1994**, *60*, 167–175. [CrossRef] [PubMed]
104. Churchward-Venne, T.A.; Tieland, M.; Verdijk, L.B.; Leenders, M.; Dirks, M.L.; de Groot, L.C.; van Loon, L.J. There Are No Nonresponders to Resistance-Type Exercise Training in Older Men and Women. *J. Am. Med. Dir. Assoc.* **2015**, *16*, 400–411. [CrossRef]
105. Snijders, T.; Leenders, M.; de Groot, L.; van Loon, L.J.C.; Verdijk, L.B. Muscle mass and strength gains following 6months of resistance type exercise training are only partly preserved within one year with autonomous exercise continuation in older adults. *Exp. Gerontol.* **2019**, *121*, 71–78. [CrossRef]
106. Majchrzak, K.M.; Pupim, L.B.; Flakoll, P.J.; Ikizler, T.A. Resistance exercise augments the acute anabolic effects of intradialytic oral nutritional supplementation. *Nephrol. Dial. Transplant.* **2008**, *23*, 1362–1369. [CrossRef]
107. Bessa, B.; de Oliveira Leal, V.; Moraes, C.; Barboza, J.; Fouque, D.; Mafra, D. Resistance training in hemodialysis patients: A review. *Rehabil. Nurs.* **2015**, *40*, 111–126. [CrossRef]
108. Saitoh, M.; Ogawa, M.; Dos Santos, M.R.; Kondo, H.; Suga, K.; Itoh, H.; Tabata, Y. Effects of Intradialytic Resistance Exercise on Protein Energy Wasting, Physical Performance and Physical Activity in Ambulatory

Patients on Dialysis: A Single-Center Preliminary Study in a Japanese Dialysis Facility. *Ther. Apher. Dial.* **2016**, *20*, 632–638. [CrossRef]

109. Gomes Neto, M.; de Lacerda, F.F.R.; Lopes, A.A.; Martinez, B.P.; Saquetto, M.B. Intradialytic exercise training modalities on physical functioning and health-related quality of life in patients undergoing maintenance hemodialysis: Systematic review and meta-analysis. *Clin. Rehabil.* **2018**, *32*, 1189–1202. [CrossRef]
110. Salhab, N.; Alrukhaimi, M.; Kooman, J.; Fiaccadori, E.; Aljubori, H.; Rizk, R.; Karavetian, M. Effect of Intradialytic Exercise on Hyperphosphatemia and Malnutrition. *Nutrients* **2019**, *11*, 2464. [CrossRef]
111. Chan, D.; Cheema, B.S. Progressive Resistance Training in End-Stage Renal Disease: Systematic Review. *Am. J. Nephrol.* **2016**, *44*, 32–45. [CrossRef] [PubMed]
112. Cheema, B.; Abas, H.; Smith, B.; O'Sullivan, A.; Chan, M.; Patwardhan, A.; Kelly, J.; Gillin, A.; Pang, G.; Lloyd, B.; et al. Progressive exercise for anabolism in kidney disease (PEAK): A randomized, controlled trial of resistance training during hemodialysis. *J. Am. Soc. Nephrol.* **2007**, *18*, 1594–1601. [CrossRef] [PubMed]
113. Kopple, J.D.; Wang, H.; Casaburi, R.; Fournier, M.; Lewis, M.I.; Taylor, W.; Storer, T.W. Exercise in maintenance hemodialysis patients induces transcriptional changes in genes favoring anabolic muscle. *J. Am. Soc. Nephrol.* **2007**, *18*, 2975–2986. [CrossRef] [PubMed]
114. Kirkman, D.L.; Mullins, P.; Junglee, N.A.; Kumwenda, M.; Jibani, M.M.; Macdonald, J.H. Anabolic exercise in haemodialysis patients: A randomised controlled pilot study. *J. Cachexia Sarcopenia Muscle* **2014**, *5*, 199–207. [CrossRef]
115. Van den Ham, E.C.; Kooman, J.P.; Schols, A.M.; Nieman, F.H.; Does, J.D.; Akkermans, M.A.; Janssen, P.P.; Gosker, H.R.; Ward, K.A.; MacDonald, J.H.; et al. The functional, metabolic, and anabolic responses to exercise training in renal transplant and hemodialysis patients. *Transplantation* **2007**, *83*, 1059–1068. [CrossRef]
116. Martin-Alemany, G.; Valdez-Ortiz, R.; Olvera-Soto, G.; Gomez-Guerrero, I.; Aguire-Esquivel, G.; Cantu-Quintanilla, G.; Lopez-Alvarenga, J.C.; Miranda-Alatriste, P.; Espinosa-Cuevas, A. The effects of resistance exercise and oral nutritional supplementation during hemodialysis on indicators of nutritional status and quality of life. *Nephrol. Dial. Transplant.* **2016**, *31*, 1712–1720. [CrossRef]
117. Molsted, S.; Harrison, A.P.; Eidemak, I.; Andersen, J.L. The effects of high-load strength training with protein- or nonprotein-containing nutritional supplementation in patients undergoing dialysis. *J. Ren. Nutr.* **2013**, *23*, 132–140. [CrossRef]
118. Martin-Alemany, G.; Espinosa-Cuevas, M.L.A.; Perez-Navarro, M.; Wilund, K.R.; Miranda-Alatriste, P.; Cortes-Perez, M.; Garcia-Villalobos, G.; Gomez-Guerrero, I.; Cantu-Quintanilla, G.; Ramirez-Mendoza, M.; et al. Effect of Oral Nutritional Supplementation With and Without Exercise on Nutritional Status and Physical Function of Adult Hemodialysis Patients: A Parallel Controlled Clinical Trial (AVANTE-HEMO Study). *J. Ren. Nutr.* **2019**. [CrossRef]
119. Molsted, S.; Bjorkman, A.S.D.; Lundstrom, L.H. Effects of strength training to patients undergoing dialysis: A systematic review. *Dan. Med. J.* **2019**, *66*, A5526.
120. Witard, O.C.; Wardle, S.L.; Macnaughton, L.S.; Hodgson, A.B.; Tipton, K.D. Protein Considerations for Optimising Skeletal Muscle Mass in Healthy Young and Older Adults. *Nutrients* **2016**, *8*, 181. [CrossRef]
121. Trommelen, J.; Betz, M.W.; van Loon, L.J.C. The Muscle Protein Synthetic Response to Meal Ingestion Following Resistance-Type Exercise. *Sports Med.* **2019**, *49*, 185–197. [CrossRef] [PubMed]
122. Oquendo, L.G.; Asencio, J.M.M.; de Las Nieves, C.B. Contributing factors for therapeutic diet adherence in patients receiving haemodialysis treatment: An integrative review. *J. Clin. Nurs.* **2017**, *26*, 3893–3905. [CrossRef] [PubMed]

12

Poor Oral Health as a Determinant of Malnutrition and Sarcopenia

Domenico Azzolino [1,2,*,†], Pier Carmine Passarelli [3,†], Paolo De Angelis [3], Giovan Battista Piccirillo [3], Antonio D'Addona [3] and Matteo Cesari [1,2]

1 Geriatric Unit, Fondazione IRCCS Ca' Granda Ospedale Maggiore Policlinico, 20122 Milan, Italy; matteo.cesari@unimi.it
2 Department of Clinical Sciences and Community Health, University of Milan, 20122 Milan, Italy
3 Department of Head and Neck, Oral Surgery and Implantology Unit, Institute of Clinical Dentistry, Catholic University of Sacred Hearth, Fondazione Policlinico Universitario Gemelli, 00168 Rome, Italy; piercarminepassarelli@hotmail.it (P.C.P.); dr.paolodeangelis@gmail.com (P.D.A.); giovanbpiccirillo@gmail.com (G.B.P.); antonio.daddona@unicatt.it (A.D.)
* Correspondence: domenico.azzolino@policlinico.mi.it
† These authors contributed equally to this work.

Abstract: Aging is accompanied by profound changes in many physiological functions, leading to a decreased ability to cope with stressors. Many changes are subtle, but can negatively affect nutrient intake, leading to overt malnutrition. Poor oral health may affect food selection and nutrient intake, leading to malnutrition and, consequently, to frailty and sarcopenia. On the other hand, it has been highlighted that sarcopenia is a whole-body process also affecting muscles dedicated to chewing and swallowing. Hence, muscle decline of these muscle groups may also have a negative impact on nutrient intake, increasing the risk for malnutrition. The interplay between oral diseases and malnutrition with frailty and sarcopenia may be explained through biological and environmental factors that are linked to the common burden of inflammation and oxidative stress. The presence of oral problems, alone or in combination with sarcopenia, may thus represent the biological substratum of the disabling cascade experienced by many frail individuals. A multimodal and multidisciplinary approach, including personalized dietary counselling and oral health care, may thus be helpful to better manage the complexity of older people. Furthermore, preventive strategies applied throughout the lifetime could help to preserve both oral and muscle function later in life. Here, we provide an overview on the relevance of poor oral health as a determinant of malnutrition and sarcopenia.

Keywords: sarcopenia; nutrition; oral health; older people; malnutrition; swallowing; life course approach

---

1. Introduction

Advancing age is characterized by a progressive decline in multiple physiological functions, leading to an increased vulnerability to stressors and augmented risk of adverse outcomes [1–3]. During the aging process, several factors may affect body shape from both clinical and functional perspectives. Reduction in smell and taste senses, poor appetite (the so-called "anorexia of aging"), and decreased energy expenditure may all contribute to poor nutrition. Moreover, illnesses, medications, as well as poor oral health (for example, due to teeth loss and poorly fitting dentures) can exacerbate anorexia [4–6]. Nutritional status among older people may be also influenced by living or eating alone, poor financial status, dismobility, and decreased ability to shop or prepare meals [7,8]. Psychosocial factors including loneliness, sleep disorders, dementia, and depression are also recognized to have a negative impact on the dietary intake of older subjects [9].

Furthermore, with aging, there is a progressive loss in muscle mass and strength, whereas fat mass and fat infiltration of muscle increase [10,11]. Sarcopenia is the term, introduced for the first time in 1988 by Irwin Rosenberg, to indicate the pathologic reduction in muscle mass and strength leading to a poor function [12,13]. Interestingly, in recent years, it has been highlighted that sarcopenia is not limited to lower limbs, but is a whole-body process [14–16], also affecting the muscles devoted to chewing and swallowing [10,17], with a negative impact on food intake. In fact, atrophy of muscles critical for the respiratory and swallowing functions has been reported [14,18–22].

The variety of dental problems experienced by older people can result in chewing difficulties determining changes in food selection, thus leading to malnutrition and consequently to frailty [23] and sarcopenia [10,23]. Poor oral status may also predispose one to a chronic low-grade systemic inflammation through periodontal disease [24,25], which has an increased prevalence in those who are not able to perform the daily oral hygiene procedures [26], and it is a well-known risk factor in the pathogenesis of frailty [27] and sarcopenia [28]. Furthermore, periodontal disease has been associated with faster decline in handgrip strength [29], and recent studies showed an association between chewing difficulties and frailty [24].

Therefore, a hypothetical triangle oral status–nutrition–sarcopenia, exposing the older person to the frailty disabling cascade, may be suggested, as seen in Figure 1.

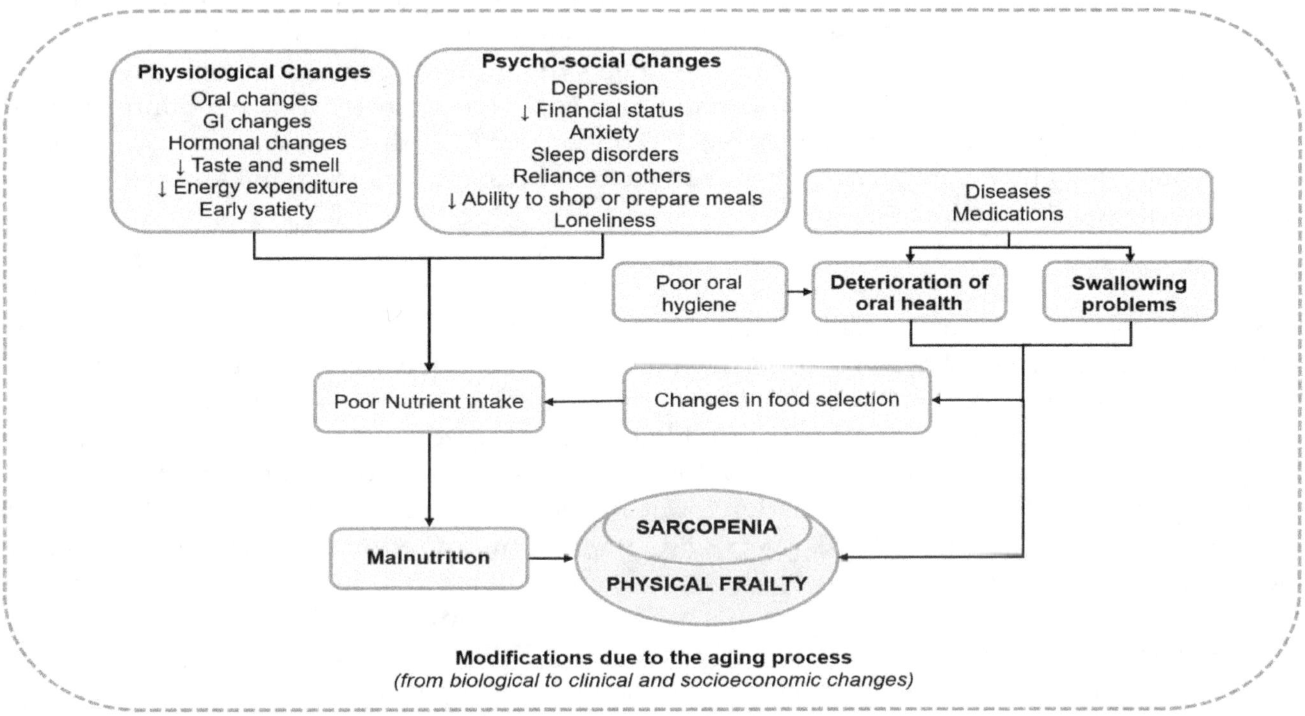

Figure 1. Overview of the interplay between poor oral status, malnutrition, and sarcopenia. GI—gastrointestinal.

2. Oral Changes with Aging

Poor oral health is not an inevitable part of aging since good care throughout the life course can result in the maintenance of functional teeth later in life [24]. Throughout a lifetime, the oral cavity experiences a variety of physiological modifications, such as enamel changes, fractures lines and stains, as well as dentin exposure and darkening of the tooth. At the same time, in the inner part of the tooth, several changes, such as the deposition of secondary dentin reducing the size of the pulp chamber and canals, may also occur [30]. Furthermore, in older people, tooth wear is frequently observed, affecting more than 85% of all the teeth groups in both the mandible and maxilla [31]. Additionally, a loss in terms of elastic fibers in the connective tissue has been documented and, subsequently, the oral mucosa becomes less resilient [32].

However, older people, especially those who are institutionalized or with limited financial resources, may experience problems to access oral care. Furthermore, it has been documented that older people frequently have difficulty expressing complaints and assign low priority to oral health until dental problems become intolerable [33]. Oral problems among older people have been implicated in a high prevalence of tooth loss, dental caries, periodontal disease, xerostomia, and oral precancer/cancer lesions [34]. Periodontitis and dental caries are very common diseases, especially in older people, and are considered the main cause of tooth loss [35].

Around the age of 70, there is also a peak of root/cementum caries, as a result of both tooth retention and major exposure of these surfaces following periodontal support loss. Moreover, older people are at higher risk of periodontitis since it is a cumulative disease, especially with regard to the multirooted teeth [36].

2.1. Edentulism

Edentulism is a pathological condition characterized by multiple missing teeth; it can be partial or total. The etiology of tooth loss includes factors such as predisposition, diet, hormonal status, coexisting diseases, hygiene habits, and use of dental clinics. Additionally, edentulism may result from an unsuccessful periodontal treatment or important carious lesions [37,38]. Dental disease and loss of teeth are not part of normal aging, but if this occurs, it is probably a result of neglected oral hygiene and/or an inadequate treatment [39,40]. Edentulism is exacerbated when masticatory function is not restored with dental prostheses [41]. Tooth loss affects the individual ability to chew determining an alteration of food choices [42]. Indeed, edentulous people are at greater risk of malnutrition than dentate or partially dentate individuals [43], and, consequently, with an increased susceptibility to sarcopenia and frailty [25]. Tooth loss is also a risk factor for disability, since it impedes self-sufficiency and worsens the quality of life [42].

2.2. Dry Mouth

Saliva is pivotal for bolus formation and consequently is also related to the sensory and textural experience. Xerostomia is a clinical condition characterized by an excessive sensation of dryness in the mouth, which is not necessarily linked to salivary gland hypofunction [30,44]. Xerostomia is estimated to affect 25–50% of older individuals [45]. Etiologic factors include polypharmacy (especially with antihypertensives, antidepressants, and antipsychotics) [46], diseases, poor general health, female sex, and older age [47,48]. Furthermore, radiation for head and neck cancers can damage salivary glands, leading to permanent xerostomia [49]. With aging, there is also a reduced salivary flow in salivary glands, which cannot be explained only on the basis of medications [50]. In fact, salivary hypofunction and xerostomia are two distinct constructs that are frequently improperly used interchangeably [33].

However, it has been reported that nearly one third of older adults complaining of xerostomia do not present any reduction of the salivary flow or saliva secretion. This suggests a psychological component may be involved when reporting the symptom [30]. Nonetheless, hyposalivation may seriously compromise chewing function and early digestive process. A reduced quantity of saliva can, in fact, affect the preparation of the alimentary bolus and the swallowing [51].

2.3. Periodontal Disease

Periodontitis is described as a chronic inflammatory disease that affects the supporting tissues of the teeth, leading to a progressive destruction of the periodontium [52]. It can also cause mobility and displacement of the remaining teeth and is often linked to difficulty in chewing. Prevalence of periodontal disease, considering a periodontal index score of 4 (deep pockets), ranges from approximately 5% to 70% among older people [53]. Periodontitis is a cumulative disease; therefore, it becomes increasingly severe as the person ages [30]. Poor oral hygiene is a critical determinant of periodontitis since it leads to the formation of dental plaque containing microorganisms [54]. Systemic risk factors for periodontal disease also include other behaviors, such as smoking, medical conditions (i.e., poorly controlled diabetes, obesity, stress, osteopenia), and inadequate dietary consumption of calcium and vitamin D [55]. Since periodontitis share some characteristics with other systemic inflammatory diseases, a relationship between periodontitis and other inflammatory pathologies (i.e., diabetes, cardiovascular diseases, adverse pregnancy outcomes, and rheumatoid arthritis) has been proposed [56].

In recent years, the role of the diet in periodontitis has been highlighted. To date, it has been documented that a diet poor in fruit and vegetables and therefore in micronutrients may lead to a greater inflammatory response of periodontal tissues that support the tooth. Interestingly, a recent systematic review of the relationship between dietary intake and periodontal health in community-dwelling older adults, reported positive associations between periodontal disease and lower intakes of docosahexaenoic acid, vitamin C, vitamin E, β-carotene, milk, fermented dairy products, dietary fiber, fruits and vegetables, and higher intakes of omega-6/omega-3 ratio and saturated fatty acids [57]. Additionally, micronutrient deficiencies can negatively affect healing following periodontal surgery [58]. At the same time, the loss of dental elements due to periodontitis can negatively affect the nutritional status of the patient, resulting in a discomfort during chewing and leading to a selection of soft and easy-to-chew foods.

2.4. *Dental Caries*

Dental caries is a multifactorial infectious disease characterized by the demineralization and destruction of the dental substance: enamel, in fact, is susceptible to acid dissolution over time. The pathological changes of the dental structure may have serious consequences, ultimately leading to the breakdown of the teeth themselves [59]. The prevalence of dental caries varies between 20% and 60% in community-dwelling older people and 60% and 80% in care home settings [60–64]. Various predisposing conditions to dental caries have been reported, including carbohydrate (especially simple sugars) consumption, diabetes, and poor socioeconomic conditions [60,65–68].

With increasing age, people may experience physical and cognitive decline, which may result in poor oral hygiene, leading to an increased incidence of caries. Over time, small lesions already filled can need a larger dental restoration, that can lead to a tooth fracture or an endodontic treatment [30]. Endodontic therapy (also known as root canal treatment) is a necessary procedure in case of inflamed or infected dental pulp. It consists in the removal of the pulp, both in the coronal and radicular part of the tooth, and in its replacement with a gutta-percha permanent filling (a substance of vegetable origin such as natural rubber). Xerostomia is closely related to a higher risk for developing caries since loss of saliva may lead to an increased acidity of the mouth. This leads to different situations that may contribute to the development of the dental caries: the proliferation of bacteria, the loss of minerals from the tooth surfaces, and the loss of lubrication [69].

2.5. *Impact of Oral Health on Nutritional Status*

Nutrition is a key modulator of health in older persons. Inadequate intake of nutrients is a well-known contributing factor in the progression of many diseases. This also has a significant impact in the complex etiology of sarcopenia and frailty [70–72]. Due to a decline in many functions, including poor oral status, dietary intake is often compromised in older people and the risk of malnutrition is increased. Particularly, acute and chronic illnesses and medications as well as poor dentition can exacerbate anorexia [5,70,73]. Oral problems in older individuals are associated with modifications in food selection and, therefore, in nutrient intake [25]. Deterioration of oral health can ultimately lead to the development of chronic conditions such as diabetes [74] and cardiovascular problems [75–77]. Masticatory performance is affected by the number of teeth in functional occlusion [78–80], the maximal biting force [81,82], denture wearing [83] and xerostomia [84]. The functional occlusion during mandibular closure is provided by the even and simultaneous contact of all remaining teeth (at least 20 with 10 contiguous teeth in each arch) [85].

Tooth loss has been implicated in the reduction of chewing ability and in difficulties in bolus formation [86]. To date, it has been reported that as number of remaining teeth decrease, the bolus size increases leading to a dysfunctional swallowing [87]. Edentulous individuals, even when using well-made dentures, may experience more chewing difficulties than dentate people [88]. Therefore, they may be considered as the group more prone to changing their diet [89,90]. Older people who experience dental problems frequently avoid harder foods such as meats, fruits, and vegetables which are typically major sources of proteins, fiber, vitamins, and minerals [41,88,91]. The lack of these latter key nutrients may expose older individuals to an increased risk for malnutrition, frailty, and sarcopenia [24,92]. In addition, it is well established that micronutrient deficiencies, even subtle, may lead to oxidative stress and consequently to inflammation. Therefore, these processes can further exacerbate sarcopenia and frailty and become a clear risk factor for periodontitis. Nutritional deficiencies may also negatively affect the mineralization process, increasing the susceptibility to dental caries [93]. Furthermore, undernutrition can exacerbate the severity of oral infections [94]. Indeed, with advancing age, people show a tendency to select soft foods due to difficulty and fatigue of chewing [10,95]. However, these latter are frequently processed foods that are high in fat and sugar and with a poor content of vitamins and minerals, leading to fat deposition, oxidative stress, inflammation, and, consequently, increased risk of cardiovascular disease and metabolic syndrome [88,95–97]. In fact, it is well established that obesity leads to chronic low-grade inflammation, increasing the susceptibility to dental caries, periodontal disease, and tooth loss [98]. The excess of energy is stored in adipocytes and leads to both hypertrophy and hyperplasia, resulting in an abnormal adipocyte function. This may increase mitochondrial stress and altered endoplasmatic reticulum function. Furthermore, adipocyte-associated inflammatory macrophages can also induce oxidative stress [99]. On the other hand, it is widely recognized that an excessive consumption of simple sugars is a major risk factor for dental caries [100,101].

Large epidemiological studies, such as the UK National Diet and Nutrition Survey (NDNS) [102] and the US National Health and Nutritional Examination Surveys (NHANES) [103,104], reported an association between poor dental status and inadequate dietary intake in older people. In particular, they reported that edentulous subjects, with and without prosthesis, consumed less fruits and vegetables. Moreover, decreased protein and micronutrient intake, together with increased carbohydrate consumption, has been reported in people with less than 21 teeth [104].

3. Sarcopenia and Oral Status

Sarcopenia, defined as the progressive and accelerated loss of muscle mass and function, is a major determinant of several adverse outcomes including frailty, disability, and mortality [13,105]. Although sarcopenia is a condition commonly observed with the aging process, it can also occur earlier in life [106]. Since 2016, sarcopenia has been recognized as an independent condition with an International Classification of Disease, 10th Revision, Clinical Modification (ICD-10-CM) Diagnosis Code [107]. Recently, the European Working Group on Sarcopenia in Older People (EWGSOP) [106] updated their consensus on definition and diagnosis (EWGSOP2). In this revised consensus, low muscle strength is considered a key characteristic of sarcopenia, and poor physical performance is identified as indicative of severe sarcopenia. Moreover, EWGSOP2 have recommended specific cut-off points to identify and characterize the sarcopenic condition, and provide an algorithm that can be used for case-finding.

Sarcopenia has a complex multifactorial pathogenesis, which involves lifestyle habits (i.e., malnutrition, physical inactivity), disease triggers, and age-dependent biological changes (i.e., chronic inflammation, mitochondrial abnormalities, loss of neuromuscular junctions, reduced satellite cell numbers, hormonal alterations) [108,109]. Sarcopenia is a whole-body process, affecting not only lower extremities, but also muscles dedicated to breathing, mastication, and swallowing [14,18–22]. In particular, swallowing is a complex mechanism involving several head and neck muscles simultaneously and in conjunction to coordinate the entire process [110]. Several age-related changes, such as as reduction of tissue elasticity, changes of the head and neck anatomy, reduced oral and pharyngeal sensitivity, and impaired dental status, may contribute to different degrees to a subtle swallowing impairment, the so called "presbyphagia". It is usually an asymptomatic condition in which swallowing function is preserved, but tends to slowly worsen as the aging process advances [16,111]. Presbyphagia may increase the risk of dysphagia and aspiration in older people, especially during acute illnesses and other stressors [112]. Moreover, reductions in muscle mass of the geniohyoid, pterygoid, masseter, tongue, and pharyngeal muscles have been documented in older individuals [20,113–115]. Several authors also reported a decline in the strength of the swallowing muscles with aging or sarcopenia [116]. Maximal tongue strength decreases with aging [116–119], and there is some evidence that aging leads to a decreased jaw-opening force in older men. Several authors also reported an association between tongue strength and handgrip strength [120,121]. A decrease in tongue strength has been associated with a decline of activities of daily living [122], and a reduced tongue thickness has been noted in people with low body weight [20].

Lip function is also important for feeding. In fact, poor lip muscle closure may cause leakage through the corners of the mouth [123]. Additionally, decreased lip strength has been suggested to occur due to sarcopenia and to be related to difficulties in eating and drinking (i.e., dysphagia) [117]. Lip force has been associated with hand grip strength and lip pendency has been associated with aging [117,124].

Indeed, since it has been shown that skeletal muscle mass and strength decline may affect both swallowing and general muscle groups, a new condition, called "sarcopenic dysphagia" has been coined [22,124,125]. Swallowing muscles are characterized by a high percentage of type II fibers, which are more easily affected by malnutrition and sarcopenia than type I muscle fibers [22]. However, some cranial muscles, including the jaw-closers, are very different in fiber-type composition than other skeletal muscle groups (i.e., limbs or abdomen). For instance, the masseter muscle, which originates from the zygomatic arch, contains both type I and type II fibers, but shows a predominance of type I muscle fibers, which are more strongly affected by inactivity rather than aging [126,127]. Given that the meal texture of older people frequently becomes softer, less power of tongue movement and of masseter muscle is required, which may result in decreased activity of these muscles.

Interestingly, poor oral health may predispose one to a chronic low-grade inflammatory state through periodontal disease, which is a well-known risk factor for frailty and sarcopenia [25,128,129]. In fact, the detrimental effects of periodontitis are not confined solely to the oral cavity, but extend systemically, leading to metabolic alterations [130], including insulin resistance [131], diabetes [131,132], arthritis [133], and heart disease [134]. Furthermore, alterations in mitochondrial function leading to oxidative stress through the production of reactive oxygen species (ROS) have also been reported to mediate both oral and systemic pathologies (i.e., sarcopenia) [108,135–137]. Given their regulatory role as signaling molecules in autophagy, it has been speculated that elevated ROS production in periodontal disease could lead to autophagic alterations [138]. Bullon et al. [139] found high levels of mitochondrial-derived ROS, accompanied by mitochondrial dysfunction in peripheral blood mononuclear cells from patients with periodontitis. Moreover, oral gingiva seems to be highly responsive to the lipopolysaccharides (LPS), which are bacterial endotoxins prevalent in periodontal disease. In fact, gingival fibroblasts, which play an important role in remodeling periodontal soft tissues, may directly interact with LPS. In particular, LPS from *Porphyromonas gingivalis* enhances the production of inflammatory cytokines [140]. *Porphyromonas gingivalis* has been found to be responsible for high mitochondrial ROS and coenzyme Q10 levels, and for mitochondrial dysfunction, given its influence on the amount of respiratory chain complex I and III [138,139]. Indeed, LPS-mediated mitochondrial dysfunction could explain the oxidative stress onset in patients with periodontitis. Furthermore, Hamalainen et al. [29] reported an association between periodontitis and quicker declines in handgrip strength.

On the other hand, as discussed in the previous section, the variety of dental problems experienced by older people can lead to a decline in general health through poor nutrient intake, pain, and low quality of life [25]. Poor oral status has been reported to affect 71% of patients in rehabilitation settings [141] and 91% of people in acute-care hospitals [142], and has been associated with malnutrition, dysphagia, and reduced activities of daily living [17]. Hence, poor oral status may lead to sarcopenia through poor nutrient intake. Moreover, inflammation further contributes to malnutrition through various mechanisms, such as anorexia, decreased nutrient intake, altered metabolism (i.e., elevation of resting energy expenditure), and increased muscle catabolism [143]. Chronic inflammation is a common underlying factor, not only in the etiology of sarcopenia, but also for frailty. In fact, sarcopenia and frailty are closely related and show a remarkable overlap especially in the physical function domain [144–146]. The presence of oral problems, alone or in combination with sarcopenia, may thus represent the biological substratum of the disabling cascade experienced by many frail individuals.

4. Interventions

The management of older people should be multimodal and multidisciplinary, especially for those with or at risk of malnutrition [147], in order to improve different conditions (i.e., oral problems and sarcopenia). From a practical point of view, comprehensive geriatric assessment (CGA) is the multidimensional, interdisciplinary diagnostic and therapeutic process aimed at determining the medical, psychological, and functional problems of older people. The CGA's objective is the development of a coordinated and integrated plan for treatment and follow-up in order to maximize overall health with aging [148]. To date, increasing evidence suggests that prosthodontic treatment in combination with personalized dietary counselling may improve the nutritional status of patients [51]. Here, we provide an overview on the management of oral problems, malnutrition, and sarcopenia.

4.1. Oral Management

The stomatognathic system is very vulnerable over time, but with special care, it can be preserved throughout the lifetime [30]. Nevertheless, one of the major challenges in providing both restorative and preventive care for older adults is to check dental status on a regular basis [34]. Prevention is pivotal to detecting oral disease as soon as possible and requires regular patient contact. However, since it has been reported that older people frequently fail to achieve a good oral hygiene, both patients and caregivers should be made more aware about the importance to check dental status as well as oral hygiene.

The oral health-care professionals should develop a personalized program, in order to prevent all the problems related to the aging process. In some cases, it is difficult to provide dental care in the hospital setting in a short time, since in many countries there are long waiting lists (especially in publicly funded hospitals) [149]. Therefore, private dentists also need better awareness concerning the complexity of older people. There is, first and foremost, a need to understand the level of dependency, the medical condition, and the physical or cognitive impairment of the patient. Secondly, it is important to establish an oral healthcare plan that includes both professional and self-care elements [150].

The oral management of older people usually involves different aspects:

(1) For the teeth affected by carious lesions, it must be recommended that prompt treatment be provided in order to prevent tooth loss. It would be equally appropriate for endodontic treatments for teeth with endodontic problems.
(2) It is very important to monitor the periodontal status of the older patient and to provide a proper treatment plan, such as modification of general health-risk factors and oral health-specific risk factors, but professional hygiene or surgical procedures may also be necessary.
(3) Prosthetic rehabilitation of the edentulous patient may help to prevent malnutrition [151] since it restores the chewing function.
(4) In order to prevent problems related to the xerostomia and reduce exacerbation of carious lesions, it may be helpful to treat with saliva substitutes.

4.2. Nutritional Interventions

As discussed above, nutrition is an important determinant of health in older people. Thereby, it is pivotal to provide adequate amounts of energy, proteins, fluid, and micronutrients in order to prevent or treat excess or deficiencies, and therefore improve several health-related outcomes in terms of morbidity and mortality. A personalized approach is pivotal in order to respect individual preferences, needs, and to increase compliance to the diet. Nutritional status should be assessed before each intervention, and the amount of energy and proteins should be individually adjusted with regard to nutritional status, physical activity level, disease status, and tolerance [152]. The European Society for Clinical Nutrition and Metabolism (ESPEN) [152], in its guidelines on clinical nutrition and hydration in geriatrics, recommends a guiding value for energy intake of 30 kcal/kg of body weight/day. However, as stated above, it should be adapted individually. Both ESPEN [153] and the PROT-AGE study group [147] recommend providing a protein intake of at least 1.0 g/kg body weight/day in older people to maintain muscle mass, increasing the intake up to 1.2–1.5 g/kg body weight/day in presence of acute or chronic illness. Additionally, it seems that the per-meal anabolic threshold of protein intake is higher in older individuals (i.e., 25 to 30 g protein/meal, containing about 2.5 to 2.8 g leucine) than young adults [147]. However, since older people may experience difficulty of ingesting large amounts of proteins in a single meal, supplementation should be considered. Since serum vitamin D levels decline gradually with aging [154,155] and have been associated with reduced muscle mass and strength, supplementation should thus be considered in those who are deficient.

Food texture should be adapted depending on the chewing and swallowing condition in order to avoid choking risk [10]. Harder foods may be modified to soft consistencies (i.e., bite-sized, minced, pureed) requiring little chewing, as well as liquids, which may be thickened to render the swallowing process slower and safer [10,156,157]. Controlling the intake of simple sugars is pivotal to prevent both dental caries [101] and metabolic complications [158]. World Health Organization recommends to limit the intake of free sugars to less than 10% of total energy intake to minimize the risk of dental caries [159].

Fruit and vegetables are major sources of minerals and vitamins with antioxidant properties; therefore, their consumption should be promoted both for oral and general health. It has been documented that excessive antioxidant supplementation could compromise both the mechanism of adaption to exercise and have even pro-oxidant effects. Thus, supplementation in people who are not deficient should be regarded carefully [160]. Dietary consumption of fatty fish (i.e., salmon, mackerel, herring, lake trout, sardines, albacore tuna, and their oils), which are a major source of omega-3 fatty acids, has been associated with a greater fat-free mass [161]. Given their antioxidant role, omega-3 fatty acid supplementation has been suggested to improve inflammatory status both in periodontal disease [162] and sarcopenia [163]. However, more studies are needed to further elucidate the exact time and dosage of supplementation as well as long term effects [164]. Nevertheless, consumption of foods rich in omega-3, such as as fatty fish, should be promoted.

4.3. Exercise and Rehabilitative Strategies

Physical inactivity is considered one of the main causes of sarcopenia [165] because it determines a resistance to muscle anabolic stimuli [166]. Moreover, it has been proposed that physically inactive individuals may have a greater risk of periodontal disease [167]. In particular, resistance training seems to be the most effective type of exercise to counteract sarcopenia [168]. Furthermore, since sarcopenia is a systemic process [15,21], it has been recommended to perform a holistic training involving all muscle groups [15]. In fact, it has been documented that both masticatory and swallowing functions can be improved through muscle-strengthening exercises [169,170]. Several studies reported enhancements in subjective chewing ability, swallowing function, salivation, relief of oral dryness, and oral-health quality of life. Indeed, the synergistic effect of nutritional interventions coupled with physical exercise may improve both muscle [164] and oral health [167]. Recently, Kim et al. [171] reported an improvement in oral function following an exercise program which included stretching of the lip, tongue, cheek, masticatory muscle exercise, and swallowing movements. Several studies have been focused on swallowing rehabilitation. To date, a positive effect of expiratory muscle resistance training has been documented in improving suprahyoid muscle activity [172,173]. Furthermore, head lift exercises showed a beneficial impact on swallowing movements [174,175], and tongue strengthening exercises have been reported to enhance tongue strength [176,177]. Yeates et al. [178] demonstrated that isometric tongue strength exercises and tongue pressure accuracy tasks improved isometric tongue strength, tongue pressure generation accuracy, bolus control, and dietary intake by mouth. It has also been reported that tongue exercises prevented general sarcopenia [178,179]. Indeed, swallowing muscles training, despite its focus on swallowing function, may exert its beneficial effects systemically.

5. Conclusions

Aging is characterized by a progressive loss of physiological integrity, leading to a decline in many functions and increased vulnerability to stressors. Many changes in masticatory and swallowing function are subtle but can amplify disease processes seen with aging. Nevertheless, it is often difficult to clearly distinguish the effects of diseases from the underlying age-related modifications. Several stressors, including oral problems, may therefore negatively impact on the increasingly weak homeostatic reserves of older individuals. As a healthy diet may have a systemic beneficial effect, oral care also shows an important role in maintaining and improving not only oral health, but also general health and well-being.

Overall, severe tooth loss, as well as swallowing and masticatory problems, partly contribute to restricted dietary choices and poor nutritional status of older adults, leading to frailty and sarcopenia. On the other hand, oral diseases might be influenced both by frailty and sarcopenia, probably through biological and environmental factors that are linked to the common burden of inflammation and oxidative stress.

A multidisciplinary intervention of dental professionals, geriatricians, nutritionists, and dietitians may help to provide better care and preserve the functional status of older people. Increasing evidence also suggests that oral care, when offered with personalized nutritional advice, may improve the nutritional status of patients. A life course approach to prevention at a younger age, including diet optimization and oral preventive care, as well as physical activity, may help in preserving both oral and muscle function later in life.

Author Contributions: D.A. and P.C.P. equally contributed to conceptualizing and writing the manuscript. P.D.A., G.B.P., A.D. and M.C. edited and revised manuscript. D.A., P.C.P., P.D.A., G.B.P., A.D. and M.C. approved the final version of manuscript.

References

1. Bales, C.W.; Ritchie, C.S. Sarcopenia, weight loss, and nutritional frailty in the elderly. *Annu. Rev. Nutr.* **2002**, *22*, 309–323. [CrossRef]
2. Palmer, K.; Onder, G.; Cesari, M. The geriatric condition of frailty. *Eur. J. Intern. Med.* **2018**, *56*, 1–2. [CrossRef]
3. López-Otín, C.; Blasco, M.A.; Partridge, L.; Serrano, M.; Kroemer, G. The hallmarks of aging. *Cell* **2013**, *153*, 1194–1217. [CrossRef]
4. Leslie, W.; Hankey, C. Aging, Nutritional Status and Health. *Healthcare* **2015**, *3*, 648–658. [CrossRef]
5. Roberts, H.C.; Lim, S.E.R.; Cox, N.J.; Ibrahim, K. The Challenge of Managing Undernutrition in Older People with Frailty. *Nutrients* **2019**, *11*, 808. [CrossRef]
6. Hickson, M. Malnutrition and ageing. *Postgrad. Med. J.* **2006**, *82*, 2–8. [CrossRef]
7. Schilp, J.; Wijnhoven, H.A.H.; Deeg, D.J.H.; Visser, M. Early determinants for the development of undernutrition in an older general population: Longitudinal Aging Study Amsterdam. *Br. J. Nutr.* **2011**, *106*, 708–717. [CrossRef]
8. Locher, J.L.; Ritchie, C.S.; Roth, D.L.; Sen, B.; Vickers, K.S.; Vailas, L.I. Food choice among homebound older adults: Motivations and perceived barriers. *J. Nutr. Health Aging* **2009**, *13*, 659–664. [CrossRef]
9. Bloom, I.; Lawrence, W.; Barker, M.; Baird, J.; Dennison, E.; Sayer, A.A.; Cooper, C.; Robinson, S. What influences diet quality in older people? A qualitative study among community-dwelling older adults from the Hertfordshire Cohort Study, UK. *Public Health Nutr.* **2017**, *20*, 2685–2693. [CrossRef]
10. Cichero, J.A.Y. Age-Related Changes to Eating and Swallowing Impact Frailty: Aspiration, Choking Risk, Modified Food Texture and Autonomy of Choice. *Geriatrics* **2018**, *3*, 69. [CrossRef]

11. Calvani, R.; Miccheli, A.; Landi, F.; Bossola, M.; Cesari, M.; Leeuwenburgh, C.; Sieber, C.C.; Bernabei, R.; Marzetti, E. Current nutritional recommendations and novel dietary strategies to manage sarcopenia. *J. Frailty Aging* **2013**, *2*, 38–53.
12. Rosenberg, I.H. Sarcopenia: Origins and clinical relevance. *J. Nutr.* **1997**, *127* (Suppl. S5), 990S–991S. [CrossRef]
13. Cruz-Jentoft, A.J.; Landi, F. Sarcopenia. *Clin. Med.* **2014**, *14*, 183–186. [CrossRef]
14. Komatsu, R.; Okazaki, T.; Ebihara, S.; Kobayashi, M.; Tsukita, Y.; Nihei, M.; Sugiura, H.; Niu, K.; Ebihara, T.; Ichinose, M. Aspiration pneumonia induces muscle atrophy in the respiratory, skeletal, and swallowing systems. *J. Cachexia Sarcopenia Muscle* **2018**, *9*, 643–653. [CrossRef]
15. Beckwée, D.; Delaere, A.; Aelbrecht, S.; Baert, V.; Beaudart, C.; Bruyere, O.; de Saint-Hubert, M.; Bautmans, I. Exercise Interventions for the Prevention and Treatment of Sarcopenia. A Systematic Umbrella Review. *J. Nutr. Health Aging* **2019**, *23*, 494–502. [CrossRef]
16. Azzolino, D.; Damanti, S.; Bertagnoli, L.; Lucchi, T.; Cesari, M. Sarcopenia and swallowing disorders in older people. *Aging. Clin. Exp. Res.* **2019**, *22*, 1–7. [CrossRef]
17. Shiraishi, A.; Yoshimura, Y.; Wakabayashi, H.; Tsuji, Y. Prevalence of stroke-related sarcopenia and its association with poor oral status in post-acute stroke patients: Implications for oral sarcopenia. *Clin. Nutr.* **2018**, *37*, 204–207. [CrossRef]
18. Iee Shin, H.; Kim, D.-K.; Seo, K.M.; Kang, S.H.; Lee, S.Y.; Son, S. Relation Between Respiratory Muscle Strength and Skeletal Muscle Mass and Hand Grip Strength in the Healthy Elderly. *Ann. Rehabil. Med.* **2017**, *41*, 686–692. [CrossRef]
19. Fujishima, I.; Fujiu-Kurachi, M.; Arai, H.; Hyodo, M.; Kagaya, H.; Maeda, K.; Mori, T.; Nishioka, S.; Oshima, F.; Ogawa, S.; et al. Sarcopenia and dysphagia: Position paper by four professional organizations. *Geriatr. Gerontol. Int.* **2019**, *19*, 91–97. [CrossRef]
20. Tamura, F.; Kikutani, T.; Tohara, T.; Yoshida, M.; Yaegaki, K. Tongue thickness relates to nutritional status in the elderly. *Dysphagia* **2012**, *27*, 556–561. [CrossRef]
21. Cruz-Jentoft, A.J.; Sayer, A.A. Sarcopenia. *Lancet* **2019**, *393*, 2636–2646. [CrossRef]
22. Wakabayashi, H.; Sakuma, K. Rehabilitation nutrition for sarcopenia with disability: A combination of both rehabilitation and nutrition care management. *J. Cachexia Sarcopenia Muscle* **2014**, *5*, 269–277. [CrossRef] [PubMed]
23. Castrejón-Pérez, R.C.; Jiménez-Corona, A.; Bernabé, E.; Villa-Romero, A.R.; Arrivé, E.; Dartigues, J.-F.; Gutiérrez-Robledo, L.M.; Borges-Yáñez, S.A. Oral Disease and 3-Year Incidence of Frailty in Mexican Older Adults. *J. Gerontol. Ser. A* **2017**, *72*, 951–957. [CrossRef] [PubMed]
24. Woo, J.; Tong, C.; Yu, R. Chewing Difficulty Should be Included as a Geriatric Syndrome. *Nutrients* **2018**, *10*, 2019. Available online: https://www.ncbi.nlm.nih.gov/pmc/articles/PMC6315631/ (accessed on 11 October 2019). [CrossRef] [PubMed]
25. Castrejón-Pérez, R.C.; Borges-Yáñez, S.A.; Gutiérrez-Robledo, L.M.; Avila-Funes, J.A. Oral health conditions and frailty in Mexican community-dwelling elderly: A cross sectional analysis. *BMC Public Health* **2012**, *12*, 773. [CrossRef] [PubMed]
26. Lertpimonchai, A.; Rattanasiri, S.; Arj-Ong Vallibhakara, S.; Attia, J.; Thakkinstian, A. The association between oral hygiene and periodontitis: A systematic review and meta-analysis. *Int. Dent. J.* **2017**, *67*, 332–343. [CrossRef]
27. Dent, E.; Kowal, P.; Hoogendijk, E.O. Frailty measurement in research and clinical practice: A review. *Eur. J. Intern. Med.* **2016**, *31*, 3–10. [CrossRef]
28. Rolland, Y.; Czerwinski, S.; Abellan Van Kan, G.; Morley, J.E.; Cesari, M.; Onder, G.; Woo, J.; Baumgartner, R.; Pillard, F.; Boirie, Y.; et al. Sarcopenia: Its assessment, etiology, pathogenesis, consequences and future perspectives. *J. Nutr. Health Aging* **2008**, *12*, 433–450. [CrossRef]
29. Hämäläinen, P.; Rantanen, T.; Keskinen, M.; Meurman, J.H. Oral health status and change in handgrip strength over a 5-year period in 80-year-old people. *Gerodontology* **2004**, *21*, 155–160. [CrossRef]
30. Lamster, I.B.; Asadourian, L.; Del Carmen, T.; Friedman, P.K. The aging mouth: Differentiating normal aging from disease. *Periodontol 2000* **2016**, *72*, 96–107. [CrossRef]
31. Liu, B.; Zhang, M.; Chen, Y.; Yao, Y. Tooth wear in aging people: An investigation of the prevalence and the influential factors of incisal/occlusal tooth wear in northwest China. *BMC Oral Health* **2014**, *14*, 65. [CrossRef] [PubMed]
32. Klein, D.R. Oral soft tissue changes in geriatric patients. *Bull. N. Y. Acad. Med.* **1980**, *56*, 721–727. [PubMed]
33. MacEntee, M.I.; Donnelly, L.R. Oral health and the frailty syndrome. *Periodontology 2000* **2016**, *72*, 135–141. [CrossRef] [PubMed]

34. Razak, P.A.; Richard, K.M.J.; Thankachan, R.P.; Hafiz, K.A.A.; Kumar, K.N.; Sameer, K.M. Geriatric Oral Health: A Review Article. *J. Int. Oral Health* **2014**, *6*, 110–116. [PubMed]
35. Chapple, I.L.C.; Bouchard, P.; Cagetti, M.G.; Campus, G.; Carra, M.-C.; Cocco, F.; Nibali, L.; Hujoel, P.; Laine, M.L.; Lingstrom, P.; et al. Interaction of lifestyle, behaviour or systemic diseases with dental caries and periodontal diseases: Consensus report of group 2 of the joint EFP/ORCA workshop on the boundaries between caries and periodontal diseases. *J. Clin. Periodontol.* **2017**, *44* (Suppl S18), S39–S51. [CrossRef]
36. Hirotomi, T.; Yoshihara, A.; Yano, M.; Ando, Y.; Miyazaki, H. Longitudinal study on periodontal conditions in healthy elderly people in Japan. *Community Dent. Oral Epidemiol.* **2002**, *30*, 409–417. [CrossRef] [PubMed]
37. Burt, B.A.; Ismail, A.I.; Morrison, E.C.; Beltran, E.D. Risk factors for tooth loss over a 28-year period. *J. Dent. Res.* **1990**, *69*, 1126–1130. [CrossRef]
38. Bahrami, G.; Vaeth, M.; Kirkevang, L.-L.; Wenzel, A.; Isidor, F. Risk factors for tooth loss in an adult population: A radiographic study. *J. Clin. Periodontol.* **2008**, *35*, 1059–1065. [CrossRef]
39. Singh, K.A.; Brennan, D.S. Chewing disability in older adults attributable to tooth loss and other oral conditions. *Gerodontology* **2012**, *29*, 106–110. [CrossRef]
40. Zhang, Q.; Witter, D.J.; Bronkhorst, E.M.; Creugers, N.H. Chewing ability in an urban and rural population over 40 years in Shandong Province, China. *Clin. Oral Investig.* **2013**, *17*, 1425–1435. [CrossRef]
41. Gil-Montoya, J.A.; Ferreira de Mello, A.L.; Barrios, R.; Gonzalez-Moles, M.A.; Bravo, M. Oral health in the elderly patient and its impact on general well-being: A nonsystematic review. *Clin. Interv. Aging* **2015**, *10*, 461–467. [CrossRef] [PubMed]
42. Musacchio, E.; Perissinotto, E.; Binotto, P.; Sartori, L.; Silva-Netto, F.; Zambon, S.; Manzato, E.; Corti, M.C.; Baggio, G.; Crepaldi, G. Tooth loss in the elderly and its association with nutritional status, socio-economic and lifestyle factors. *Acta Odontol. Scand.* **2007**, *65*, 78–86. [CrossRef] [PubMed]
43. Felton, D.A. Complete Edentulism and Comorbid Diseases: An Update. *J. Prosthodont.* **2016**, *25*, 5–20. [CrossRef] [PubMed]
44. Xu, F.; Laguna, L.; Sarkar, A. Aging-related changes in quantity and quality of saliva: Where do we stand in our understanding? *J. Texture Stud.* **2019**, *50*, 27–35. [CrossRef]
45. Nagler, R.M. Salivary glands and the aging process: Mechanistic aspects, health-status and medicinal-efficacy monitoring. *Biogerontology* **2004**, *5*, 223–233. [CrossRef]
46. Scully, C. Drug effects on salivary glands: Dry mouth. *Oral Dis.* **2003**, *9*, 165–176. [CrossRef]
47. Singh, M.L.; Papas, A. Oral implications of polypharmacy in the elderly. *Dent. Clin.* **2014**, *58*, 783–796. [CrossRef]
48. Mortazavi, H.; Baharvand, M.; Movahhedian, A.; Mohammadi, M.; Khodadoustan, A. Xerostomia Due to Systemic Disease: A Review of 20 Conditions and Mechanisms. *Ann. Med. Health Sci. Res.* **2014**, *4*, 503–510.
49. Dumic, I.; Nordin, T.; Jecmenica, M.; Stojkovic Lalosevic, M.; Milosavljevic, T.; Milovanovic, T. Gastrointestinal Tract Disorders in Older Age. *Can. J. Gastroenterol. Hepatol.* **2019**. Available online: https://www.hindawi.com/journals/cjgh/2019/6757524/ (accessed on 11 October 2019). [CrossRef]
50. Affoo, R.H.; Foley, N.; Garrick, R.; Siqueira, W.L.; Martin, R.E. Meta-Analysis of Salivary Flow Rates in Young and Older Adults. *J. Am. Geriatr. Soc.* **2015**, *63*, 2142–2151. [CrossRef]
51. Kossioni, A.E. The Association of Poor Oral Health Parameters with Malnutrition in Older Adults: A Review Considering the Potential Implications for Cognitive Impairment. *Nutrients* **2018**, *10*, 1709. [CrossRef] [PubMed]
52. Saini, R.; Marawar, P.P.; Shete, S.; Saini, S. Periodontitis, a true infection. *J. Glob. Infect. Dis.* **2009**, *1*, 149–150. [CrossRef] [PubMed]
53. WHO. WHO Oral Health Country Area Profile Programe. Available online: https://www.who.int/oral_health/databases/malmo/en/ (accessed on 11 October 2019).
54. Ashimoto, A.; Chen, C.; Bakker, I.; Slots, J. Polymerase chain reaction detection of 8 putative periodontal pathogens in subgingival plaque of gingivitis and advanced periodontitis lesions. *Oral Microbiol. Immunol.* **1996**, *11*, 266–273. [CrossRef] [PubMed]
55. Genco, R.J.; Borgnakke, W.S. Risk factors for periodontal disease. *Periodontol 2000* **2013**, *62*, 59–94. [CrossRef] [PubMed]
56. Hasturk, H.; Kantarci, A. Activation and Resolution of Periodontal Inflammation and Its Systemic Impact. *Periodontol 2000* **2015**, *69*, 255–273. [CrossRef] [PubMed]
57. O'Connor, J.-L.P.; Milledge, K.L.; O'Leary, F.; Cumming, R.; Eberhard, J.; Hirani, V. Poor dietary intake of nutrients and food groups are associated with increased risk of periodontal disease among community-dwelling older adults: A systematic literature review. *Nutr. Rev.* **2019**. [CrossRef]

58. Najeeb, S.; Zafar, M.S.; Khurshid, Z.; Zohaib, S.; Almas, K. The Role of Nutrition in Periodontal Health: An Update. *Nutrients* **2016**, *8*, 530. Available online: https://www.ncbi.nlm.nih.gov/pmc/articles/PMC5037517/ (accessed on 11 October 2019). [CrossRef]
59. Kunin, A.A.; Evdokimova, A.Y.; Moiseeva, N.S. Age-related differences of tooth enamel morphochemistry in health and dental caries. *EPMA J.* **2015**, *6*, 3. [CrossRef]
60. Avlund, K.; Holm-Pedersen, P.; Morse, D.E.; Viitanen, M.; Winblad, B. Tooth loss and caries prevalence in very old Swedish people: The relationship to cognitive function and functional ability. *Gerodontology* **2004**, *21*, 17–26. [CrossRef]
61. Banting, D.W.; Ellen, R.P.; Fillery, E.D. Prevalence of root surface caries among institutionalized older persons. *Community Dent. Oral Epidemiol.* **1980**, *8*, 84–88. [CrossRef]
62. Ellefsen, B.; Holm-Pedersen, P.; Morse, D.E.; Schroll, M.; Andersen, B.B.; Waldemar, G. Caries prevalence in older persons with and without dementia. *J. Am. Geriatr. Soc.* **2008**, *56*, 59–67. [CrossRef] [PubMed]
63. Fure, S.; Zickert, I. Prevalence of root surface caries in 55, 65, and 75-year-old Swedish individuals. *Community Dent. Oral Epidemiol.* **1990**, *18*, 100–105. [CrossRef] [PubMed]
64. Johanson, C.N.; Osterberg, T.; Steen, B.; Birkhed, D. Prevalence and incidence of dental caries and related risk factors in 70- to 76-year-olds. *Acta Odontol. Scand.* **2009**, *67*, 304–312. [CrossRef] [PubMed]
65. Wiktorsson, A.M.; Martinsson, T.; Zimmerman, M. Salivary levels of lactobacilli, buffer capacity and salivary flow rate related to caries activity among adults in communities with optimal and low water fluoride concentrations. *Swed. Dent. J.* **1992**, *16*, 231–237.
66. Lundberg, J.O. Nitrate transport in salivary glands with implications for NO homeostasis. *Proc. Natl. Acad. Sci. USA* **2012**, *109*, 13144–13145. [CrossRef]
67. Guivante-Nabet, C.; Berenholc, C.; Berdal, A. Caries activity and associated risk factors in elderly hospitalised population – 15-months follow-up in French institutions. *Gerodontology* **1999**, *16*, 47–58. [CrossRef]
68. Fure, S. Ten-year cross-sectional and incidence study of coronal and root caries and some related factors in elderly Swedish individuals. *Gerodontology* **2004**, *21*, 130–140. [CrossRef]
69. Su, N.; Marek, C.L.; Ching, V.; Grushka, M. Caries prevention for patients with dry mouth. *J. Can. Dent. Assoc.* **2011**, *77*, 1–8.
70. Morley, J.E. Anorexia of ageing: A key component in the pathogenesis of both sarcopenia and cachexia. *J. Cachexia Sarcopenia Muscle* **2017**, *8*, 523–526. [CrossRef]
71. Clegg, A.; Young, J.; Iliffe, S.; Rikkert, M.O.; Rockwood, K. Frailty in elderly people. *Lancet* **2013**, *381*, 752–762. [CrossRef]
72. Cruz-Jentoft, A.J.; Baeyens, J.P.; Bauer, J.M.; Boirie, Y.; Cederholm, T.; Landi, F.; Martin, F.C.; Michel, J.-P.; Rolland, Y.; Schneider, S.M.; et al. Sarcopenia: European consensus on definition and diagnosis: Report of the European Working Group on Sarcopenia in Older People. *Age Ageing* **2010**, *39*, 412–423. [CrossRef] [PubMed]
73. Agarwal, E.; Miller, M.; Yaxley, A.; Isenring, E. Malnutrition in the elderly: A narrative review. *Maturitas* **2013**, *76*, 296–302. [CrossRef] [PubMed]
74. Mealey, B.L.; Ocampo, G.L. Diabetes mellitus and periodontal disease. *Periodontol 2000* **2007**, *44*, 127–153. [CrossRef] [PubMed]
75. Karnoutsos, K.; Papastergiou, P.; Stefanidis, S.; Vakaloudi, A. Periodontitis as a risk factor for cardiovascular disease: The role of anti-phosphorylcholine and anti-cardiolipin antibodies. *Hippokratia* **2008**, *12*, 144.
76. Syrjälä, A.-M.H.; Ylöstalo, P.; Hartikainen, S.; Sulkava, R.; Knuuttila, M. Number of teeth and selected cardiovascular risk factors among elderly people. *Gerodontology* **2010**, *27*, 189–192. [CrossRef]
77. Touger-Decker, R. Diet, cardiovascular disease and oral health: Promoting health and reducing risk. *J. Am. Dent. Assoc.* **2010**, *141*, 167–170. [CrossRef]
78. Helkimo, E.; Carlsson, G.E.; Helkimo, M. Chewing efficiency and state of dentition. A methodologic study. *Acta Odontol. Scand.* **1978**, *36*, 33–41. [CrossRef]
79. Akeel, R.; Nilner, M.; Nilner, K. Masticatory efficiency in individuals with natural dentition. *Swed. Dent. J.* **1992**, *16*, 191–198.
80. Naka, O.; Anastassiadou, V.; Pissiotis, A. Association between functional tooth units and chewing ability in older adults: A systematic review. *Gerodontology* **2014**, *31*, 166–177. [CrossRef]
81. Tate, G.S.; Throckmorton, G.S.; Ellis, E.; Sinn, D.P. Masticatory performance, muscle activity, and occlusal force in preorthognathic surgery patients. *J. Oral Maxillofac. Surg.* **1994**, *52*, 476–482; discussion 482. [CrossRef]

82. Fontijn-Tekamp, F.A.; Slagter, A.P.; Van Der Bilt, A.; Van 'T Hof, M.A.; Witter, D.J.; Kalk, W.; Jansen, J.A. Biting and chewing in overdentures, full dentures, and natural dentitions. *J. Dent. Res.* **2000**, *79*, 1519–1524. [CrossRef] [PubMed]
83. Kapur, K.K.; Soman, S.D. Masticatory performance and efficiency in denture wearers. *J. Prosthet. Dent.* **2006**, *95*, 407–411. [CrossRef] [PubMed]
84. Pedersen, A.M.; Bardow, A.; Jensen, S.B.; Nauntofte, B. Saliva and gastrointestinal functions of taste, mastication, swallowing and digestion. *Oral Dis.* **2002**, *8*, 117–129. [CrossRef] [PubMed]
85. Clark, J.R.; Evans, R.D. Functional occlusion: I. A review. *J. Orthod.* **2001**, *28*, 76–81. [CrossRef]
86. Furuta, M.; Yamashita, Y. Oral Health and Swallowing Problems. *Curr. Phys. Med. Rehabil. Rep.* **2013**, *1*, 216–222. [CrossRef]
87. Mishellany, A.; Woda, A.; Labas, R.; Peyron, M.-A. The challenge of mastication: Preparing a bolus suitable for deglutition. *Dysphagia* **2006**, *21*, 87–94. [CrossRef]
88. Hutton, B.; Feine, J.; Morais, J. Is there an association between edentulism and nutritional state? *J. Can. Dent. Assoc.* **2002**, *68*, 182–187.
89. Fontijn-Tekamp, F.A.; van 't Hof, M.A.; Slagter, A.P.; van Waas, M.A. The state of dentition in relation to nutrition in elderly Europeans in the SENECA Study of 1993. *Eur. J. Clin. Nutr.* **1996**, *50* (Suppl. S2), S117–S122.
90. Greksa, L.P.; Parraga, I.M.; Clark, C.A. The dietary adequacy of edentulous older adults. *J. Prosthet. Dent.* **1995**, *73*, 142–145. [CrossRef]
91. Hung, H.-C.; Colditz, G.; Joshipura, K.J. The association between tooth loss and the self-reported intake of selected CVD-related nutrients and foods among US women. *Community Dent. Oral Epidemiol.* **2005**, *33*, 167–173. [CrossRef]
92. Takahashi, M.; Maeda, K.; Wakabayashi, H. Prevalence of sarcopenia and association with oral health-related quality of life and oral health status in older dental clinic outpatients. *Geriatr. Gerontol. Int.* **2018**, *18*, 915–921. [CrossRef] [PubMed]
93. Alvarez, J.O. Nutrition, tooth development, and dental caries. *Am. J. Clin. Nutr.* **1995**, *61*, 410S–416S. [CrossRef] [PubMed]
94. Enwonwu, C.O.; Phillips, R.S.; Falkler, W.A. Nutrition and oral infectious diseases: State of the science. *Compend. Contin. Educ. Dent.* **2002**, *23*, 431–434. [PubMed]
95. Friedlander, A.H.; Weinreb, J.; Friedlander, I.; Yagiela, J.A. Metabolic syndrome: Pathogenesis, medical care and dental implications. *J. Am. Dent. Assoc.* **2007**, *138*, 179–187. [CrossRef] [PubMed]
96. Tan, B.L.; Norhaizan, M.E.; Liew, W.-P.-P. Nutrients and Oxidative Stress: Friend or Foe? *Oxid. Med. Cell. Longev.* **2018**, *2018*. Available online: https://www.ncbi.nlm.nih.gov/pmc/articles/PMC5831951/ (accessed on 11 October 2019). [CrossRef]
97. Manzel, A.; Muller, D.N.; Hafler, D.A.; Erdman, S.E.; Linker, R.A.; Kleinewietfeld, M. Role of "Western Diet" in Inflammatory Autoimmune Diseases. *Curr. Allergy Asthma Rep.* **2014**, *14*, 404. Available online: http://link.springer.com/10.1007/s11882-013-0404-6 (accessed on 7 June 2019). [CrossRef]
98. Kang, J.; Smith, S.; Pavitt, S.; Wu, J. Association between central obesity and tooth loss in the non-obese people: Results from the continuous National Health and Nutrition Examination Survey (NHANES) 1999–2012. *J. Clin. Periodontol.* **2019**, *46*, 430–437. [CrossRef]
99. Codoñer-Franch, P.; Valls-Bellés, V.; Arilla-Codoñer, A.; Alonso-Iglesias, E. Oxidant mechanisms in childhood obesity: The link between inflammation and oxidative stress. *Transl. Res.* **2011**, *158*, 369–384. [CrossRef]
100. Hujoel, P.P.; Lingström, P. Nutrition, dental caries and periodontal disease: A narrative review. *J. Clin. Periodontol.* **2017**, *44* (Suppl. S18), S79–S84. [CrossRef]
101. Moynihan, P.J. The role of diet and nutrition in the etiology and prevention of oral diseases. *Bull. World Health Org.* **2005**, *83*, 694–699.
102. Sheiham, A.; Steele, J.G.; Marcenes, W.; Lowe, C.; Finch, S.; Bates, C.J.; Prentice, A.; Walls, A.W. The relationship among dental status, nutrient intake, and nutritional status in older people. *J. Dent. Res.* **2001**, *80*, 408–413. [CrossRef] [PubMed]
103. Nowjack-Raymer, R.E.; Sheiham, A. Numbers of natural teeth, diet, and nutritional status in US adults. *J. Dent. Res.* **2007**, *86*, 1171–1175. [CrossRef] [PubMed]
104. Zhu, Y.; Hollis, J.H. Tooth loss and its association with dietary intake and diet quality in American adults. *J. Dent.* **2014**, *42*, 1428–1435. [CrossRef] [PubMed]

105. Cruz-Jentoft, A.J.; Landi, F.; Topinková, E.; Michel, J.-P. Understanding sarcopenia as a geriatric syndrome. *Curr. Opin. Clin. Nutr. Metab. Care* **2010**, *13*, 1–7. [CrossRef]
106. Cruz-Jentoft, A.J.; Bahat, G.; Bauer, J.; Boirie, Y.; Bruyère, O.; Cederholm, T.; Cooper, C.; Landi, F.; Rolland, Y.; Sayer, A.A.; et al. Sarcopenia: Revised European consensus on definition and diagnosis. *Age Ageing* **2019**, *48*, 16–31. [CrossRef]
107. Anker, S.D.; Morley, J.E.; von Haehling, S. Welcome to the ICD-10 code for sarcopenia. *J. Cachexia Sarcopenia Muscle* **2016**, *7*, 512–514. [CrossRef]
108. Landi, F.; Calvani, R.; Cesari, M.; Tosato, M.; Martone, A.M.; Ortolani, E.; Savera, G.; Salini, S.; Sisto, A.; Picca, A.; et al. Sarcopenia: An Overview on Current Definitions, Diagnosis and Treatment. *Curr. Protein Pept. Sci.* **2018**, *19*, 633–638. [CrossRef]
109. Liguori, I.; Russo, G.; Aran, L.; Bulli, G.; Curcio, F.; Della-Morte, D.; Gargiulo, G.; Testa, G.; Cacciatore, F.; Bonaduce, D.; et al. Sarcopenia: Assessment of disease burden and strategies to improve outcomes. *Clin. Interv. Aging* **2018**, *13*, 913–927. [CrossRef]
110. McCulloch, T.M.; Jaffe, D. Head and neck disorders affecting swallowing. *GI Motil. Online* **2006**. Available online: https://www.nature.com/gimo/contents/pt1/full/gimo36.html (accessed on 11 October 2019).
111. Wirth, R.; Dziewas, R.; Beck, A.M.; Clavé, P.; Hamdy, S.; Heppner, H.J.; Langmore, S.; Leischker, A.H.; Martino, R.; Pluschinski, P.; et al. Oropharyngeal dysphagia in older persons—From pathophysiology to adequate intervention: A review and summary of an international expert meeting. *Clin. Interv. Aging* **2016**, *11*, 189–208. [CrossRef]
112. Robbins, J.; Bridges, A.D.; Taylor, A. Oral, pharyngeal and esophageal motor function in aging. *GI Motil. Online* **2006**. Available online: https://www.nature.com/gimo/contents/pt1/full/gimo39.html (accessed on 11 October 2019).
113. Feng, X.; Todd, T.; Lintzenich, C.R.; Ding, J.; Carr, J.J.; Ge, Y.; Browne, J.D.; Kritchevsky, S.B.; Butler, S.G. Aging-related geniohyoid muscle atrophy is related to aspiration status in healthy older adults. *J. Gerontol. Ser. A* **2013**, *68*, 853–860. [CrossRef] [PubMed]
114. Newton, J.P.; Yemm, R.; Abel, R.W.; Menhinick, S. Changes in human jaw muscles with age and dental state. *Gerodontology* **1993**, *10*, 16–22. [CrossRef] [PubMed]
115. Wakabayashi, H.; Takahashi, R.; Watanabe, N.; Oritsu, H.; Shimizu, Y. Prevalence of skeletal muscle mass loss and its association with swallowing function after cardiovascular surgery. *Nutrition* **2017**, *38*, 70–73. [CrossRef] [PubMed]
116. Machida, N.; Tohara, H.; Hara, K.; Kumakura, A.; Wakasugi, Y.; Nakane, A.; Minakuchi, S. Effects of aging and sarcopenia on tongue pressure and jaw-opening force. *Geriatr. Gerontol. Int.* **2017**, *17*, 295–301. [CrossRef]
117. Sakai, K.; Nakayama, E.; Tohara, H.; Kodama, K.; Takehisa, T.; Takehisa, Y.; Ueda, K. Relationship between tongue strength, lip strength, and nutrition-related sarcopenia in older rehabilitation inpatients: A cross-sectional study. *Clin. Interv. Aging* **2017**, *12*, 1207–1214. [CrossRef]
118. Sporns, P.B.; Muhle, P.; Hanning, U.; Suntrup-Krueger, S.; Schwindt, W.; Eversmann, J.; Warnecke, T.; Wirth, R.; Zimmer, S.; Dziewas, R. Atrophy of Swallowing Muscles Is Associated with Severity of Dysphagia and Age in Patients with Acute Stroke. *J. Am. Med. Dir. Assoc.* **2017**, *18*, 635.e1–635.e7. [CrossRef]
119. Maeda, K.; Akagi, J. Decreased tongue pressure is associated with sarcopenia and sarcopenic dysphagia in the elderly. *Dysphagia* **2015**, *30*, 80–87. [CrossRef]
120. Butler, S.G.; Stuart, A.; Leng, X.; Wilhelm, E.; Rees, C.; Williamson, J.; Kritchevsky, S.B. The relationship of aspiration status with tongue and handgrip strength in healthy older adults. *J. Gerontol. Ser. A* **2011**, *66*, 452–458. [CrossRef]
121. Buehring, B.; Hind, J.; Fidler, E.; Krueger, D.; Binkley, N.; Robbins, J. Tongue strength is associated with jumping mechanography performance and handgrip strength but not with classic functional tests in older adults. *J. Am. Geriatr. Soc.* **2013**, *61*, 418–422. [CrossRef]
122. Tsuga, K.; Yoshikawa, M.; Oue, H.; Okazaki, Y.; Tsuchioka, H.; Maruyama, M.; Yoshida, M.; Akagawa, Y. Maximal voluntary tongue pressure is decreased in Japanese frail elderly persons. *Gerodontology* **2012**, *29*, e1078–e1085. [CrossRef] [PubMed]
123. Ertekin, C.; Aydogdu, I. Neurophysiology of swallowing. *Clin. Neurophysiol.* **2003**, *114*, 2226–2244. [CrossRef]
124. Sakai, K.; Sakuma, K. Sarcopenic Dysphagia as a New Concept. *Frailty Sarcopenia Onset Dev. Clin. Chall.* **2017**. Available online: https://www.intechopen.com/books/frailty-and-sarcopenia-onset-development-and-clinical-challenges/sarcopenic-dysphagia-as-a-new-concept (accessed on 11 October 2019).

125. Wakabayashi, H. Presbyphagia and Sarcopenic Dysphagia: Association between Aging, Sarcopenia, and Deglutition Disorders. *J. Frailty Aging* **2014**, *3*, 97–103. [PubMed]
126. Rowlerson, A.; Raoul, G.; Daniel, Y.; Close, J.; Maurage, C.-A.; Ferri, J.; Sciote, J.J. Fiber-type differences in masseter muscle associated with different facial morphologies. *Am. J. Orthod. Dentofac. Orthop.* **2005**, *127*, 37–46. [CrossRef] [PubMed]
127. Yamaguchi, K.; Tohara, H.; Hara, K.; Nakane, A.; Kajisa, E.; Yoshimi, K.; Minakuchi, S. Relationship of aging, skeletal muscle mass, and tooth loss with masseter muscle thickness. *BMC Geriatr.* **2018**, *18*, 67. [CrossRef]
128. Ferrucci, L.; Fabbri, E. Inflammageing: Chronic inflammation in ageing, cardiovascular disease, and frailty. *Nat. Rev. Cardiol.* **2018**, *15*, 505–522. [CrossRef]
129. Yao, X.; Li, H.; Leng, S.X. Inflammation and immune system alterations in frailty. *Clin. Geriatr. Med.* **2011**, *27*, 79–87. [CrossRef]
130. Napa, K.; Baeder, A.C.; Witt, J.E.; Rayburn, S.T.; Miller, M.G.; Dallon, B.W.; Gibbs, J.L.; Wilcox, S.H.; Winden, D.R.; Smith, J.H.; et al. LPS from, P. gingivalis Negatively Alters Gingival Cell Mitochondrial Bioenergetics. *Int. J. Dent.* **2017**, *2017*. Available online: https://www.ncbi.nlm.nih.gov/pmc/articles/PMC5448046/ (accessed on 11 October 2019). [CrossRef]
131. Taylor, G.W.; Burt, B.A.; Becker, M.P.; Genco, R.J.; Shlossman, M.; Knowler, W.C.; Pettitt, D.J. Severe periodontitis and risk for poor glycemic control in patients with non-insulin-dependent diabetes mellitus. *J. Periodontol.* **1996**, *67* (Suppl. S10), 1085–1093. [CrossRef]
132. Chee, B.; Park, B.; Bartold, P.M. Periodontitis and type II diabetes: A two-way relationship. *Int. J. Evid. Based Healthc.* **2013**, *11*, 317–329. [CrossRef] [PubMed]
133. Fuggle, N.R.; Smith, T.O.; Kaul, A.; Sofat, N. Hand to Mouth: A Systematic Review and Meta-Analysis of the Association between Rheumatoid Arthritis and Periodontitis. *Front. Immunol.* **2016**, *7*, 80. [CrossRef] [PubMed]
134. Beck, J.D.; Offenbacher, S.; Williams, R.; Gibbs, P.; Garcia, R. Periodontitis: A risk factor for coronary heart disease? *Ann. Periodontol.* **1998**, *3*, 127–141. [CrossRef] [PubMed]
135. D'Aiuto, F.; Nibali, L.; Parkar, M.; Patel, K.; Suvan, J.; Donos, N. Oxidative stress, systemic inflammation, and severe periodontitis. *J. Dent. Res.* **2010**, *89*, 1241–1246. [CrossRef]
136. Borges, I.; Moreira, E.A.M.; Filho, D.W.; de Oliveira, T.B.; da Silva, M.B.S.; Fröde, T.S. Proinflammatory and oxidative stress markers in patients with periodontal disease. *Mediat. Inflamm.* **2007**, *2007*, 45794. [CrossRef]
137. Horton, A.L.; Boggess, K.A.; Moss, K.L.; Beck, J.; Offenbacher, S. Periodontal disease, oxidative stress, and risk for preeclampsia. *J. Periodontol.* **2010**, *81*, 199–204. [CrossRef]
138. Bullon, P.; Cordero, M.D.; Quiles, J.L.; del Carmen Ramirez-Tortosa, M.; Gonzalez-Alonso, A.; Alfonsi, S.; García-Marín, R.; de Miguel, M.; Battino, M. Autophagy in periodontitis patients and gingival fibroblasts: Unraveling the link between chronic diseases and inflammation. *BMC Med.* **2012**, *10*, 122. [CrossRef]
139. Bullon, P.; Cordero, M.D.; Quiles, J.L.; Morillo, J.M.; del Carmen Ramirez-Tortosa, M.; Battino, M. Mitochondrial dysfunction promoted by Porphyromonas gingivalis lipopolysaccharide as a possible link between cardiovascular disease and periodontitis. *Free Radic. Biol. Med.* **2011**, *50*, 1336–1343. [CrossRef]
140. Wang, P.-L.; Ohura, K. Porphyromonas gingivalis lipopolysaccharide signaling in gingival fibroblasts-CD14 and Toll-like receptors. *Crit. Rev. Oral Biol. Med.* **2002**, *13*, 132–142. [CrossRef]
141. Andersson, P.; Hallberg, I.R.; Lorefält, B.; Unosson, M.; Renvert, S. Oral health problems in elderly rehabilitation patients. *Int. J. Dent. Hyg.* **2004**, *2*, 70–77. [CrossRef]
142. Hanne, K.; Ingelise, T.; Linda, C.; Ulrich, P.P. Oral status and the need for oral health care among patients hospitalised with acute medical conditions. *J. Clin. Nurs.* **2012**, *21*, 2851–2859. [CrossRef] [PubMed]
143. Cederholm, T.; Jensen, G.L.; Correia, M.I.T.D.; Gonzalez, M.C.; Fukushima, R.; Higashiguchi, T.; Baptista, G.; Barazzoni, R.; Blaauw, R.; Coats, A.; et al. GLIM criteria for the diagnosis of malnutrition—A consensus report from the global clinical nutrition community. *Clin. Nutr.* **2019**, *38*, 1–9. [CrossRef] [PubMed]
144. Cesari, M.; Landi, F.; Vellas, B.; Bernabei, R.; Marzetti, E. Sarcopenia and Physical Frailty: Two Sides of the Same Coin. *Front. Aging Neurosci* **2014**, *6*, 192. Available online: https://www.ncbi.nlm.nih.gov/pmc/articles/PMC4112807/ (accessed on 5 November 2019). [CrossRef] [PubMed]
145. Cruz-Jentoft, A.J.; Kiesswetter, E.; Drey, M.; Sieber, C.C. Nutrition, frailty, and sarcopenia. *Aging Clin. Exp. Res.* **2017**, *29*, 43–48. [CrossRef] [PubMed]
146. Landi, F.; Cherubini, A.; Cesari, M.; Calvani, R.; Tosato, M.; Sisto, A.; Martone, A.M.; Bernabei, R.; Marzetti, E. Sarcopenia and frailty: From theoretical approach into clinical practice. *Eur. Geriatr. Med.* **2016**, *7*, 197–200.

Available online: https://moh-it.pure.elsevier.com/en/publications/sarcopenia-and-frailty-from-theoretical-approach-into-clinical-pr (accessed on 11 October 2019). [CrossRef]

147. Bauer, J.; Biolo, G.; Cederholm, T.; Cesari, M.; Cruz-Jentoft, A.J.; Morley, J.E.; Phillips, S.; Sieber, C.; Stehle, P.; Teta, D.; et al. Evidence-Based Recommendations for Optimal Dietary Protein Intake in Older People: A Position Paper from the PROT-AGE Study Group. *J. Am. Med. Dir. Assoc.* **2013**, *14*, 542–559. [CrossRef]
148. Ellis, G.; Whitehead, M.A.; O'Neill, D.; Langhorne, P.; Robinson, D. Comprehensive geriatric assessment for older adults admitted to hospital. *Cochrane. Database. Syst. Rev.* **2011**, *7*, CD006211.
149. Bollero, P.; Passarelli, P.C.; D'Addona, A.; Pasquantonio, G.; Mancini, M.; Condò, R.; Cerroni, L. Oral management of adult patients undergoing hematopoietic stem cell transplantation. *Eur. Rev. Med. Pharmacol. Sci.* **2018**, *22*, 876–887.
150. Tonetti, M.S.; Bottenberg, P.; Conrads, G.; Eickholz, P.; Heasman, P.; Huysmans, M.-C.; López, R.; Madianos, P.; Müller, F.; Needleman, I.; et al. Dental caries and periodontal diseases in the ageing population: Call to action to protect and enhance oral health and well-being as an essential component of healthy ageing—Consensus report of group 4 of the joint EFP/ORCA workshop on the boundaries between caries and periodontal diseases. *J. Clin. Periodontol.* **2017**, *44* (Suppl. S18), S135–S144.
151. Andreas Zenthöfer, A.; Rammelsberg, P.; Cabrera, T.; Hassel, A. Prosthetic rehabilitation of edentulism prevents malnutrition in nursing home residents. *Int. J. Prosthodont.* **2015**, *28*, 198–200. [CrossRef]
152. Volkert, D.; Beck, A.M.; Cederholm, T.; Cruz-Jentoft, A.; Goisser, S.; Hooper, L.; Kiesswetter, E.; Maggio, M.; Raynaud-Simon, A.; Sieber, C.C.; et al. ESPEN guideline on clinical nutrition and hydration in geriatrics. *Clin. Nutr.* **2019**, *38*, 10–47. [CrossRef] [PubMed]
153. Deutz, N.E.P.; Bauer, J.M.; Barazzoni, R.; Biolo, G.; Boirie, Y.; Bosy-Westphal, A.; Cederholm, T.; Cruz-Jentoft , A.; Krznariç, Z.; Nair, K.S.; et al. Protein intake and exercise for optimal muscle function with aging: Recommendations from the ESPEN Expert Group. *Clin. Nutr.* **2014**, *33*, 929–936. [CrossRef] [PubMed]
154. Johnson, M.A.; Kimlin, M.G. Vitamin D, aging, and the 2005 Dietary Guidelines for Americans. *Nutr. Rev.* **2006**, *64*, 410–421. [CrossRef] [PubMed]
155. Visser, M.; Deeg, D.J.H.; Lips, P. Longitudinal Aging Study Amsterdam. Low vitamin D and high parathyroid hormone levels as determinants of loss of muscle strength and muscle mass (sarcopenia): The Longitudinal Aging Study Amsterdam. *J. Clin. Endocrinol. Metab.* **2003**, *88*, 5766–5772. [CrossRef] [PubMed]
156. Ney, D.M.; Weiss, J.M.; Kind, A.J.H.; Robbins, J. Senescent Swallowing: Impact, Strategies, and Interventions. *Nutr. Clin. Pract.* **2009**, *24*, 395–413. [CrossRef] [PubMed]
157. Sura, L.; Madhavan, A.; Carnaby, G.; Crary, M.A. Dysphagia in the elderly: Management and nutritional considerations. *Clin. Interv. Aging* **2012**, *7*, 287–298.
158. Lutsey, P.L.; Steffen, L.M.; Stevens, J. Dietary intake and the development of the metabolic syndrome: The Atherosclerosis Risk in Communities study. *Circulation* **2008**, *117*, 754–761. [CrossRef]
159. Guideline: Sugars Intake for Adults and Children. Available online: https://apps.who.int/iris/handle/10665/149782 (accessed on 22 October 2019).
160. Gutteridge, J.M.C.; Halliwell, B. Antioxidants: Molecules, medicines, and myths. *Biochem. Biophys. Res. Commun.* **2010**, *393*, 561–564. [CrossRef]
161. Welch, A.A.; MacGregor, A.J.; Minihane, A.-M.; Skinner, J.; Valdes, A.A.; Spector, T.D.; Cassidy, A. Dietary fat and fatty acid profile are associated with indices of skeletal muscle mass in women aged 18-79 years. *J. Nutr.* **2014**, *144*, 327–334. [CrossRef]
162. Woelber, J.P.; Bremer, K.; Vach, K.; König, D.; Hellwig, E.; Ratka-Krüger, P.; Al-Ahmad, A.; Tennert, C. An oral health optimized diet can reduce gingival and periodontal inflammation in humans—A randomized controlled pilot study. *BMC Oral Health* **2016**, *17*, 28. [CrossRef]
163. Dupont, J.; Dedeyne, L.; Dalle, S.; Koppo, K.; Gielen, E. The role of omega-3 in the prevention and treatment of sarcopenia. *Aging Clin. Exp. Res.* **2019**, *31*, 825–836. [CrossRef] [PubMed]
164. Damanti, S.; Azzolino, D.; Roncaglione, C.; Arosio, B.; Rossi, P.; Cesari, M. Efficacy of Nutritional Interventions as Stand-Alone or Synergistic Treatments with Exercise for the Management of Sarcopenia. *Nutrients* **2019**, *11*, 1991. [CrossRef] [PubMed]
165. Dickinson, J.M.; Volpi, E.; Rasmussen, B.B. Exercise and nutrition to target protein synthesis impairments in aging skeletal muscle. *Exerc. Sport Sci. Rev.* **2013**, *41*, 216–223. [CrossRef] [PubMed]

166. Glover, E.I.; Phillips, S.M.; Oates, B.R.; Tang, J.E.; Tarnopolsky, M.A.; Selby, A.; Smith, K.; Rennie, M.J. Immobilization induces anabolic resistance in human myofibrillar protein synthesis with low and high dose amino acid infusion. *J. Physiol.* **2008**, *586*, 6049–6061. [CrossRef]
167. Bawadi, H.A.; Khader, Y.S.; Haroun, T.F.; Al-Omari, M.; Tayyem, R.F. The association between periodontal disease, physical activity and healthy diet among adults in Jordan. *J. Periodont. Res.* **2011**, *46*, 74–81. [CrossRef]
168. Cruz-Jentoft, A.J.; Landi, F.; Schneider, S.M.; Zúñiga, C.; Arai, H.; Boirie, Y.; Chen, L.-K.; Fielding, R.A.; Martin, F.C.; Michel, J.-P.; et al. Prevalence of and interventions for sarcopenia in ageing adults: A systematic review. Report of the International Sarcopenia Initiative (EWGSOP and IWGS). *Age Ageing* **2014**, *43*, 748–759. [CrossRef]
169. Sugiyama, T.; Ohkubo, M.; Honda, Y.; Tasaka, A.; Nagasawa, K.; Ishida, R.; Sakurai, K. Effect of swallowing exercises in independent elderly. *Bull. Tokyo. Dent. Coll.* **2013**, *54*, 109–115. [CrossRef]
170. Argolo, N.; Sampaio, M.; Pinho, P.; Melo, A.; Nóbrega, A.C. Do swallowing exercises improve swallowing dynamic and quality of life in Parkinson's disease? *NeuroRehabilitation* **2013**, *32*, 949–955.
171. Kim, H.-J.; Lee, J.-Y.; Lee, E.-S.; Jung, H.-J.; Ahn, H.-J.; Kim, B.-I. Improvements in oral functions of elderly after simple oral exercise. *Clin. Interv. Aging* **2019**, *14*, 915–924. [CrossRef]
172. Park, J.S.; Oh, D.H.; Chang, M.Y.; Kim, K.M. Effects of expiratory muscle strength training on oropharyngeal dysphagia in subacute stroke patients: A randomised controlled trial. *J. Oral Rehabil.* **2016**, *43*, 364–372. [CrossRef]
173. Park, J.-S.; Oh, D.-H.; Chang, M.-Y. Effect of expiratory muscle strength training on swallowing-related muscle strength in community-dwelling elderly individuals: A randomized controlled trial. *Gerodontology* **2017**, *34*, 121–128. [CrossRef] [PubMed]
174. Park, J.S.; Hwang, N.K.; Oh, D.H.; Chang, M.Y. Effect of head lift exercise on kinematic motion of the hyolaryngeal complex and aspiration in patients with dysphagic stroke. *J. Oral Rehabil.* **2017**, *44*, 385–391. [CrossRef] [PubMed]
175. Antunes, E.B.; Lunet, N. Effects of the head lift exercise on the swallow function: A systematic review. *Gerodontology* **2012**, *29*, 247–257. [CrossRef] [PubMed]
176. Steele, C.M.; Bayley, M.T.; Peladeau-Pigeon, M.; Nagy, A.; Namasivayam, A.M.; Stokely, S.L.; Wolkin, T. A Randomized Trial Comparing Two Tongue-Pressure Resistance Training Protocols for Post-Stroke Dysphagia. *Dysphagia* **2016**, *31*, 452–461. [CrossRef] [PubMed]
177. Kim, H.D.; Choi, J.B.; Yoo, S.J.; Chang, M.Y.; Lee, S.W.; Park, J.S. Tongue-to-palate resistance training improves tongue strength and oropharyngeal swallowing function in subacute stroke survivors with dysphagia. *J. Oral Rehabil.* **2017**, *44*, 59–64. [CrossRef] [PubMed]
178. Yeates, E.M.; Molfenter, S.M.; Steele, C.M. Improvements in tongue strength and pressure-generation precision following a tongue-pressure training protocol in older individuals with dysphagia: Three case reports. *Clin. Interv. Aging* **2008**, *3*, 735–747. [CrossRef]
179. Robbins, J.; Gangnon, R.E.; Theis, S.M.; Kays, S.A.; Hewitt, A.L.; Hind, J.A. The effects of lingual exercise on swallowing in older adults. *J. Am. Geriatr. Soc.* **2005**, *53*, 1483–1489. [CrossRef]

13

Antiosteoporotic Activity of Genistein Aglycone in Postmenopausal Women: Evidence from a Post-Hoc Analysis of a Multicenter Randomized Controlled Trial

Vincenzo Arcoraci [1,†], Marco Atteritano [1,*,†], Francesco Squadrito [1], Rosario D'Anna [2], Herbert Marini [1], Domenico Santoro [1], Letteria Minutoli [1], Sonia Messina [2], Domenica Altavilla [3] and Alessandra Bitto [1]

1 Department of Clinical and Experimental Medicine, University of Messina, 98100 Messina, Italy; varcoraci@unime.it (V.A.); fsquadrito@unime.it (F.S.); hrmarini@unime.it (H.M.); santisi@hotmail.com (D.S.); lminutoli@unime.it (L.M.); abitto@unime.it (A.B.)

2 Department of Neurosciences and Nemo Sud Clinical Center, University of Messina, 98100 Messina, Italy; rdannna@unime.it (R.D.); smessina@unime.it (S.M.)

3 Department of Paediatric, Gynaecological, Microbiological and Biomedical Sciences, University of Messina, 98100 Messina, Italy; daltavilla@unime.it

* Correspondence: matteritano@unime.it

† These authors contributed equally to this work.

Abstract: Genistein has a preventive role against bone mass loss during menopause. However, experimental data in animal models of osteoporosis suggest an anti-osteoporotic potential for this isoflavone. We performed a post-hoc analysis of a previously published trial investigating the effects of genistein in postmenopausal women with low bone mineral density. The parent study was a randomized, double-blind, placebo-controlled trial involving postmenopausal women with a femoral neck (FN) density <0.795 g/cm^2. A cohort of the enrolled women was, in fact, identified at the baseline as osteoporotic (n = 121) on the basis of their T-score and analyzed thereafter for the 24 months' treatment with either 1000 mg of calcium and 800 IU vitamin D3 (placebo; n = 59); or calcium, vitamin D3, and Genistein aglycone (54 mg/day; genistein; n = 62). According to the femoral neck T-scores, 31.3% of the genistein and 30.9% of the placebo recipients were osteoporotic at baseline. In the placebo and genistein groups, the 10-year hip fracture probability risk assessed by Fracture Risk Assessment tool (FRAX) was 4.1 ± 1.9 (SD) and 4.2 ± 2.1 (SD), respectively. Mean bone mineral density (BMD) at the femoral neck increased from 0.62 g/cm^2 at baseline to 0.68 g/cm^2 at 1 year and 0.70 g/cm^2 at 2 years in genistein recipients, and decreased from 0.61 g/cm^2 at baseline to 0.60 g/cm^2 at 1 year and 0.57 g/cm^2 at 2 years in placebo recipients. At the end of the study only 18 postmenopausal women had osteoporosis in the genistein group with a prevalence of 12%, whereas in the placebo group the number of postmenopausal women with osteoporosis was unchanged, after 24 months. This post-hoc analysis is a proof-of concept study suggesting that genistein may be useful not only in postmenopausal osteopenia but also in osteoporosis. However, this proof-of concept study needs to be confirmed by a large, well designed, and appropriately focused randomized clinical trial in a population at high risk of fractures.

Keywords: bone mineral density; genistein; postemenopausal osteoporosis

1. Introduction

Estrogen deficiency is a major cause of osteoporosis worldwide. Hormone Replacement Therapy (HRT) increases the bone mineral density (BMD) and decreases the fracture risk, but the adverse effects limit its use in a large cohort of subjects [1–3]. In the last few years, many researchers have focused their attention on natural alternatives to HRT, such as phytoestrogen. Epidemiological data indicate that women consuming high amounts of phytoestrogens, in the form of soy-derived dietary products, have less menopausal symptoms than those on Western diets, and consequently, it was assumed that bone mineral density may be favorably influenced by phytoestrogens [4,5]. A major phytoestrogen is genistein, which prevents bone mass loss and improves quality of life without the harmful estrogenic activity on reproductive tissues, or genotoxic effects in postmenopausal women, at least at the dose of 54 mg/day [6–12]. We have studied the effects of pure genistein (in its aglycone form) on BMD and bone metabolism in a large cohort of postmenopausal women [6], showing that a long-term intake of genistein produced a positive effect on bone metabolism with no clinically significant adverse effects on the breast and uterus [7–9]. Overall, these results agree with previous intervention trials in which >40 mg/day of genistein equivalents yielded the most positive effects on bone mineral density and bone markers when compared to other trials with lower amounts of genistein [13–16]. Animal studies suggest that genistein has an antiosteoporotic activity, improving bone morphology parameters in osteoporotic ovarictomized mice [17] and preventing bone fragility in rats with glucocorticoid-induced osteoporosis [18]. To date, no data are available on osteoporotic subjects, however a re-analysis of the 389 postmenopausal women enrolled in our previous trial, evaluating the efficacy of genistein in osteopenic women, revealed that a significant number was actually osteoporotic, according to the T-score. The aim of this study was to perform a post-hoc analysis to evaluate the efficacy of genistein aglycone on bone mineral density in women with osteoporosis.

2. Materials and Methods

2.1. Design Overview, Setting, Participants

A post-hoc analysis was carried out using data from the main multicenter randomized controlled trial "Effects of the phytoestrogen genistein on bone metabolism in osteopenic postmenopausal women". The study subjects and methods are described in detail elsewhere [6–8]. The protocol is consistent with the principles of the Declaration of Helsinki, was approved by the Ethics Committee of Palermo University (RODA-12254) and the participants gave their written informed consent. The trial included 389 postmenopausal women, randomly assigned to receive the isoflavone genistein (n = 198), or placebo (n = 191). Placebo and genistein (54 mg/day) tablets were identical in appearance and taste. The purity of genistein was >98%. All patients were co-prescribed with 1000 mg calcium carbonate and 800 IU vitamin D3, in two tablets. The bone mineral density was assumed as the primary outcome. The femoral neck (FN), lumbar spine (LN), and total hip (TH) bone mineral density, were measured by Dual-Energy X-ray Absorptiometry (DXA; Hologic QDR 4500 W, Technologic Srl, Turin, Italy) at baseline and after 12 and 24 months of treatment as previously published [6–8]. In addition, the ten-year fracture probability was assessed with the Fracture Risk Assessment (FRAX) tool, as a secondary outcome.

2.2. Study Population

This primary analysis included all postmenopausal women with osteoporosis at the femoral neck. A cohort of the enrolled postmenopausal women was identified at the baseline as osteoporotic (n = 121) on the basis of their T-score on the femoral neck and were analyzed thereafter for the 24 months' treatment with either placebo (n = 59) or genistein (n = 62). Data from postmenopausal women with osteopenia are also shown to assess whether these patients had similar beneficial effects on BMD and incidence of adverse events.

2.3. Assessment of Fracture Risk

The ten-year fracture probability was assessed with the FRAX tool (version 2.0; University of Sheffield, South Yorkshire, England) in osteoporotic and osteopenic patients. FRAX is a computer-based algorithm [19] that provides models for the assessment of fracture probability in men and women. In this analysis, FN BMD was included since fracture risk prediction is enhanced with the input of BMD.

The probability of fracture is calculated in women according to age, body mass index, and dichotomized risk variables that comprise: a prior fragility fracture, parental history of hip fracture, current tobacco smoking, ever long-term use of oral glucocorticoids, rheumatoid arthritis, other causes of secondary osteoporosis, and alcohol consumption of three or more units daily [20].

2.4. Statistical Analysis

Descriptive statistical analyses were performed to evaluate basal demographic and clinical characteristics. All results were expressed as mean with standard deviation (SD) for continuous variables, and absolute and percentage frequencies for categorical variables. All variables were evaluated at basal time and after 12 and 24 months of treatment and absolute values were evaluated in both genistein and placebo patients to verify differences between the groups. The primary efficacy data on BMD were analyzed as already described [6–8]. The significance of differences in mean values between placebo and genistein groups at year 1 and 2 was assessed by two-way analysis of variance (2-way ANOVA). A p value of 0.05 or less was considered statistically significant and 95% confidence intervals were calculated wherever possible. Statistical analysis was performed by using SAS software, version 9.1 (SAS Institute, Inc., Cary, NC, USA).

3. Results

Of the 389 postmenopausal women who were enrolled in the main study, 121 (31.1%) were osteoporotic and were included in this analysis. The baseline characteristics of the osteoporotic and osteopenic women are shown in Table 1. The number of osteoporotic women was similar in both groups: 59 (30.9%) in the placebo group and 62 (31.3%) in the genistein group.

Table 1. Baseline characteristics of postmenopausal women with osteoporosis and osteopenia in both groups.

Variable	Osteoporotic		Osteopenic	
	Placebo (59)	Genistein (62)	Placebo (132)	Genistein (136)
Mean age (SD), year	54.3 (2.4)	54.5 (2.9)	54.6 (2.7)	54.8 (2.2)
Mean body mass index (SD), Kg/m^2	25.2 (3.0)	25.5 (2.8)	25.4 (3.9)	24.8 (3.7)
Mean time since menopause (SD), m	69.4 (44.7)	68.3 (39.2)	69.1 (35.9)	66.4 (38.3)
Mean BMD Femoral neck (SD), g/cm^2	0.61 (0.07)	0.62 (0.05)	0.79 (0.04)	0.78 (0.05)
Mean BMD Lumbar Spine (SD), g/cm^2	0.81 (0.10)	0.82 (0.08)	0.85 (0.10	0.85 (0.08)
Mean BMD Total hip (SD), g/cm^2	0.72 (0.08)	0.73 (0.06)	0.93 (0.04)	0.92 (0.05)
B-ALP (μg/L)	10.8 (1.79)	10.0 (2.21)	10.0 (1.87)	10.6 (2.09)
D-Pyr (pmol/μmol of urinary creatinine)	22.0 (6.92)	22.7 (7.86)	20.6 (5.19)	21.2 (3.97)
FRAX index				
Major fractures (SD)	6.5 (2.8)	6.6 (2.4)	3.3 (0.5)	3.4 (0.5)
Femur fractures (SD)	4.1 (1.9)	4.2 (2.1)	0.7 (0.1)	0.7 (0.1)

BMD: Mean bone mineral density.

Mean bone mineral density (BMD) at the femoral neck increased from 0.62 g/cm^2 $\pm$ 0.05 (SD) at baseline to 0.68 g/cm^2 $\pm$ 0.06 (SD) at 1 year and to 0.70 g/cm^2 $\pm$ 0.07 (SD) at 2 years in the genistein recipients. Conversely, in the placebo group, BMD decreased from 0.61 g/cm^2 $\pm$ 0.07 (SD) at baseline to 0.60 g/cm^2 $\pm$ 0.06 (SD) at 1 year and to 0.57 g/cm^2 $\pm$ 0.07 (SD) at 2 years. Over time the BMD significantly improved in the genistein group compared to the placebo group (p = 0.0046).

Moreover, a significant time effect ($p = 0.0068$) and treatment-time interaction ($p = 0.0073$) were also observed. Similar trends, on bone mineral density at the femoral neck, were observed in osteopenic patients when considering treatment ($p = 0.0130$) and treatment-time interaction ($p = 0.0241$), while no significance was found for the time effect ($p = 0.4929$) (Figure 1). In genistein-treated osteoporotic patients, a significant increase of BMD at the lumbar spine (from 0.82 ± 0.08 at baseline to 0.85 ± 0.09 at 1 year and to 0.88 ± 0.08 at 2 years) and total hip (from 0.73 ± 0.06 at baseline to 0.80 ± 0.07 at 1 year and to 0.82 ± 0.08 at 2 years) was observed.

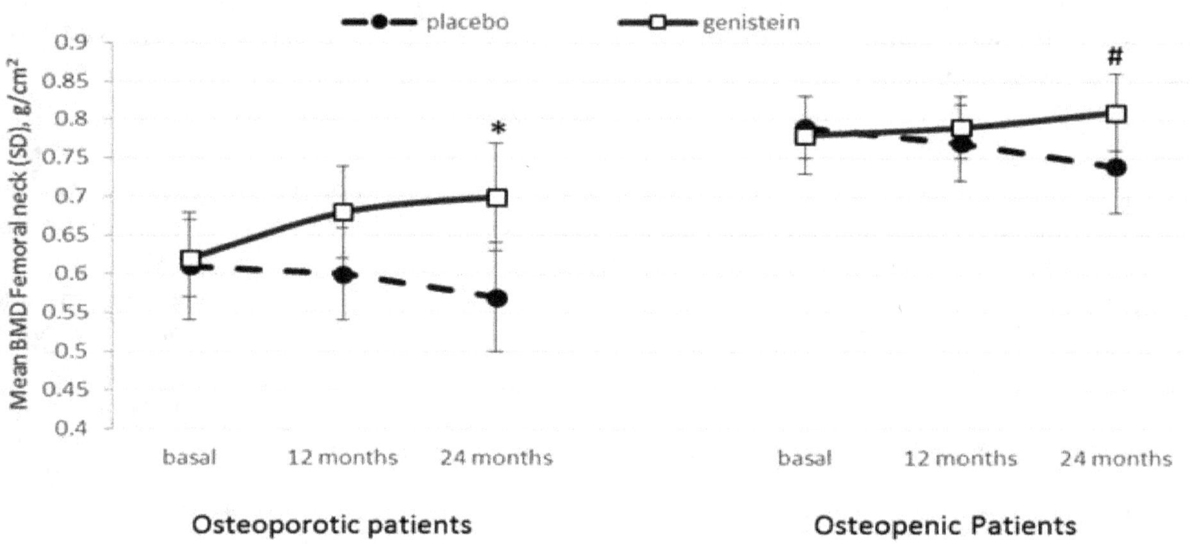

Figure 1. Femoral Neck Bone mineral density changes in absolute values over time in placebo and genistein group. (**left**) Femoral neck Bone Mineral Density changes in osteoporotic postmenopausal women groups; (**right**) Femoral neck Bone Mineral Density changes in osteopenic postmenopausal women groups. 2-way ANOVA: Over time, genistein vs. placebo: * Treatment $p = 0.0046$; # Treatment $p = 0.0130$; * Time $p = 0.0068$; # Time $p = 0.4929$; * Interaction $p = 0.0073$; # Interaction $p = 0.0241$.

Treatment also affected the bone turnover rate. Indeed, in genistein-treated osteoporotic women, B-ALP increased from 10.0 ± 2.2 at baseline to 13.8 ± 2.3 after 1 year and to 14.6 ± 2.2 at 2 years, while no differences were observed in the placebo group (basal: 10.8 ± 1.8; 1 year 10.3 ± 1.6; 2 year 10.4 ± 1.6).

Over time a significant treatment effect ($p < 0.01$), time effect ($p < 0.01$), and treatment-time interaction ($p < 0.01$) were observed using the 2-way ANOVA. Similar results were observed in osteopenic women. D-Pyr excretion in osteoporotic patients was affected only by time ($p = 0.002$).

According to the World Health Organization (WHO) classification criteria, at baseline, the number of postmenopausal women with osteoporosis was 62 in the genistein group and 59 in the placebo group. At the end of the study only 18 (29%) genistein-treated subjects were osteoporotic, while no changes were observed in the placebo group.

Gastrointestinal side effects were the most common reason for dropout, possibly because of the presence of calcium. There were no significant changes in routine biochemistry, liver function, or hematology results. The daily administration of 54 mg of genistein did not cause any significant change in the endometrial thickness.

4. Discussion

In a cohort of postmenopausal osteoporotic subjects, we confirmed the protective effects of genistein treatment on bone loss, as previously observed in osteopenic women. Postmenopausal osteoporosis significantly increases the risk of fractures and requires adequate prevention and appropriate medical treatment [21]. Since the lack of estrogen is the main etiopathogenetic element of postmenopausal bone loss, as a result, estrogen replacement therapy represents an established treatment for the prevention of osteoporosis [22]. However, the possibility of side-effects related to the estrogenic treatment requires therapeutic alternatives [23].

We previously showed that a daily administration of genistein aglycone produced a net gain in bone mass after 2 years of therapy in postmenopausal women with low bone mineral density and low fracture risk [6,7]. Although BMD and the bone markers previously assessed in our clinical trial are considered good surrogates of bone strength and bone quality, they may not correlate perfectly with a reduction in fracture risk. Fracture risk can be assessed more accurately by considering more variables than BMD alone, by using the FRAX tool. In this post-hoc analysis, our population had a medium-high fracture risk according to the FRAX scores; in fact, at baseline a 10-year fracture probability at the femur was 4.1 (1.9) in the placebo group and 4.2 (2.1) in the genistein group. This post-hoc comparison was made between the two treatment groups, showing for the first time that genistein aglycone (54 mg/day) plus calcium and vitamin D3 compared to only calcium and vitamin D3 supplementation significantly reduced the rate of osteoporosis, increasing BMD in postmenopausal women with medium-high 10-year fracture risk at the femur site. This analysis shows novel and additional findings distinct from those previously published [6–8]. More specifically, it appears that genistein has possible implications for the reduction of fracture risk in postmenopausal women with osteoporosis.

We believe that these data are particularly intriguing: in fact, this surrogate result on fractures overcomes one of the main limitations of our previous study, which was the lack of data on this major outcome. Additionally, the possibility to include, through the FRAX calculation, different risk factors in every patient enrolled in our clinical trial represents a strong advantage in terms of analysis for therapeutic efficacy.

Women enrolled in the parent trial were osteopenic rather than osteoporotic and this might represent a limitation for the current analysis; nevertheless, our study [6] remains, to date, the largest double-blind, placebo-controlled trial on genistein aglycone in the literature. To fill this gap, additional trials involving osteoporotic women are needed to further confirm the present results.

5. Conclusions

In conclusion, genistein plus calcium and vitamin D3 treatment demonstrated similar effects in terms of BMD increase at the femur versus placebo over 2 years in the subgroup of patients with osteoporosis. Collectively, these data confirm the positive and unique role of genistein aglycone, suggesting that it may be the most active isoflavone for treating postmenopausal bone loss, with a time-dependent effect, and suggesting that a long-term intake of genistein produces ongoing effects on bone health. This post-hoc analysis represents a proof-of concept study: it points out that genistein may counteract osteoporosis in postmenopausal women. However, this proof-of concept study needs to be confirmed by a large, well designed, and appropriately focused randomized clinical trial in a population at high risk of fractures. Currently, a clinical trial is investigating the effects of genistein on the fracture rate in glucocorticoid-induced osteoporosis and the final results are expected to be released in late 2018. These results will definitely clarify whether genistein may be useful not only in osteopenia but also in osteoporosis.

Acknowledgments: The authors are thankful to Bruce Burnett for his support in performing the analysis. Funding sources: Grant of the Italian Ministry of Education, University and Research, Code: 20073XZSR3; liberal donation from Primus Pharmaceuticals, Inc., Scottsdale, AZ, USA.

Author Contributions: V.A., M.A., F.S. and A.B. conceived and designed the experiments; M.A., R.D., H.M., D.S., L.M., S.M., D.A. performed the experiments; V.A., M.A., F.S. and A.B. analyzed the data; F.S., R.D., H.M., D.S., L.M., S.M., D.A. contributed reagents/materials/analysis tools; V.A., M.A., F.S., A.B. wrote the paper. All authors approved the final version of the manuscript.

References

1. Writing Group for the Women's Health Initiative Investigators. Risks and benefits of estrogen plus progestin in healthy postmenopausal women: Principal results from the Women's Health Initiative randomized controlled trial. *JAMA* **2002**, *288*, 321–333.
2. Collaborative group on Hormonal Factors in Breast Cancer. Breast Cancer and hormone replacement therapy: Collaborative reanalysis of data from 51 epidemiological studies of 52,705 women with breast cancer and 108,411 women without breast cancer. *Lancet* **1997**, *350*, 1047–1059.
3. Beral, V.; Million Women Study Collaborators. Breast cancer and hormone replacement therapy in the Million Women Study. *Lancet* **2003**, *362*, 419–427. [CrossRef]
4. Adlecreutz, H.L.; Mazur, W. Phyto-estrogen and western disease. *Ann. Med.* **1997**, *29*, 95–120. [CrossRef]
5. Horiuchi, T.; Onouchi, T.; Takahashi, M.; Ito, H.; Orimo, H. Effect of soy protein on bone metabolism in postmenopausal Japanese women. *Osteoporos. Int.* **2000**, *11*, 721–724. [CrossRef] [PubMed]
6. Marini, H.; Minutoli, L.; Polito, F.; Bitto, A.; Altavilla, D.; Atteritano, M.; Gaudio, A.; Mazzaferro, S.; Frisina, A.; Frisina, N.; et al. Effects of the phytoestrogen genistein on bone metabolism in osteopenic postmenopausal women: A randomized trial. *Ann. Intern. Med.* **2007**, *146*, 839–847. [CrossRef] [PubMed]
7. Marini, H.; Minutoli, L.; Polito, F.; Bitto, A.; Altavilla, D.; Atteritano, M.; Gaudio, A.; Mazzaferro, S.; Frisina, A.; Frisina, N.; et al. OPG and sRANKL serum concentrations in osteopenic, postmenopausal women after 2-year genistein administration. *J. Bone Miner. Res.* **2008**, *23*, 715–720. [CrossRef] [PubMed]
8. Marini, H.; Bitto, A.; Altavilla, D.; Burnett, B.P.; Polito, F.; Di Stefano, V.; Minutoli, L.; Atteritano, M.; Levy, R.M.; D'Anna, R.; et al. Breast safety and efficacy of genistein aglycone for postmenopausal bone loss: A follow-up study. *J. Clin. Endocrinol. Metab.* **2008**, *93*, 4787–4796. [CrossRef] [PubMed]
9. Bitto, A.; Polito, F.; Squadrito, F.; Marini, H.; D'Anna, R.; Irrera, N.; Minutoli, L.; Granese, R.; Altavilla, D. Genistein Aglycone: A Dual Mode of Action Anti-Osteoporotic Soy Isoflavone Rebalancing Bone Turnover Towards Bone Formation. *Curr. Med. Chem.* **2010**, *27*, 3007–3018. [CrossRef]
10. Atteritano, M.; Mazzaferro, S.; Frisina, A.; Cannata, M.L.; Bitto, A.; D'Anna, R.; Squadrito, F.; Macrì, I.; Frisina, N.; Buemi, M. Genistein effects on quantitative ultrasound parameters and bone mineral density in osteopenic postmenopausal women. *Osteoporos. Int.* **2009**, *20*, 1947–1954. [CrossRef] [PubMed]
11. Atteritano, M.; Mazzaferro, S.; Bitto, A.; Cannata, M.L.; D'Anna, R.; Squadrito, F.; Macrì, I.; Frisina, A.; Frisina, N.; Bagnato, G. Genistein effects on quality of life and depression symptoms in osteopenic postmenopausal women: A 2-year randomized, double-blind, controlled study. *Osteoporos. Int.* **2014**, *25*, 1123–1129. [CrossRef] [PubMed]
12. Atteritano, M.; Pernice, F.; Mazzaferro, S.; Mantuano, S.; Frisina, A.; D'Anna, R.; Cannata, M.L.; Bitto, A.; Squadrito, F.; Frisina, N.; et al. Effects of phytoestrogen genistein on cytogenetic biomarkers in postmenopausal women: 1 year randomized, placebo-controlled study. *Eur. J. Pharmacol.* **2008**, *28*, 22–26. [CrossRef] [PubMed]
13. Harkness, L.S.; Fiedler, K.; Sehgal, A.R.; Oravec, D.; Lerner, E. Decreased bone resorption with soy isoflavone supplementation in postmenopausal women. *J. Womens Health* **2004**, *13*, 1000–1007. [CrossRef] [PubMed]
14. Kreijkamp-Kaspers, S.; Kok, L.; Grobbee, D.E.; de Haan, E.H.; Aleman, A.; Lampe, J.W.; van der Schouw, Y.T. Effect of soy protein containing isoflavones on cognitive function, bone mineral density, and plasma lipids in postmenopausal women: A randomized controlled trial. *JAMA* **2004**, *292*, 65–74. [CrossRef] [PubMed]
15. Lydeking-Olsen, E.; Beck-Jensen, J.E.; Setchell, K.D.; Holm-Jensen, T. Soymilk or progesterone for prevention of bone loss—A 2 years randomized, placebo-controlled trial. *Eur. J. Nutr.* **2004**, *43*, 246–257. [CrossRef] [PubMed]
16. Newton, K.M.; LaCroix, A.Z.; Levy, L.; Li, S.S.; Qu, P.; Potter, J.D.; Lampe, J.W. Soy protein and bone mineral density in older men and women: A randomized trial. *Maturitas* **2006**, *55*, 270–277. [CrossRef] [PubMed]
17. Sehmisch, S.; Uffenorde, J.; Maehlmeyer, S.; Tezval, M.; Jarry, H.; Stuermer, K.M.; Stuermer, E.K. Evaluation of bone quality and quantity in osteoporotic mice—The effects of genistein and equol. *Phytomedicine* **2010**, *17*, 424–430. [CrossRef] [PubMed]
18. Bitto, A.; Burnett, B.P.; Polito, F.; Levy, R.M.; Marini, H.; Di Stefano, V.; Irrera, N.; Armbruster, M.A.; Minutoli, L.; Altavilla, D.; et al. Genistein aglycone reverses glucocorticoid-induced osteoporosis and increases bone breaking strength in rats: A comparative study with alendronate. *Br. J. Pharmacol.* **2009**, *156*, 1287–1295. [CrossRef] [PubMed]

19. FRAX. Fracture Risk Assessment Tool. Available online: http://www.shef.ac.uk/FRAX (accessed on 7–11 March 2016).
20. Kanis, J.A.; Johnell, O.; Oden, A.; Johansson, H.; McCloskey, E. FRAX and the assessment of fracture probability in men and women from the UK. *Osteoporos. Int.* **2008**, *19*, 385–397. [CrossRef] [PubMed]
21. Kanis, J.A.; Burlet, N.; Cooper, C. European Society for Clinical and Economic Aspects of Osteoporosis and Osteoarthritis (ESCEO) European guidance for the diagnosis and management of osteoporosis in postmenopausal women. *Osteoporos. Int.* **2008**, *19*, 399–428. [CrossRef] [PubMed]
22. Kanis, J.A.; Johnell, O. Requirements for DXA for the management of osteoporosis in Europe. *Osteoporos. Int.* **2005**, *16*, 229–238. [CrossRef] [PubMed]
23. Palacios, S. Advances in hormone replacement therapy: Making the menopause manageable. *BMC Womens Health* **2008**, *8*, 22. [CrossRef] [PubMed]

14

Maternal Consumption of Hesperidin and Naringin Flavanones Exerts Transient Effects to Tibia Bone Structure in Female CD-1 Offspring

Sandra M. Sacco [1,2], Caitlin Saint [2,3], Paul J. LeBlanc [2,3] and Wendy E. Ward [1,2,3,*]

1 Department of Kinesiology, Faculty of Applied Health Sciences, Brock University, St. Catharines, ON L2S 3A1, Canada; ssacco@brocku.ca

2 Centre for Bone and Muscle Health, Brock University, St. Catharines, ON L2S 3A1, Canada; caitlinsaint@trentu.ca (C.S.); pleblanc@brocku.ca (P.J.L.)

3 Department of Health Sciences, Faculty of Applied Health Sciences, Brock University, St. Catharines, ON L2S 3A1, Canada

* Correspondence: wward@brocku.ca

Abstract: Hesperidin (HSP) and naringin (NAR), flavanones rich in citrus fruits, support skeletal integrity in adult and aging rodent models. This study determined whether maternal consumption of HSP and NAR favorably programs bone development, resulting in higher bone mineral density (BMD) and greater structure and biomechanical strength (i.e., peak load) in female offspring. Female CD-1 mice were fed a control diet or a HSP + NAR diet five weeks before pregnancy and throughout pregnancy and lactation. At weaning, female offspring were fed a control diet until six months of age. The structure and BMD of the proximal tibia were measured longitudinally using in vivo micro-computed tomography at 2, 4, and 6 months of age. The trabecular bone structure at two and four months and the trabecular BMD at four months were compromised at the proximal tibia in mice exposed to HSP and NAR compared to the control diet ($p < 0.001$). At six months of age, these differences in trabecular structure and BMD at the proximal tibia had disappeared. At 6 months of age, the tibia midpoint peak load, BMD, structure, and the peak load of lumbar vertebrae and femurs were similar ($p > 0.05$) between the HSP + NAR and control groups. In conclusion, maternal consumption of HSP and NAR does not enhance bone development in female CD-1 offspring.

Keywords: bone development; flavanones; hesperidin; mice; naringin; structure

---

1. Introduction

Bioactives, naturally present in foods, may provide a dietary strategy to support healthy bone development. In a developing mouse model, exposure to soy isoflavones during early postnatal life, but not maternal exposure, sets a trajectory for higher bone mineral density (BMD), improved bone structure, and greater bone strength in female offspring at adulthood [1–4]. Other bioactives such as citrus flavanones (i.e., hesperidin (HSP) and naringin (NAR)) have been shown to exert bone-sparing effects in adult and aging rodents [5–11], but whether maternal consumption of citrus flavanones during pregnancy and lactation changes the trajectory of bone development of offspring, resulting in stronger, healthier bones at adulthood has not been investigated. Given that the metabolites of citrus flavanones (i.e., hesperetin and naringenin) can be transferred to human offspring via mother's milk [12], it is of interest to examine whether maternal exposure to HSP and NAR programs the bone tissue in adult female mouse offspring.

HSP (hesperetin-7-rutinoside) and NAR (naringenin-7-neohesperidoside) are flavanone glycosides found in high amounts in citrus fruits. HSP is found in particularly rich amounts in oranges while

NAR is present at high levels in grapefruits [13–15]. When consumed by humans and rodents, HSP and NAR are hydrolyzed into the aglycones, hesperetin and naringenin, and metabolized mainly into glucuronide forms by intestinal and liver conjugation [9,13,14,16,17]. The conjugated and aglycone metabolites circulate the body and modulate bone cell activity; in rat primary osteoblasts, hesperetin and hesperitin-7-*O*-glucuronide, at levels that are physiologically achievable through dietary consumption, increased osteoblast differentiation [18,19], and increased the mRNA expression of bone morphogenic proteins (BMPs) [18,19], runt-related transcription factor 2 (Runx2) [19], and osterix [18,19] that promote osteoblast differentiation. In murine MC3T3-E1 osteoblast cells [20] and rat [10] and human [21] bone mesenchymal stem cells, NAR increased osteoblast differentiation and proliferation and increased the expression of BMP-2 [20], osteopontin [21], and osteocalcin [10]. No data exists on the ability for HSP, NAR, or their metabolites to epigenetically regulate the transcriptions of genes involved in bone development. However, that HSP and NAR stimulate signaling pathways implicated in stimulating bone formation provides biological plausibility for HSP and NAR to support bone development and skeletal integrity.

The majority of our knowledge on the positive effects of HSP and NAR on bone is derived from rodent models of bone loss (i.e., ovariectomy, orchidectomy) [5–8,10,11] and aging (i.e., senescence) [9]. While intake of HSP and NAR is reported to benefit bone health in male and female rodents, most research has been performed in females. These studies demonstrate that dietary HSP and NAR protect against the loss of bone mineral and the deterioration of bone structure and strength during ovariectomy [6–8,10,11]. However, one study [7] in younger (3 months old) intact female rats reported gains in femoral BMD, which agrees with other work demonstrating that HSP supports bone cell function via modulating signaling proteins and bone cell differentiation to increase bone formation [18]. However, no studies have assessed whether maternal consumption of HSP and NAR affects bone development in growing and adult offspring. Given that treatment with HSP, NAR, or their combination stimulates bone formation [10,18], supports bone mineral accrual [7], and protects against bone loss in ovariectomized [6–8,10,11] female rodents, we hypothesized that maternal consumption of HSP and NAR before and during pregnancy and throughout lactation would set a trajectory for better bone health in female offspring. Thus, the objective of the present study was to determine whether maternal consumption of HSP and NAR results in higher BMD, improved bone structure, and greater bone strength in female CD-1 offspring at adulthood.

2. Materials and Methods

2.1. Animals and Diets

The experimental protocol (AUP 14-04-01, 2014) was approved by the Animal Care Committee at Brock University, St. Catharines, ON, Canada. Five-week-old female (n = 17) and 8-week-old male (n = 8) CD-1 mice were purchased from Charles River Canada (St. Constant, QC, Canada) and housed with 4–5 mice per cage at 22 °C–24 °C, 50% humidity with a 12:12-h light:dark cycle. Female mice were randomized to the American Institute of Nutrition-93 (AIN-93G) control diet (CON, n = 9) for growth, pregnancy and lactation [22] or the CON diet supplemented with 0.5% HSP + 0.25% NAR (HSP + NAR, n = 8). These doses reflect a moderate (400 mL) to high (1 L) daily intake of orange or grapefruit juices in humans [14,17] and represent doses that have been shown to exert protection to bone health in adult and aging rodents [5–9]. The AIN-93G diet used in the present study was modified to contain alcohol-extracted casein (TD. 06706, Harlan Teklad, Mississauga, ON, Canada) to remove vitamins that are naturally-occurring in casein and that may influence bone development. HSP (H5254, Sigma Aldrich, Oakville, ON, Canada) and NAR (N1376, Sigma Aldrich, Oakville, ON, Canada) were added to the CON diet at the expense of cornstarch. All mice had free access to food and water throughout the study, and food intake was measured twice per week using an electronic scale.

2.2. *Study Design*

At 10 weeks of age, mice were mated harem-style by housing 2–3 females with one male. Mating pairs were maintained on the female's respective diets, and, once identified as pregnant, female mice were housed individually and remained on their respective diets during the remainder of pregnancy and throughout lactation. Offspring were weighed at post-natal day (PND) 9, PND 16, and PND 21 using an electronic scale. At weaning, female offspring were housed with five mice per cage and switched to the CON diet for the remainder of the study duration. Food intake was measured twice per week and body weights measured weekly to monitor growth.

2.3. *In Vivo Analysis of Structure of Tibias by μCT*

At 2, 4, and 6 months of age, mouse offspring were anesthetized using 2%–5% isoflurane dissolved in 100% oxygen, and the right tibias were scanned in vivo using micro-computed tomography scanning (μCT) (Skyscan 1176, Bruker microCT, Kontich, Belgium) and host software (1176 version 1.1, Skyscan 1176, Bruker microCT, Kontich, Belgium), as previously described [23]. Scanning of the right proximal tibia was performed using an isotropic voxel size of 9 μm^3, 1 mm aluminum filter, 40 kV tube voltage, 300 μA amperage, a rotation step of 0.8°, 3350 ms integration time, and over 180° with no frame averaging. Each scan lasted 16 min 23 s and resulted in 460 mGy exposure per scan to the scanned tibias (TN-502RD-H, Best Medical Canada, Ottawa, ON, Canada). This dose of radiation does not affect tibial bone structure when tibias are repeatedly exposed at 2, 4, and 6 months of age [23]. At 6 months of age, animals were euthanized within five days after receiving their last scan by exsanguination under anesthesia (5% isoflurane dissolved in 100% oxygen), followed by cervical dislocation. Tibias, femurs, and lumbar vertebrae (LV 1–6) were excised, cleaned of soft tissue, and then wrapped in saline soaked gauze and stored at −80 °C for future analyses.

2.4. *Ex Vivo Analysis of Structure of Femurs and Lumbar Vertebrae by μCT*

Right femurs and the second lumber vertebra (LV2) were scanned ex vivo using μCT scanning (Skyscan 1176, Bruker microCT, Kontich, Belgium). These sites were scanned ex vivo to minimize the level of radiation exposure to each mouse. The bones were wrapped in parafilm to retain moisture during scanning and placed axially in a foam holder. The foam holder containing the bones was then secured to a mouse bed for ex vivo scanning using a 9 μm^3 isotropic voxel size, 0.25 mm aluminum filter, voltage of 45 kVp, tube current of 545 μA, 850 ms exposure time, and 0.2° rotation step. Scans were performed over 180° without using frame averaging.

2.5. *Reconstruction of In Vivo and Ex Vivo Images Obtained Using μCT*

Graphics Processing Unit (GPU)-acceleration (GPUReconServer, Skyscan, Bruker microCT, Kontich, Belgium) and NRecon Reconstruction 64-bit software (Skyscan, Bruker microCT, Kontich, Belgium) were used to reconstruct scanned images. Except for variable misalignment compensations, all scanned samples within each skeletal site received the same corrections to smoothing, ring artifacts, beam hardening, and defect pixel masking. Reconstructed images were then reoriented (DataViewer software, version 1.5.0, Skyscan, Bruker microCT, Kontich, Belgium), and the transaxial images were saved.

2.6. *Regions of Interest (ROI) and Segmentation of In Vivo and Ex Vivo Images Obtained Using μCT*

ROIs were selected from transaxial images and saved as new datasets using CTAnalyzer software (Skyscan Bruker microCT, Kontich, Belgium). At the proximal tibia, the ROI consisted of the trabecular and cortical bone and began 0.967 mm (110 slices) away from the metaphyseal side of the growth plate and extended 0.510 mm (58 transaxial slices) towards the ankle [23]. At the femur neck, an ROI of the trabecular region was manually drawn to a few pixels away from the endocortical boundary and consisted of 1.680 mm (191 slices), starting at the distal edge of the femur head and extending towards the diaphysis of the femur. At the distal femur, the ROI of the trabecular region was manually drawn a few pixels away from the endocortical boundary and consisted of 0.879 mm (100 slices), starting 0.616 (70 slices) proximal to the metaphyseal edge of the growth plate and extending toward the femur neck. Another ROI was manually drawn around the midpoint region of the femur, rich in cortical bone, and consisted of 0.879 mm (100 slices) spanning above and below the femur midpoint. At the LV2, ROIs of the trabecular and cortical regions of the vertebral bodies were manually and consisted of 115 transverse slices (1.011 mm), spanning above and below the midpoint of LV2.

Task lists were generated and applied (CTAnalyzer software, Skyscan Bruker microCT, Kontich, Belgium) to the saved datasets to segment bone from the background and to analyze trabecular or cortical bone structure at each skeletal site. At the proximal tibia, an automated task list was generated [23] to segment the trabecular bone from the cortical bone. Trabecular and cortical bone were then segmented as previously described [23]. At the femur neck, femur midpoint, distal femur, and LV, task lists were generated to segment the trabecular and cortical bones from the background. Local thresholding was used to segment the trabecular bone from the background (femur neck: lower threshold = 74, upper threshold = 255, radius = 6, constant = 0; distal femur: lower threshold = 71, upper threshold = 255, radius = 6, constant = 0; LV: lower threshold = 80, upper threshold = 255, radius = 7, constant = 0) and global thresholding (femur: lower threshold = 124, upper threshold = 255; LV2: lower threshold = 122, upper threshold = 255) for segmenting the cortical bone from the background at the femur midpoint and LV2 [24].

The trabecular bone outcome measures determined at the proximal tibia, femur neck, distal femur, and LV included bone volume (BV, mm^3), total volume (TV, mm^3), bone volume fraction (BV/TV, %), trabecular thickness (Tb.Th, mm), trabecular number (Tb.N, mm-1), trabecular separation (Tb.Sp, mm), degree of anisotropy (DA, no unit), and connectivity density (Conn.D, $1/mm^3$). Cortical bone outcome measures at the tibia, femur midpoint and LV included total cross-sectional area inside the periosteal envelope (Tt.Ar, mm^2), cortical bone area (Ct.Ar, mm^2), cortical area fraction (Ct.Ar/Tt.Ar, %), average cortical thickness (Ct.Th, mm), periosteal perimeter (Ps.Pm, mm), endocortical perimeter (Ec.Pm, mm), marrow area (Ma.Ar, mm^2), and eccentricity (no unit).

2.7. *Bone Mineral Density (BMD) and Peak Load of Tibias, Femurs and LV1-3*

To determine the trabecular BMD and cortical tissue mineral density (TMD) at the proximal tibia that were scanned in vivo at 2, 4, and 6 months of age, calibration phantoms consisting of 0.25 and 0.75 g/cm^3 calcium hydroxyapatite were scanned and reconstructed using the exact same parameters as all in vivo scans. BMD was then calibrated against the attenuation coefficient, and the trabecular BMD and cortical TMD at the proximal tibia were then measured against the attenuation coefficient [25]. Since measurement of BMD using μCT scanning is often not possible in excised samples due to the introduction of air bubbles from storage [25], BMD of the right femurs and LV1-3 was measured by dual energy X-ray absorptiometry (DXA) (Orthometrix, White Plains, NY, USA) and a specialized software program (Host Software version 3.9.4; Scanner Software version 1.2.0, Orthometrix, White Plains, NY, USA). Calibration of the DXA was performed daily using a calibration phantom. Femurs and LV1-3 were scanned using a resolution of 0.01 mm $\times$ 0.01 mm and at a speed of 2 mm/s. To determine bone strength at skeletal sites rich in cortical bone, the peak load at the midpoint of the right tibia and right femur was determined by 3-point bending using a Materials Testing System (Model 4442, Instron Corp., Norwood, MA, USA) and specialized software (Bluehill 2, Instron Corp., Norwood, MA, USA) [26]. The peak load at skeletal sites rich in trabecular bone was determined by compression testing at the femur neck and LV2 [26].

2.8. *Statistical Analyses*

All statistical analyses were performed using SPSS Statistics (version 22, IBM, Armonk, NY, USA). The effects of diet, age, and their interaction on food intake, body weight, and in vivo trabecular and cortical bone structure were determined using a repeated measures analysis of variance (ANOVA) (general linear model). Comparisons on all bone outcome measures between CON and HSP + NAR groups within each time point were assessed by unpaired two-tailed *t*-tests. A repeated measures ANOVA (general linear model) with a Bonferroni post-hoc test was used to determine longitudinal changes within the trabecular and cortical bone structural outcomes within each group. The primary outcome included BV/TV at the proximal tibia, with a total of seven mice per treatment group required to achieve a power of 0.8 and an alpha of 0.5. Missing values that resulted from mouse leg movement during the scan or due to computer error were replaced with the series mean. This occurred a total of four times (once in the CON group at 2 months of age, twice in the CON group at 4 months of age, and once in the HSP + NAR group at 4 months of age). Results are expressed as mean ± standard error of the mean (SEM) and the significance level was set at $p < 0.05$.

3. Results

3.1. Food Intake and Body Weight

Litter sizes (CON = 14 ± 2 pups/L, HSP + NAR= 13 ± 2 pups/L) were similar between the CON and HSP + NAR groups (p > 0.05). In addition, no differences (p > 0.05) in litter weight at PND9 (CON = 83 ± 10 g, HSP + NAR = 82 ± 6 g), PND16 (CON = 118 ± 10 g, HSP + NAR = 118 ± 5 g), or at weaning (PND21, CON = 162 ± 17 g, HSP + NAR = 160 ± 13 g) were observed between the groups. These results demonstrate that maternal consumption of HSP + NAR does not affect the growth patterns of female CD-1 offspring during suckling.

After weaning, an effect of time was observed for the mean daily food intake ($p < 0.01$) (Figure 1A) and weekly body weight ($p < 0.001$) (Figure 1B), which was expected because the mice were growing. There was no diet or time x diet effect on daily food intake or body weight throughout the study ($p > 0.05$). At the end of the study, the final body weights in 6-month-old offspring did not differ between CON and HSP + NAR groups. Thus, the food intake or growth characteristics of female offspring from weaning until six months of age were not affected by maternal and suckling exposure to HSP + NAR.

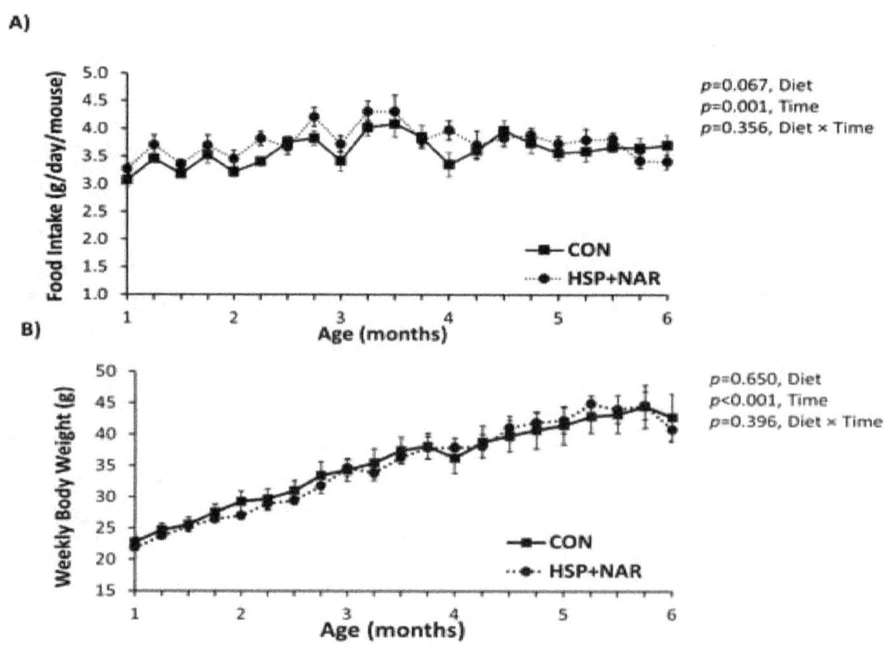

Figure 1. Mean daily food intake (**A**) and body weight (**B**) of female mice whose mothers were fed a control diet (CON) or a diet consisting of a combination of 0.5% hesperidin (HSP) and 0.25% naringin (NAR) before and during pregnancy and lactation, $n = 8–9$ per group. Mean ± standard error of the mean (SEM).

3.2. *In Vivo Measurements of Trabecular and Cortical Bone Mineral Density (BMD) and Bone Structure at the Proximal Tibia*

At the proximal tibia, a significant effect of diet ($p < 0.05$) was observed for several trabecular structural outcomes, whereby HSP + NAR resulted in lower BV, BV/TV, Tb.N, and Conn.D and higher Tb.Sp compared to CON at both 2 and 4 months of age (Table 1, Figure 2). A significant interaction between diet and time ($p < 0.05$) was observed for BMD and Tb.Sp, whereby HSP + NAR resulted in lower BMD at 4 months of age and higher Tb.Sp at 2 and 4 months of age compared to the CON group. No effects of diet on the trabecular bone structure at the proximal tibia was observed at 6 months of age. Thus, maternal consumption of HSP + NAR during pregnancy and lactation compromises trabecular BMD and bone structure at the proximal tibia in developing female CD-1 offspring; however, this effect does not persist into adulthood. In addition to an effect of diet, an effect of time ($p < 0.001$) was observed, whereby offspring from both the CON and HSP + NAR groups experienced a decrease in TV, BV, BV/TV, Tb.N, and Conn.D and an increase in Tb.Th and Tb.Sp from 2 to 4 months of age (Table 1, Figure 2). Similar to these changes, trabecular BMD from HSP + NAR exposure decreased from 2 to 4 months of age, while BMD decreased in the CON group after 4 months of age ($p < 0.001$). Diminutions in BV, BV/TV, Tb.N, and Conn.D within the CON group persisted to 6 months of age, resulting in trabecular bone structural outcomes that were significantly lower compared to both the 2- and 4-month time points ($p < 0.05$). In the HSP + NAR group, changes in trabecular BMD and bone structure were maintained from 4 to 6 months of age. Thus, female CD-1 offspring achieve peak trabecular BMD and bone structure before 4 months of age, a finding that agrees with previous work [23].

With regards to the cortical bone structure at the proximal tibia, Ct.Ar was significantly lower ($p < 0.05$) in the HSP + NAR group compared to the CON group at 4 months of age (Table 1, Figure 2). In addition, a time x diet effect was observed ($p < 0.05$) for Ps.Pm at the proximal tibia, whereby HSP + NAR resulted in lower Ps.Pm at 2 months of age compared to CON ($p < 0.05$). However, this effect was not apparent at 4 and 6 months of age. No effects ($p > 0.05$) from HSP + NAR exposure on cortical TMD were observed. Thus, maternal exposure during pregnancy and lactation to a combined 0.5% HSP and 0.25% NAR diet delays some characteristics of cortical bone development in female CD-1 offspring. In addition to an effect of diet on cortical bone structure, an effect of time ($p < 0.001$) was observed, whereby augments to the cortical bone TMD and structure, including Ct.Ar, Ct.Ar/Tt.Ar, and Ct.Th, were observed from 2 to 6 months of age in the CON and HSP + NAR groups (Table 1, Figure 2). In addition, diminution of Tt.Ar, Ec.Pm, and Ma.Ar were observed in both groups. These findings agree with our previous work showing that cortical bone structure reaches its peak at a later time point compared to trabecular bone in female CD-1 mice [23].

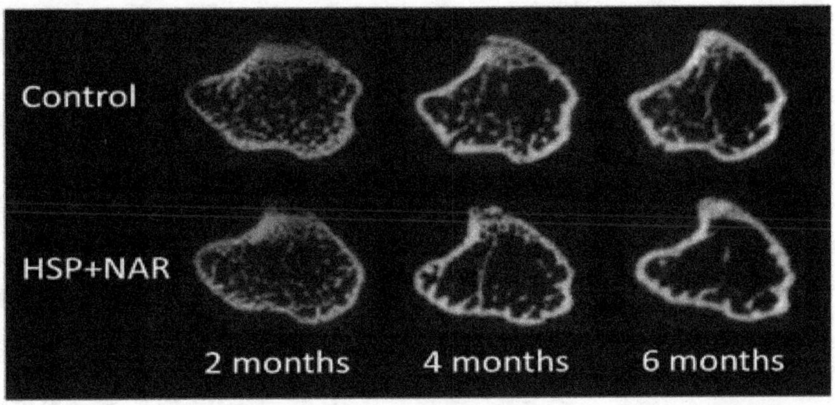

Figure 2. Representative grayscale transaxial images of right proximal tibias of female CD-1 mouse offspring at 2, 4, and 6 months of age.

Table 1. Bone mineral density (BMD) and structure at the proximal tibia at 2, 4, and 6 months of age in female CD-1 mice whose mothers were exposed to control (CON) or 0.5% hesperidin (HSP) and 0.25% naringin (NAR) diets through pregnancy and lactation.

Outcomes	CON			HSP + NAR			p Value		
	Age (Months)								
	2	4	6	2	4	6	Time	Diet	Time × Diet
Trabecular Structure									
BMD (g/cm^3)	0.212 ± 0.007 ^{a}	0.198 ± 0.003 ^{a}	0.154 ± 0.006 ^{b}	0.190 ± 0.010 ^{a}	0.162 ± 0.008 ^{†,b}	0.142 ± 0.008 ^{b}	<0.001	0.007	0.015
TV (mm^3)	1.185 ± 0.064 ^{a}	0.936 ± 0.045 ^{b}	0.898 ± 0.046 ^{b}	1.022 ± 0.065 ^{a}	0.853 ± 0.052 ^{b}	0.831 ± 0.058 ^{b}	<0.001	0.184	0.151
BV (mm^3)	0.097 ± 0.010 ^{a}	0.050 ± 0.006 ^{b}	0.025 ± 0.004 ^{c}	0.061 ± 0.009 ^{†,a}	0.029 ± 0.005 ^{†,b}	0.017 ± 0.004 ^{b}	<0.001	0.013	0.099
BV/TV (%)	8.177 ± 0.645 ^{a}	5.282 ± 0.464 ^{b}	2.764 ± 0.298 ^{c}	5.782 ± 0.698 ^{†,a}	3.260 ± 0.434 ^{†,b}	2.018 ± 0.526 ^{b}	<0.001	0.011	0.161
Tb.Th (mm)	0.059 ± 0.001 ^{b}	0.070 ± 0.001 ^{a}	0.073 ± 0.001 ^{a}	0.059 ± 0.001 ^{b}	0.068 ± 0.002 ^{a}	0.069 ± 0.002 ^{a}	<0.001	0.243	0.406
Tb.N (1/mm)	1.386 ± 0.105 ^{a}	0.751 ± 0.058 ^{b}	0.379 ± 0.42 ^{c}	0.976 ± 0.104 ^{†,a}	0.479 ± 0.063 ^{†,b}	0.284 ± 0.071 ^{b}	<0.001	0.009	0.094
Tb.Sp (mm)	0.297 ± 0.010 ^{c}	0.386 ± 0.003 ^{b}	0.429 ± 0.006 ^{a}	0.350 ± 0.015 ^{†,b}	0.430 ± 0.008 ^{†,a}	0.445 ± 0.006 ^{a}	<0.001	0.002	0.004
DA (no unit)	2.334 ± 0.095 ^{a}	1.970 ± 0.072 ^{b}	2.150 ± 0.116 ^{a,b}	2.562 ± 0.087	2.212 ± 0.126	2.962 ± 0.401	<0.001	0.030	0.305
Conn.D (1/mm^3)	46.6 ± 4.7 ^{a}	20.0 ± 2.1 ^{b}	7.9 ± 1.8 ^{c}	30.1 ± 2.1 ^{†,a}	11.3 ± 3.1 ^{†,b}	8.5 ± 2.3 ^{b}	<0.001	0.004	0.051
Cortical Structure									
TMD (g/cm^3)	0.802 ± 0.007 ^{c}	0.941 ± 0.112 ^{b}	0.996 ± 0.010 ^{a}	0.810 ± 0.007 ^{c}	0.932 ± 0.004 ^{b}	0.995 ± 0.007 ^{a}	<0.001	0.969	0.298
Ct.Ar (mm^2)	1.295 ± 0.041 ^{b}	1.396 ± 0.025 ^{a,b}	1.456 ± 0.021 ^{a}	1.230 ± 0.035 ^{b}	1.299 ± 0.037 ^{†,a}	1.367 ± 0.049 ^{a}	<0.001	0.061	0.798
Tt.Ar (mm^2)	3.951 ± 0.127 ^{a}	3.493 ± 0.104 ^{b}	3.517 ± 0.107 ^{b}	3.544 ± 0.158 ^{a}	3.236 ± 0.137 ^{b}	3.284 ± 0.159 ^{b}	<0.001	0.119	0.085
Ct.Ar/Tt.Ar (%)	33.1 ± 1.6 ^{b}	40.2 ± 1.1 ^{a}	41.6 ± 1.1 ^{a}	35.0 ± 1.0 ^{b}	40.4 ± 0.9 ^{a}	41.9 ± 1.2 ^{a}	<0.001	0.634	0.384
Ct.Th (mm)	0.110 ± 0.005 ^{c}	0.164 ± 0.005 ^{b}	0.187 ± 0.004 ^{a}	0.120 ± 0.004 ^{c}	0.167 ± 0.005 ^{b}	0.185 ± 0.003 ^{a}	<0.001	0.492	0.139
Ps.Pm (mm)	8.231 ± 0.123 ^{a}	7.851 ± 0.104 ^{b}	7.939 ± 0.097 ^{b}	7.780 ± 0.169 †	7.609 ± 0.159	7.731 ± 0.179	<0.001	0.135	0.046
Ec.Pm (mm)	6.535 ± 0.178 ^{a}	5.804 ± 0.153 ^{b}	5.724 ± 0.154 ^{b}	6.005 ± 0.193 ^{a}	5.457 ± 0.184 ^{b}	5.440 ± 0.214 ^{b}	<0.001	0.134	0.231
Ma.Ar (mm^2)	2.656 ± 0.139 ^{a}	2.097 ± 0.097 ^{b}	2.061 ± 0.099 ^{b}	2.314 ± 0.131 ^{a}	1.937 ± 0.106 ^{b}	1.917 ± 0.125 ^{b}	<0.001	0.196	0.116
Ecc (no unit)	0.459 ± 0.032 ^{a,b}	0.370 ± 0.026 ^{b}	0.426 ± 0.021 ^{a}	0.459 ± 0.028	0.458 ± 0.034	0.502 ± 0.034	0.041	0.054	0.452

† denotes significantly different ($p < 0.05$) compared to CON within the same month. Different letters in a row denote statistical significance ($p < 0.05$) within a group over time by repeated measures analysis of variance (ANOVA). Data are expressed as mean ± standard error of the mean (SEM), n = 8–9/group. BV = bone volume, BV/TV = bone volume fraction, Conn.D = connectivity density, Ct.Ar = cortical bone area, Ct.Ar/Tt.Ar = cortical area fraction, Ct.Th = cortical thickness, DA = degree of anisotropy, Ecc = mean eccentricity, Ec.Pm = endocortical perimeter, Ma.Ar = marrow area, Ps.Pm = periosteal perimeter, Tb.Th = trabecular thickness, Tb.N = trabecular number, Tb.Sp = trabecular separation, TMD = tissue mineral density, Tt.Ar = total cross sectional area inside the periosteal envelope, and TV = total volume.

3.3. Ex Vivo Measurements of Trabecular and Cortical Bone Structure

At the femur neck, there were no significant differences between the CON and HSP + NAR groups for BV/TV, Tb.Th, Tb.N, and Tb.Sp (Table 2, Figure 3A). Other trabecular parameters including BV, TV, Conn.D, and DA did not differ between groups. In addition, no differences in trabecular bone properties ($p > 0.05$) were observed at the distal metaphyseal region of the femur (Table 2). At the femur midpoint, there were no differences in cortical bone properties including Ct.Ar and Ct.Th (Table 2, Figure 3A), as well as Tt.Ar, Ct.Ar/Tt.Ar, Ps.Pm, Ec.Pm, Ma.Ar, or Ecc between the CON and HSP + NAR groups.

Table 2. Ex vivo bone mineral density (BMD), structure and peak load of the femur in 6-month-old female mice whose mothers were exposed to control (CON) or 0.5% hesperidin (HSP) + 0.25% naringin (NAR) diets through pregnancy and lactation.

	CON	HSP + NAR	*p* Value
Femur BMD (g/cm^2)	0.092 ± 0.002	0.090 ± 0.003	0.427
Femur Neck Trabecular Structure			
BV/TV (%)	15.6 ± 0.7	15.0 ± 0.9	0.621
Tb.Th (mm)	0.098 ± 0.002	0.099 ± 0.002	0.835
Tb.N (1/mm)	1.591 ± 0.083	1.523 ± 0.102	0.610
Tb.Sp (mm)	0.426 ± 0.014	0.440 ± 0.013	0.462
Femur Midpoint Cortical Structure			
Ct.Ar (mm^2)	1.312 ± 0.034	1.181 ± 0.076	0.101
Ct.Th (mm)	0.264 ± 0.009	0.252 ± 0.010	0.422
Distal Femur Trabecular Structure			
BV/TV (%)	11.0 ± 0.9	10.8 ± 2.8	0.932
Tb.Th (mm)	0.081 ± 0.002	0.078 ± 0.005	0.520
Tb.N (1/mm)	1.361 ± 0.105	1.294 ± 0.292	0.813
Tb.Sp (mm)	0.463 ± 0.031	0.544 ± 0.069	0.324
Femur Neck Peak Load (N)	23.5 ± 1.2	24.3 ± 1.8	0.697
Midpoint Peak Load (N)	25.5 ± 1.1	25.4 ± 2.4	0.602

There were no significant differences in femur outcomes between CON and HSP + NAR groups. Data are expressed as mean ± standard error of the mean (SEM), n = 5–9/group. BV/TV = bone volume fraction, Ct.Ar = cortical bone area, Ct.Th = cortical thickness, Tb.Th = trabecular thickness, Tb.N = trabecular number, Tb.Sp = trabecular separation.

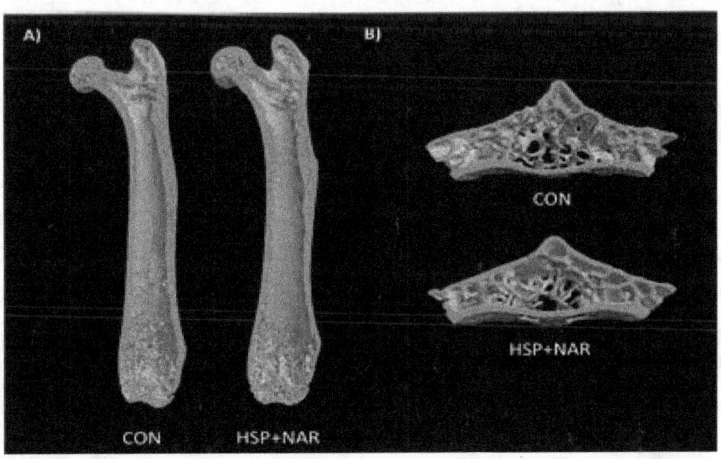

Figure 3. Representative images of the right femur (**A**) and the second lumbar vertebra (LV2) (**B**) of 6-month-old female mice whose mothers were exposed to control (CON) or 0.5% hesperidin (HSP) and 0.25% naringin (NAR) diets through pregnancy and lactation. Coronal sections consisting of the ventral half of the femur are depicted in (**A**); Transverse sections consisting of 1.011 mm of the vertebral body midsection are depicted in (**B**).

At LV2, there were no significant differences between CON and HSP + NAR with regards to BV/TV, Tb.Th, Tb.N, Tb.Sp (Table 3, Figure 3B), or other trabecular parameters. Similar to the trabecular bone, the cortical bone structural properties at LV2, including Ct.Ar and Ct.Th, were similar ($p < 0.05$) between the CON and HSP + NAR groups (Table 3). No other differences in cortical bone structure were observed between the groups. Collectively, these data indicate that maternal exposure to HSP and NAR does not result in long-term consequences to the trabecular or cortical bone structure at multiple skeletal sites in female CD-1 offspring.

Table 3. Ex vivo bone mineral density (BMD), structure and peak load of the lumbar vertebra (LV) in 6-month-old female CD-1 mice whose mothers were exposed to control (CON) or 0.5% hesperidin (HSP) + 0.25% naringin (NAR) diets through pregnancy and lactation.

	CON	HSP + NAR	*p* Value
LV1-3 BMD (g/cm^2)	0.075 ± 0.002	0.078 ± 0.004	0.490
LV2 Trabecular Structure			
BV/TV (%)	25.1 ± 1.6	22.5 ± 2.3	0.360
Tb.Th (mm)	0.081 ± 0.001	0.087 ± 0.005	0.304
Tb.N (1/mm)	3.106 ± 0.179	2.619 ± 0.228	0.110
Tb.Sp (mm)	0.296 ± 0.012	0.315 ± 0.017	0.359
LV2 Cortical Structure			
Ct.Ar (mm^2)	0.525 ± 0.013	0.523 ± 0.032	0.957
Ct.Th (mm)	0.083 ± 0.002	0.085 ± 0.005	0.706
LV2 Peak Load (N)	32.2 ± 2.7	35.8 ± 6.3	0.544

There were no significant differences in bone structure or strength between CON and HSP + NAR groups. Data are expressed as mean ± standard error of the mean (SEM), n = 5–9/group. BV/TV = bone volume fraction, Ct.Ar = cortical bone area, Ct.Th = cortical thickness, Tb.Th = trabecular thickness, Tb.N = trabecular number, Tb.Sp = trabecular separation.

3.4. Ex Vivo Measurement of Bone Mineral Density (BMD) and Peak Load

No significant differences ($p > 0.05$) in BMD at the whole femur (Table 2) or LV1-3 (Table 3) were observed between the CON and HSP + NAR groups at six months of age. The peak load at the tibia midpoint (CON = 18.1 ± 1.3 N, HSP + NAR= 18.1 ± 1.2) and at the femur midpoint, femur neck, and LV2 did not differ ($p > 0.05$) between the CON and HSP + NAR groups (Tables 2 and 3).

4. Discussion

Our data demonstrates that maternal consumption of HSP and NAR compromises trabecular structure at the proximal tibia in female CD-1 offspring at two and four months of age and trabecular BMD at four months of age; however, these differences do not persist to six months of age. At the femur and LV, the trabecular and cortical BMD and structure were not affected by dietary HSP and NAR. Moreover, the peak load was not altered by dietary HSP and NAR at the three skeletal sites measured (i.e. tibia midpoint, femur midpoint, and LV2). Thus, maternal consumption of HSP and NAR during pregnancy and lactation exerts transient effects on trabecular BMD and bone structure in female CD-1 offspring post-weaning, but these effects do not result in long-term detriments to skeletal integrity and strength at adulthood.

A novel aspect of this study included the timing of exposure to HSP and NAR. Previous studies have not investigated the effect of maternal exposure to these citrus flavanones on offspring. Thus, findings from the present study suggest that there is a critical period before and/or during pregnancy and/or lactation that transiently compromises the trabecular bone structure in female offspring. Determining which of these period(s) are critical for the effects of HSP and/or NAR on skeletal development is an area of future research interest. In addition, our findings suggest that HSP + NAR exerts differential effects on bone tissue that is dependent on the timing of exposure, as others have demonstrated that HSP, NAR, or their aglycones support bone health in mouse and rat models of adulthood, aging, or surgically- or senescent-induced bone loss [5–11]. For example, in 3-month-old female rats, a daily intake of 0.5% HSP increased femoral BMD by six months of age [7]. In ovariectomized mouse [8,11] and rat [6,7,10] models of postmenopausal bone loss, HSP, NAR or their combination protected against the deterioration of BMD, bone structure, and biomechanical strength. The protective effects of HSP and NAR on the trabecular bone have also been observed in orchidectomized mice [5] and senescent rats [9]. Collectively, these studies demonstrate that HSP, NAR, or their combination support the accrual and maintenance of BMD, bone structure, and strength in both adult and aging rodents at doses [5–9] similar to those used in the present study.

The mechanism of action is currently unknown. Studies have not investigated the effects of HSP, NAR, or their metabolites on their potential to regulate the transcription of genes involved in bone development through epigenetic mechanisms. The action of HSP and NAR on bone cell function is largely positive and attributed to their aglycone or glucuronide forms acting to increase the mRNA expression of BMP-2, BMP-4, Runx2, and osterix, which are involved in driving osteoblast differentiation and facilitating bone formation [18–20]. HSP and NAR may also decrease osteoclast activity and bone resorption [9,11]. While some literature has indicated HSP and NAR metabolites as exhibiting estrogenic properties [11,27], others have demonstrated that they do not activate estrogen receptor-alpha- (ER-alpha) or ER-beta-mediated transcription of genes [11] and that their binding affinities to estrogen receptors are low [28]. Thus, the estrogenic or anti-estrogenic potential of HSP and NAR is uncertain. Moreover, whether HSP and/or NAR metabolites can cross the placenta or be transferred to the offspring via the mother's milk in CD-1 mice is an area of future investigation. It is possible that maternal exposure to HSP and/or NAR modulates circulating levels of calciotropic hormones in the mother to result in alterations to calcium availability to the fetus in utero or to offspring during suckling; however, this remains to be determined. Further investigation is necessary to determine the mechanisms whereby HSP + NAR compromises trabecular bone structure at the proximal tibia in two- and four-month-old female offspring. Moreover, further investigation is warranted to determine whether the skeletal tissue of male offspring also responds to maternal exposure to HSP + NAR.

Among the strengths of the present study is the comprehensive assessment that was performed on BMD, structure, and strength at multiple skeletal sites. That HSP + NAR exposure did not induce effects at 6 months of age on bone mineral, structure, and biomechanical strength at the tibias, femurs, and LV demonstrates consistency among all skeletal sites examined and provides strong evidence that HSP + NAR does not have long lasting effects on skeletal integrity in female CD-1 offspring when mothers are exposed before and during pregnancy and throughout lactation. Another strength is that that changes in tibial BMD and bone structure were evaluated within the same mice throughout the course of the study. This longitudinal evaluation of BMD and bone structure within the same mice resulted in a statistically powerful design and reduced the number of animals required to conduct the present study. A limitation of the present study is the uncertainty of whether the compromised bone structure with HSP + NAR treatment at two and four months of age is due to the combined action of HSP and NAR or if one of these flavanones is responsible for these observed effects. As we are the first to examine the efficacy HSP and NAR in a programming model of bone development, we chose to provide HSP and NAR in combination at levels that have established effects in aging rodent models [8,9,11] as a proof of efficacy. Moreover, identifying whether the critical period is preconception, and/or during pregnancy, and/or lactation remains unknown.

5. Conclusions

In conclusion, maternal consumption of HSP + NAR exerts transient effects on trabecular bone development at the proximal tibia in female CD-1 offspring. That BMD, structure, and strength at the tibia, femur, and LV were similar between the CON and HSP + NAR groups at six months of age suggests that maternal consumption of HSP + NAR does not favorably program bone health in female CD-1 offspring.

Acknowledgments: W.E.W. holds a Canada Research Chair in Bone and Muscle Development. We thank the Canadian Institutes of Health Research for funding this research (grant number 130544) and the Canada Foundation for Innovation (grant number 222084) for the purchase of the micro-computed tomography system.

Author Contributions: S.M.S. and W.E.W. conceptualized the study and designed the experiments. S.M.S. and C.S. conducted the in vivo portion of the study, including the in vivo micro-computed tomography scanning of mice. P.J.L. provided insight into the study. S.M.S. performed the bone analyses. S.M.S. wrote the initial drafts of the manuscript with W.E.W., and all authors contributed to and approved the final version.

References

1. Kaludjerovic, J.; Ward, W.E. Bone-specific gene expression patterns and whole bone tissue of female mice are programmed by early life exposure to soy isoflavones and folic acid. *J. Nutr. Biochem.* **2015**, *26*, 1068–1076. [CrossRef] [PubMed]
2. Kaludjerovic, J.; Ward, W.E. Neonatal administration of isoflavones attenuates deterioration of bone tissue in female but not male mice. *J. Nutr.* **2010**, *140*, 766–772. [CrossRef] [PubMed]
3. Dinsdale, E.C.; Kaludjerovic, J.; Ward, W.E. Isoflavone exposure throughout suckling results in improved adult bone health in mice. *J. Dev. Orig. Health Dis.* **2012**, *3*, 271–275. [CrossRef] [PubMed]
4. Kaludjerovic, J.; Ward, W.E. Neonatal exposure to daidzein, genistein, or the combination modulates bone development in female CD-1 mice. *J. Nutr.* **2009**, *139*, 467–473. [CrossRef] [PubMed]
5. Chiba, H.; Kim, H.; Matsumoto, A.; Akiyama, S.; Ishimi, Y.; Suzuki, K.; Uehara, M. Hesperidin prevents androgen deficiency-induced bone loss in male mice. *Phytother. Res.* **2014**, *28*, 289–295. [CrossRef] [PubMed]
6. Habauzit, V.; Nielsen, I.L.; Gil-Izquierdo, A.; Trzeciakiewicz, A.; Morand, C.; Chee, W.; Barron, D.; Lebecque, P.; Davicco, M.J.; Williamson, G.; et al. Increased bioavailability of hesperetin-7-glucoside compared with hesperidin results in more efficient prevention of bone loss in adult ovariectomised rats. *Br. J. Nutr.* **2009**, *102*, 976–984. [CrossRef] [PubMed]
7. Horcajada, M.N.; Habauzit, V.; Trzeciakiewicz, A.; Morand, C.; Gil-Izquierdo, A.; Mardon, J.; Lebecque, P.; Davicco, M.J.; Chee, W.S.; Coxam, V.; et al. Hesperidin inhibits ovariectomized-induced osteopenia and shows differential effects on bone mass and strength in young and adult intact rats. *J. Appl. Physiol. (1985)* **2008**, *104*, 648–654. [CrossRef] [PubMed]
8. Chiba, H.; Uehara, M.; Wu, J.; Wang, X.; Masuyama, R.; Suzuki, K.; Kanazawa, K.; Ishimi, Y. Hesperidin, a citrus flavonoid, inhibits bone loss and decreases serum and hepatic lipids in ovariectomized mice. *J. Nutr.* **2003**, *133*, 1892–1897. [PubMed]
9. Habauzit, V.; Sacco, S.M.; Gil-Izquierdo, A.; Trzeciakiewicz, A.; Morand, C.; Barron, D.; Pinaud, S.; Offord, E.; Horcajada, M.N. Differential effects of two citrus flavanones on bone quality in senescent male rats in relation to their bioavailability and metabolism. *Bone* **2011**, *49*, 1108–1116. [CrossRef] [PubMed]
10. Li, N.; Jiang, Y.; Wooley, P.H.; Xu, Z.; Yang, S.Y. Naringin promotes osteoblast differentiation and effectively reverses ovariectomy-associated osteoporosis. *J. Orthop. Sci.* **2013**, *18*, 478–485. [PubMed]
11. Pang, W.Y.; Wang, X.L.; Mok, S.K.; Lai, W.P.; Chow, H.K.; Leung, P.C.; Yao, X.S.; Wong, M.S. Naringin improves bone properties in ovariectomized mice and exerts oestrogen-like activities in rat osteoblast-like (UMR-106) cells. *Br. J. Pharmacol.* **2010**, *159*, 1693–1703. [CrossRef] [PubMed]
12. Song, B.J.; Jouni, Z.E.; Ferruzzi, M.G. Assessment of phytochemical content in human milk during different stages of lactation. *Nutrition* **2013**, *29*, 195–202. [CrossRef] [PubMed]
13. Zeng, X.; Bai, Y.; Peng, W.; Su, W. Identification of naringin metabolites in human urine and feces. *Eur. J. Drug Metab. Pharmacokinet.* **2016**. [CrossRef] [PubMed]
14. Manach, C.; Morand, C.; Gil-Izquierdo, A.; Bouteloup-Demange, C.; Remesy, C. Bioavailability in humans of the flavanones hesperidin and narirutin after the ingestion of two doses of orange juice. *Eur. J. Clin. Nutr.* **2003**, *57*, 235–242. [CrossRef] [PubMed]
15. Rouseff, R.L.; Martin, S.F.; Youtsey, C.O. Quantitative survey of narirutin, naringin, hesperidin, and neohesperidin in citrus. *J. Agric. Food Chem.* **1987**, *35*, 1027–1030. [CrossRef]

16. Booth, A.N.; Jones, F.T.; Deeds, F. Metabolic and glucosuria studies on naringin and phloridzin. *J. Biol. Chem.* **1958**, *233*, 280–282. [PubMed]
17. Erlund, I.; Meririnne, E.; Alfthan, G.; Aro, A. Plasma kinetics and urinary excretion of the flavanones naringenin and hesperetin in humans after ingestion of orange juice and grapefruit juice. *J. Nutr.* **2001**, *131*, 235–241. [PubMed]
18. Trzeciakiewicz, A.; Habauzit, V.; Mercier, S.; Lebecque, P.; Davicco, M.J.; Coxam, V.; Demigne, C.; Horcajada, M.N. Hesperetin stimulates differentiation of primary rat osteoblasts involving the bmp signalling pathway. *J. Nutr. Biochem.* **2010**, *21*, 424–431. [CrossRef] [PubMed]
19. Trzeciakiewicz, A.; Habauzit, V.; Mercier, S.; Barron, D.; Urpi-Sarda, M.; Manach, C.; Offord, E.; Horcajada, M.N. Molecular mechanism of hesperetin-7-o-glucuronide, the main circulating metabolite of hesperidin, involved in osteoblast differentiation. *J. Agric. Food Chem.* **2010**, *58*, 668–675. [CrossRef] [PubMed]
20. Wu, J.B.; Fong, Y.C.; Tsai, H.Y.; Chen, Y.F.; Tsuzuki, M.; Tang, C.H. Naringin-induced bone morphogenetic protein-2 expression via PI3K, Akt, c-Fos/c-Jun and AP-1 pathway in osteoblasts. *Eur. J. Pharmacol.* **2008**, *588*, 333–341. [CrossRef] [PubMed]
21. Zhang, P.; Dai, K.R.; Yan, S.G.; Yan, W.Q.; Zhang, C.; Chen, D.Q.; Xu, B.; Xu, Z.W. Effects of naringin on the proliferation and osteogenic differentiation of human bone mesenchymal stem cell. *Eur. J. Pharmacol.* **2009**, *607*, 1–5. [CrossRef] [PubMed]
22. Reeves, P.G.; Nielsen, F.H.; Fahey, G.C., Jr. AIN-93 purified diets for laboratory rodents: Final report of the American institute of nutrition ad hoc writing committee on the reformulation of the AIN-76A rodent diet. *J. Nutr.* **1993**, *123*, 1939–1951. [PubMed]
23. Sacco, S.M.; Saint, C.; Longo, A.B.; Wakefield, C.B.; Salmon, P.L.; LeBlanc, P.J.; Ward, W.E. Repeated irradiation from micro-computed tomography scanning at 2, 4 and 6 months of age does not induce damage to tibial bone microstructure in male and female CD-1 mice. *BoneKEy Rep.* **2017**. [CrossRef]
24. Otsu, N. A threshold selection method from gray-level histograms. *IEEE Trans. Syst. Man. Cyber.* **1979**, *9*, 62–66. [CrossRef]
25. Bruker. *Method Note: Bone Mineral Density (BMD) and Tissue Mineral Density (TMD) Calibration and Measurement by Micro-CT Using Bruker-MicroCT CT-Analyser*; Bruker microCT: Kontich, Belgium, 2014.
26. Fonseca, D.; Ward, W.E. Daidzein together with high calcium preserve bone mass and biomechanical strength at multiple sites in ovariectomized mice. *Bone* **2004**, *35*, 489–497. [CrossRef] [PubMed]
27. Breinholt, V.; Larsen, J.C. Detection of weak estrogenic flavonoids using a recombinant yeast strain and a modified MCF7 cell proliferation assay. *Chem. Res. Toxicol.* **1998**, *11*, 622–629. [CrossRef] [PubMed]
28. Kuiper, G.G.; Lemmen, J.G.; Carlsson, B.; Corton, J.C.; Safe, S.H.; van der Saag, P.T.; van der Burg, B.; Gustafsson, J.A. Interaction of estrogenic chemicals and phytoestrogens with estrogen receptor beta. *Endocrinology* **1998**, *139*, 4252–4263. [PubMed]

15

Determinants of Adherence in Time-Restricted Feeding in Older Adults

Stephanie A. Lee [1,*], Caroline Sypniewski [1], Benjamin A. Bensadon [1], Christian McLaren [1], William T. Donahoo [2], Kimberly T. Sibille [1] and Stephen Anton [1,3,*]

1 Department of Aging and Geriatric Research, Institute on Aging, University of Florida, Gainesville, FL 32610, USA; csypniewski@ufl.edu (C.S.); bensadon@ufl.edu (B.A.B.); mclaren@ufl.edu (C.M.); ksibille@ufl.edu (K.T.S.)

2 Department of Medicine, University of Florida, Gainesville, FL 32610, USA; troy.donahoo@medicine.ufl.edu

3 Department of Clinical and Health Psychology, University of Florida, Gainesville, FL 32610, USA

* Correspondence: Stephanie.lee2@valpo.edu (S.A.L.); santon@ufl.edu (S.A.)

Abstract: Time-restricted feeding (TRF) is a type of intermittent fasting in which no calories are commonly consumed for approximately 12–18 hours on a daily basis. The health benefits of this eating pattern have been shown in overweight adults, with improvements in cardiometabolic risk factors as well as the preservation of lean mass during weight loss. Although TRF has been well studied in younger and middle-aged adults, few studies have evaluated the effects of TRF in older adults. Thus, the goal of this study was to evaluate older-adult perspectives regarding the real-world advantages, disadvantages, and challenges to adopting a TRF eating pattern among participants aged 65 and over. A four-week single-arm pre- and post-test design was used for this clinical pilot trial TRF intervention study. Participants were instructed to fast for approximately 16 h per day with the daily target range between 14 and 18 h. Participants were provided with the TRF protocol at a baseline visit, along with a pictorial guide that depicted food items and beverages that were allowed and not allowed during fasting windows to reinforce that calorie-containing items were to be avoided. The trial interventionist called each participant weekly to promote adherence, review the protocol, monitor for adverse events, and provide support and guidance for any challenges faced during the intervention. Participants were instructed to complete daily eating time logs by recording the times at which they first consumed calories and when they stopped consuming calories. At the end of the intervention, participants completed an exit interview and a study-specific Diet Satisfaction Survey (Table 1) to assess their satisfaction, feasibility, and overall experience with the study intervention. Of the 10 participants who commenced the study (mean age = 77.1 y; 6 women, 4 men), nine completed the entire protocol. Seven of the ten participants reported easy adjustment to a 16-hour fast and rated the difference from normal eating patterns as minimal. Eight participants reported no decrease in energy during fasting periods, with greater self-reported activity levels in yardwork and light exercise. Adverse events were rare, and included transient headaches, which dissipated with increased water intake, and dizziness in one participant, which subsided with a small snack. The findings of the current trial suggest that TRF is an eating approach that is well tolerated by most older adults. Six participants, however, did not fully understand the requirements of the fasting regimen, despite being provided with specific instructions and a pictorial guide at a baseline visit. This suggests that more instruction and/or participant contact is needed in the early stages of a TRF intervention to promote adherence.

Keywords: weight loss; intermittent fasting; fat loss; sarcopenia; body composition

1. Introduction

Aging is often associated with a host of biological changes that contribute to a progressive decline in cognitive and physical function, frequently leading to a loss of independence and increased risk of mortality. The life expectancy of adults in many industrialized countries continues to increase [1], with persons aged ≥65 years representing the fastest growing segment of the US population [2]. While prolongation of life remains an important public health goal, of even greater significance is the extension of healthspan, often defined as continued intact functional capacity, and delay of the physiological changes that result in disease and disability [3,4]. For these reasons, there is a longstanding interest in understanding the biopsychosocial and functional determinants of successful aging [5]. Although many factors can contribute to functional decline, loss of muscle mass (sarcopenia) in particular, has been consistently linked to functional decline during aging [6].

Globally, sarcopenia has become a major health challenge, and is now recognized as a medical condition across the world [7,8]. In a recent multi-ethnic study (MEMOSA—Multi-Ethnic Molecular determinants of Sarcopenia) involving participants from Singapore, the UK, and Jamaica [9], the genome-wide transcriptomic profiles of skeletal muscle biopsies in 119 older men diagnosed with sarcopenia compared with age-matched controls were examined using high-coverage RNA sequencing. The novel and important finding of this study was that mitochondrial bioenergetic dysfunction was the strongest molecular signature of sarcopenia in men irrespective of ethnicity. Specifically, sarcopenia was associated with major impairments of oxidative phosphorylation, mitochondrial dynamics, and mitochondrial quality. Such findings strongly suggest links between mitochondrial health, muscle quality, and physical function in older adults.

Exercise is widely known to improve mitochondrial health, potentially by providing a hormetic challenge that induces mitochondrial biogenesis [10]. Another potential intervention strategy for enhancing the metabolic flexibility of the mitochondria is intermittent fasting (IF), or more specifically, time-restricted feeding (TRF) [11]. This type of eating pattern involves a cessation in caloric intake commonly for 12–18 hours daily and has been shown to be sufficient to induce the metabolic switch from glucose to ketones as a source of energy for the mitochondria [12–14]. Specifically, this shift in metabolism takes place when nutrient availability is low and occurs at the point of negative energy balance when liver glycogen stores are depleted and fatty acids are mobilized (typically beyond 12 h after cessation of caloric intake) [15,16].

In contrast to traditional caloric restriction paradigms, food is not consumed during designated fasting time periods but is typically not restricted during designated eating time periods. The length of the fasting time period can also vary but is frequently 12 or more continuous hours. There are many types of intermittent fasting approaches, but the two most popular and well-studied approaches are alternate day fasting (ADF) or alternate day modified fasting (ADMF) and TRF. Alternate day or alternate day modified fasting involves consuming no or very little food on fasting days and then alternating with a day of unrestricted food intake or a "feast" day. Time-restricted feeding interventions differ from ADF interventions in that individuals engage in daily fasts between 14 and 18 hours. Findings from a recent review indicate participants generally have high levels of adherence (range = 77% to 98%) with no serious adverse events to fasting regimens ranging in duration from two weeks to one year [17].

Several clinical trials now indicate that a TRF eating pattern can reduce fat mass with retention of lean mass in younger and middle-aged adults [18–21]; however, the effects of TRF are not well understood in adults aged 65 and older. We recently reported that a four-week TRF eating pattern was sufficient to induce weight loss and produce small but clinically meaningful improvements in physical function in overweight older adults [22]. Although these findings are promising, they are limited by the short duration of the intervention. Therefore, the present study aimed to better understand factors affecting adherence and feasibility of TRF in an older adult population.

2. Methods

As described previously [22], ten overweight, sedentary, older adults aged 65 and older with mild to moderate functional limitations were recruited to participate in the *Time to Eat* pilot study. All participants were living independently in the community. Primary outcomes were feasibility, tolerability, and safety in overweight, sedentary older adults over four weeks using a single-arm pre–post design. Secondary outcomes included changes in body weight, waist circumference, cognitive and physical function, health-related quality of life, and adverse events [22]. The overarching goal of the present study was to evaluate participant perspectives who were enrolled in the *Time to Eat* pilot study regarding the real-world advantages, disadvantages, and challenges to adopting a TRF eating pattern via weekly phone interviews, a diet satisfaction survey, and an exit interview during the study.

2.1. Intervention

A four-week TRF single-arm clinical pilot trial was employed to test the study objectives. All participants were asked to abstain from any caloric intake during the targeted fasting window of 16 continuous hours and consume ad libitum during the eating window. Fasting times were chosen by the participant and were allowed to vary each day. The first week involved a gradual increase to a full 16-hour fasting period (Days 1–3 fast for 12–14 hours per day, Days 4–6 fast for 14–16 hours per day, Days 7–28 fast for 16 hours per day). Participants were encouraged to hydrate during fasting times. There were no dietary restrictions on the amount or types of food consumed during the 8-h feeding window, and participants were allowed to choose a time frame that best fit their lifestyle.

To promote adherence to the intervention, participants were provided with directions on how to follow the TRF protocol at the baseline visit. During this visit, participants received a pictorial flyer for future reference which depicted food items that were allowed and not allowed during fasting windows. On the flyer, "Go Foods" were written in green (water, diet soda, unsweetened teas, sugar free gum, black coffee) and "No Foods" were written in red (anything with calories, including coffee creamer, sweet teas, alcohol, snacks, drinks with calories). Participants also received an eating time log, which they were instructed to complete by recording the times when they first consumed calories and when they stopped consuming calories each day.

The trial interventionist called each participant weekly to promote adherence, review the protocol, monitor for adverse events, and provide support and guidance for any challenges faced during the intervention. A semi-structured, open-ended interview guide was used for the calls to inquire about daily activities, changes to normal routine, and any changes in health. During the call, the eating time log was reviewed, and support and guidance were provided for any challenges faced due to the intervention. An intervention-specific interview guide was used to routinely monitor adherence and adverse events, and to obtain direct participant feedback at multiple time points throughout the trial. The same questions were asked during each call, and calls concluded with open discussion. Participant answers and comments were documented during the phone calls. The questions asked during each phone call are displayed in Figure S1.

2.2. Adherence

Self-reported adherence to the study intervention was measured using the eating time log. Participants were considered adherent if they fasted between 14–18 hours per day during weeks two through four of the intervention. For this intervention, participants were allowed to pick the times of day in which they fasted as well as their eating window.

2.3. Outcome Measures

Diet Satisfaction Survey. At the end of the intervention, participants completed a study-specific Diet Satisfaction Survey (Table 1) to assess their satisfaction, feasibility, and overall experience with the study intervention. The Diet Satisfaction Survey contained 22 items and categorically measured respondents' attitudes by asking the extent to which they agreed or disagreed with a particular statement on a 5-point Likert scale (strongly disagree, disagree, neutral, agree, and strongly agree). The scores were summed and questions were grouped into one of three domains: biological, psychological, and socio-environmental.

Table 1. Participant responses to the Diet Satisfaction Survey.

Questions	Strongly Disagree (%)	Disagree (%)	Neutral (%)	Agree (%)	Strongly Agree (%)
Biological					
It was difficult to eat enough calories within the 8 hour window.	3(33)	4(44)	1(11)	1(11)	0(0)
I would eat more than normal amount of food during feeding period.	1(11)	5(56)	2(22)	1(11)	0(0)
I was uncomfortably hungry while fasting	0(0)	7(78)	1(11)	0(0)	1(11)
I had less energy than usual while fasting.	3(33)	5(56)	0(0)	0(0)	1(11)
I had difficulty falling asleep, staying asleep, or waking during fasting.	2(22)	3(33)	3(33)	1(11)	0(0)
Psychological					
Fasting became more difficult as study went on.	4(44)	2(22)	1(11)	1(11)	1(11)
Fasting became easier as the study went on.	0(0)	2(22)	1(11)	3(33)	3(33)
My mood improved while intermittent fasting.	0(0)	2(22)	6(67)	0(0)	1(11)
My mood worsened while intermittent fasting.	2(22)	1(11)	5(56)	1(11)	0(0)
Fasting was more difficult than others previously tried.	2(22)	3(33)	3(33)	0(0)	1(11)
My overall quality of life improved during the IF diet.	0(0)	2(22)	6(67)	1(11)	0(0)
I could continue to IF for 6 months.	1(11)	2(22)	0(0)	6(67)	0(0)
I could continue to IF for 12 months.	2(22)	2(22)	1(11)	4(44)	0(0)
I could continue to IF for 24 months.	3(33)	1(11)	3(33)	2(22)	0(0)
I plan to continue IF after this study.	0(0)	2(22)	2(22)	5(56)	0(0)
I would participate in this study again.	1(11)	1(11)	1(11)	5(56)	1(11)
Socio-environmental					
I consumed all of my calories in one sitting.	3(33)	4(44)	1(11)	1(11)	0(0)
Fasting periods made tasks and work and home more difficult.	2(22)	3(33)	2(22)	1(11)	1(11)
Fasting periods negatively impacted my Social life.	2(22)	3(33)	2(22)	2(22)	0(0)
It was inconvenient to restrict my food intake to an 8-hour time frame.	0(0)	4(44)	1(11)	3(33)	1(11)
If recommended by their doctor, I think people would follow the IF diet.	0(0)	0(0)	4(44)	5(56)	0(0)
I would recommend this study to a friend.	1(11)	0(0)	2(22)	4(44)	2(22)

Exit Interview. Exit interviews were also conducted in person by the study interventionist during the follow-up assessment visits. Interview format mirrored that of the weekly phone calls and included additional questions measuring interest and the likelihood of continuing the TRF eating pattern. The interview concluded by allowing the participant to offer future suggestions and modifications if desired. The Specific Exit Interview Questions asked are displayed in Figure S2.

2.4. Analyses

Using the information obtained during the weekly phone calls and exit interviews, participant views on the perceived advantages, disadvantages, and challenges to adopting the TRF regimen were explored through qualitative analyses to better understand how older adults can successfully adopt TRF. A constant-comparison coding process was used to categorize and compare interview data for analysis purposes [23]. A trained researcher (SL) open-coded each interview and mapped data within the three primary constructs of the biopsychosocial model (biological, psychological, socio-environmental) to systematically categorize these three primary factors in their interactions in the TRF intervention. Open coding was completed by hand instead of using data mining software in order to take on the full context of the interviews. Positive and negative categories within each of the three primary themes were documented.

3. Results

Nine of the ten participants who commenced the study (mean age = 77.1 y; 6 women, 3 men) completed the entire protocol. One participant was considered non-adherent as the participant did not complete phone calls during the intervention or post-intervention assessments. However, this participant did complete an exit interview but not the Diet Satisfaction Survey post intervention. Thus, exit interviews were completed with all 10 participants who were enrolled in this study. Four participants completed all three weekly phone calls with the interventionist, three participants completed two calls, one participant completed one call near study end due to the wrong phone number being provided, and one participant did not complete any phone calls due to being on vacation.

Self-reported mean adherence to the TRF regimen was 84%, measured by daily eating time logs [22]. Few adverse events were reported during this intervention. Specifically, two participants experienced headaches during fasting periods, which resolved following an increase in water intake. One participant experienced dizziness, which resolved after having a small snack.

Over the four-week TRF intervention, the average reported start time for the participant eating period was 10:21 AM (range = 6:56 AM–1:25 PM) and the average reported stop time was 6:38 PM (range = 5:08 PM–9:00 PM), respectively. During week 1, the average reported start time of the first meal was 9:23 AM. During weeks 2 to 4, the start time of the eating period shifted later in the morning by a little over an hour, with participants reporting an average start time of 10:33 AM during week 4. The average eating stop time occurred 27 minutes earlier over the four-week study, concluding at 6:49 PM during week 1 and at 6:22 PM during week 4. The self-selected start and stop times for each participant's eating window are displayed in Figure 1.

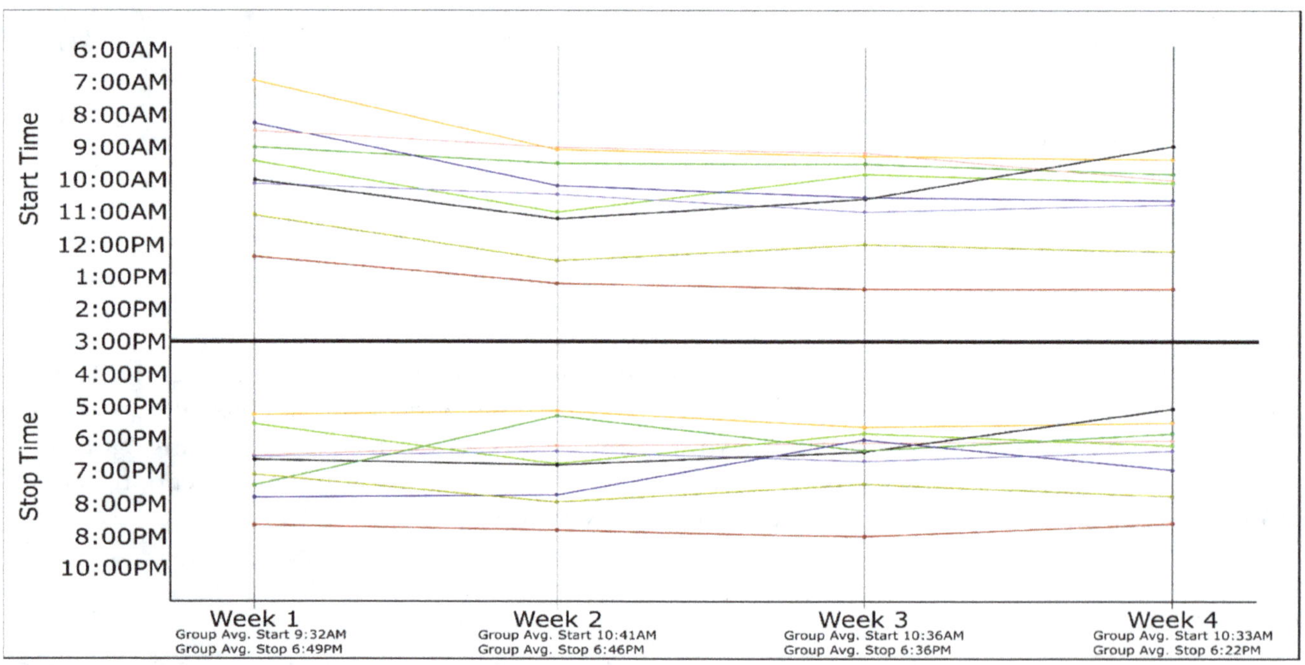

Figure 1. Self-selected start and stop times for each participant's eating window. N = 9 for each of the four weeks. Each participant's average weekly self-reported start/stop times are indicated by differing colors, with each line representing a single participant. The time between "Start Time" and "Stop Time" is indicative of each participant's eating window.

Participant answers to the questions on the Diet Satisfaction Survey revealed specific adherence-related barriers and facilitators within each of the three primary domains (biological, psychological, social) of the biopsychosocial model. Summed scores and percentages are shown in Table 1.

3.1. Biological Factors

Five participants reported easy adjustment to a 16-h fast, agreeing that fasting got easier as the study went on. Seven participants reported that it was not difficult to eat enough calories within the 8-h window. After the first few days of fasting, only one participant reported uncomfortable hunger during the study, but this participant misunderstood the protocol and was only eating one meal a day. Six of the nine participants stated that overeating was not problematic during the eating window and two participants neither agreed nor disagreed. Normal energy levels were retained throughout the intervention, with eight of the nine participants reporting "disagree" when asked if energy levels decreased while fasting. Only one participant indicated that fasting interfered with normal sleep patterns. Participant responses to the five questions within the biological domain of the Diet Satisfaction Survey are displayed in Figure S3.

3.2. Psychological Factors

Subjective mood and quality of life were unaffected in six of the nine participants, and seven participants expressed eagerness to participate in a similar study again. Despite this, participant comprehension of the TRF protocol was lower than expected, with many participants not fully understanding instructions regarding calorie consumption during fasting times. For example, during weekly phone calls, some participants stated they ate snacks in the evening before bed but did not record this in their eating window. Additionally, low-calorie foods were often confused with no-calorie foods, and not recorded even after the interventionist reiterated that any food item with calories must be documented. One participant misunderstood the regimen and only consumed one meal per day throughout the study, which was not revealed until the exit interview. Additionally, five participants thought that TRF was being examined solely for weight loss despite the interventionist explaining that other health outcomes were being evaluated. Due to this misunderstanding, two participants focused on consuming small or low-calorie foods during the eating window rather than eating as normal.

Six of nine participants agreed that they could adhere to the TRF eating pattern for six months, however, this number gradually decreased when asked about the feasibility of maintaining a TRF eating pattern for 12 or 24 months. Six of the participants agreed that fasting became easier over the study period, while two disagreed and one neither agreed nor disagreed. Five of the nine participants stated that they would continue fasting after concluding the study, while two had no preference and two indicated they would not continue. Participant responses to the ten questions within the psychological domain of the Diet Satisfaction Survey are displayed in Figure S4.

3.3. Socio-Environmental Factors

Family support was central to participant adherence. Although not formally enrolled in the trial, the spouses of participants often altered their eating patterns to accompany their partner. Seven participants were able to space out their meals during their chosen eight-hour eating window rather than consuming all daily calories in one sitting, with four participants reporting inconvenience in eating all of their meals during the eating window. Environmental challenges to TRF adherence included social events during which food was served outside the participant's eating window, as well as changes in work schedules that interfered with the timing of meals. Regular doctor appointments for the participant or their spouse requiring long commutes also extended fasting times beyond the 14-18 hour goal for a few individuals. Additionally, several participants reported that they would not want to follow this eating pattern during holidays or vacations. Notwithstanding these challenges, only one participant stated they would not recommend TRF to a friend, and five believed people would follow this eating pattern if recommended by their healthcare provider. Participant responses to the seven questions within the socio-environmental domain of the Diet Satisfaction Survey are displayed in Figure S5.

4. Discussion

The findings of the current trial suggest that TRF is an eating approach that is well tolerated by most older adults. However, six participants did not fully understand the requirements of the fasting regimen, despite being provided with specific instructions and a pictorial guide at a baseline visit. Among these six participants, three reported consuming snacks during fasting periods, two participants confused low-calorie with no-calorie items, and one participant thought they were only allowed to eat one meal a day. Thus, these findings suggest that more instruction and/or participant contact is needed in the early stages of a TRF intervention to promote adherence.

Most participants reported limited physical discomfort caused by this eating pattern. After the first few days of fasting, only one participant reported discomfort related to hunger, and this was likely due to misunderstanding the eating pattern directions. The few reported side effects included transient headaches which dissipated with increased water intake, and dizziness in one participant which subsided with a small snack.

While it is challenging to separately measure biological, psychological, and socio-environmental factors related to eating, energy, and satiety, our findings suggest each domain is relevant to TRF adherence. From a biological perspective, all but one participant perceived they were consuming the same or higher amount of calories as they did prior to beginning the intervention. It is also noteworthy that eight out of nine participants disagreed that fasting decreased energy levels, with greater self-reported activity levels in both yardwork and light exercise. Eight participants indicated on the Diet Satisfaction Survey that the TRF intervention did not negatively affect their sleep, with only one participant reporting that fasting interfered with their normal sleep patterns.

From a psychological perspective, most participants also expressed positive attitudes on the phone calls throughout the study and seven of the nine participants reported feeling eager, motivated and excited to continue with the intervention. Many had heard of IF regimens and wanted to experience this eating pattern. Despite this, participant comprehension of the TRF protocol was lower than anticipated, with six participants not fully understanding instructions regarding avoiding calorie consumption during fasting times. Two participants also had difficulty differentiating foods and beverages with low versus no calories. Additionally, participants were initially inaccurate and inconsistent when reporting their food intake times. To maximize protocol comprehension, it is recommended that future interventions provide even more frequent contact (e.g., bi-weekly) during the initial intervention period to ensure the participant understands the protocol. Similar to calorie restriction interventions, ongoing contact is advisable and can equip participants with adherence promoting behavioral modification techniques and strategies, and continued monitoring for adverse events.

Socio-environmental factors also served as both barriers and facilitators to adherence. Consistent with prior literature [24], participants were often positively influenced by their partners. Many participants reported receiving significant support from spouses, some of whom even changed their eating patterns to be in synchrony with them during the intervention. These reports were highly encouraging, as successful behavior modification requires disrupting the socio-environmental factors that cue habitual behavior [25], and spousal eating times represent an important factor that could cue eating in the participants [26]. On the other hand, a few socio-environmental factors emerged as barriers to adherence. Also consistent with previous studies [27–29], pressures from work, long commutes, vacations, and social engagements represented barriers to adherence to intervention for some participants.

Despite strong evidence indicating that lifestyle intervention programs involving diet, exercise, and behavior modification can reduce risk factors for many chronic diseases and improve physical function, long-term adherence to lifestyle interventions to date is notoriously low [30]. Consequently, the "adherence problem" represents an important challenge to weight loss interventions [30]. Findings from a recent review of 27 studies indicate that participants generally have high levels of adherence (range = 77% to 98%) to different types of fasting regimens, including ADF and TRF [17]. Thus, future trials are needed to evaluate the potential that this eating pattern may have for enhancing long-term weight loss.

There were a few notable strengths of this study. First, participants received personalized attention throughout the intervention, which allowed for discussion of individual challenges and tailored solutions to help participants adopt this new eating pattern. This contact was provided through weekly phone calls to check on their adherence and assist them in problem-solving any challenges they were experiencing following the intervention. Second, adherence was carefully tracked throughout the study, as participants reported the time of their first and last meal in an eating time log each day. The participants then reported their daily start and stop times during weekly phone calls and adjustments were discussed if needed. Third, adverse events were assessed, and potential solutions were offered during the calls. We also conducted exit interviews to obtain each participant's perspective on what challenges and what changes, if any, they would recommend the intervention in future trials.

There were also several limitations to this study, including difficulty in contacting some participants via telephone during the intervention. Additionally, only one coder was used for analysis, and triangulation was not used to cross-check data collection. In future studies, a second coder will be used to verify the coding scheme. As this was a pre–post pilot study of short duration, a small sample size was used, which limits the generalizability of the results as well as our ability to make conclusive statements. Response bias is also a possible limitation of this study, as participants may have only reported what they thought the interventionist wanted to hear in the interviews, or second-guessed what the interventionist was asking and altered their answers. Individual interpretation of the questions asked on the Diet Satisfaction Survey may have also varied. Future studies should utilize larger sample sizes to ensure sufficient power to detect both pre–post differences and between-group differences.

5. Conclusions

Most (6 of 10) participants appreciated the simplicity of the time-restricted eating pattern and reported willingness to continue this eating pattern with slight modification such as decreased daily fasting times or a weekly "unrestricted feeding" day. Comprehension of the fasting regimen and guidelines varied, indicating more participant contact and/or education is needed during the initial stages of the intervention. Additionally, baseline group instruction about the protocol with weekly in-person group sessions may enhance understanding and social support. Motivation to follow the protocol was strongly guided by weight loss, as many participants thought this was the goal of the study. Interventions with older adults should consider these factors to optimally support lifestyle modification and protocol adherence.

Clinical Implications

This study provides exciting preliminary data on the potential beneficial effects and feasibility of TRF in older adults with very few risks associated with the intervention. In addition to the previously reported weight loss outcome and high adherence to the intervention [22], most participants adjusted relatively easily to the fasting window of 14–18 hours. Adverse effects were rare and were quickly remedied. No decrease in energy during the fasting time was reported by eight participants. There was also a carry-over effect, with some family members participating and a high likelihood the participants would recommend this intervention to a friend. While these findings are promising, more work needs to be done before a TRF intervention can be effectively implemented into clinical practice. The primary challenge relates to the participants' initial misunderstanding of what they were and were not allowed to consume during the 14–18 hour fasting period. The addition of dietary monitoring in which participants record their food intake, as well as the start and stop times, may be one approach to enhance adherence levels. This approach has proven essential for most behavioral weight loss programs, so it may be beneficial to helping older adults understand the key distinction between the fasting and non-fasting time periods. Other common adherence barriers expressed by participants included program adherence during social events, changes in work schedule, or vacations.

Nevertheless, there is more opportunity to overcome these barriers due to the flexibility of TRF and the ultimate ability to focus on a yes or no behavior (eating vs. fasting) rather than consciously eating less or counting calories with traditional diets.

Author Contributions: Conceptualization, S.A.L. and S.A.; methodology, S.A.; formal analysis, S.A.L.; original draft preparation, S.A.L.; writing—Review and editing, C.S., C.M., S.A., B.A.B., K.T.S., W.T.D.; visualization, C.S., C.M.; supervision, S.A.; funding acquisition, S.A. All authors have read and agreed to the published version of the manuscript.

Acknowledgments: The authors would like to express their appreciation to the participants and research associates who made it possible to complete this research project. This research was supported by the NIH-funded Claude D. Pepper Older Americans Independence Center (P30AG028740).

References

1. Kontis, V.; Bennett, J.E.; Mathers, C.D.; Li, G.; Foreman, K.; FMedSci, M.Z. Future life expectancy in 35 industrialised countries: Projections with a Bayesian model ensemble. *Lancet* **2017**, *389*, 1323–1335. [CrossRef]
2. Reider, L. *Life Expectancy and Assessment of Functional Status in Older Patients, in Acetabular Fractures in Older Patients*; Springer: Cham, Switzerland, 2020; pp. 5–19.
3. Katz, S.; Branch, L.G.; Branson, M.H.; Papsidero, J.A.; Beck, J.C.; Greer, D.S. Active life expectancy. *N. Engl. J. Med.* **1983**, *309*, 1218–1224. [CrossRef]
4. Crimmins, E.M. Lifespan and healthspan: Past, present, and promise. *Gerontologist* **2015**, *55*, 901–911. [CrossRef] [PubMed]
5. Anton, S.D.; Woods, A.J.; Ashizawa, T.; Barb, D.; Buford, T.W.; Carter, C.S.; Clark, D.J.; Cohen, R.A.; Corbett, D.B.; Cruz-Almeida, Y.; et al. Successful aging: Advancing the science of physical independence in older adults. *Ageing Res. Rev.* **2015**, *24*, 304–327. [CrossRef] [PubMed]
6. Buford, T.W.; Anton, S.D.; Judge, A.R.; Marzetti, E.; Wohlgemuth, S.E.; Carter, C.S.; Leeuwenburgh, C.; Pahor, M.; Manini, T.M. Models of accelerated sarcopenia: Critical pieces for solving the puzzle of age-related muscle atrophy. *Ageing Res. Rev.* **2010**, *9*, 369–383. [CrossRef] [PubMed]
7. Cruz-Jentoft, A.J.; Bahat, G.; Bauer, J.; Boirie, Y.; Bruyère, O.; Cederholm, T.; Cooper, C.; Landi, F.; Rolland, Y.; Sayer, A.A. Sarcopenia: Revised European consensus on definition and diagnosis. *Age Ageing* **2019**, *48*, 601. [CrossRef]
8. Vellas, B.; Fielding, R.A.; Bens, C.; Bernabei, R.; Cawthon, P.M.; Cederholm, T.; Cruz-Jentoft, A.J.; Del Signore, S.; Donahue, S.; Morley, J.; et al. Implications of icd-10 for sarcopenia clinical practice and clinical trials: Report by the international conference on frailty and sarcopenia research task force. *J. Frailty Aging* **2018**, *7*, 2–9.
9. Migliavacca, E.; Tay, S.K.H.; Feige, J.N. Mitochondrial oxidative capacity and NAD(+) biosynthesis are reduced in human sarcopenia across ethnicities. *Nat. Commun.* **2019**, *10*, 5808. [CrossRef]
10. Musci, R.V.; Hamilton, K.L.; Linden, M.A. Exercise-induced mitohormesis for the maintenance of skeletal muscle and healthspan extension. *Sports* **2019**, *7*, 170. [CrossRef]
11. Lettieri Barbato, D.; Tatulli, G.; Aquilano, K.; Ciriolo, M.R. Mitochondrial Hormesis links nutrient restriction to improved metabolism in fat cell. *Aging* **2015**, *7*, 869–881. [CrossRef]
12. Di Francesco, A. A time to fast. *Science* **2018**, *362*, 770–775. [CrossRef] [PubMed]
13. Mattson, M.P.; Allison, D.B.; Fontana, L.; Harvie, M.; Longo, V.D.; Willy, J.; Mosley, M.M.; Notterpek, L.; Ravussin, E.; Scheer, F.A.J.K.; et al. Meal frequency and timing in health and disease. *Proc. Natl. Acad. Sci. USA* **2014**, *111*, 16647–16653. [CrossRef]
14. Anton, S.D.; Moehl, K.; Donahoo, W.T.; Marosi, K.; Lee, S.A.; Mainous, A.G., III; Leeuwenburgh, C.; Mattson, M.P. Flipping the metabolic Switch: Understanding and applying the health benefits of fasting. *Obesity* **2018**, *26*, 254–268. [CrossRef] [PubMed]
15. Longo, V.D.; Mattson, M.P. Fasting: Molecular mechanisms and clinical applications. *Cell Metab.* **2014**, *19*, 181–192. [CrossRef] [PubMed]

16. Klein, S.; Wolfe, R.R. Carbohydrate restriction regulates the adaptive response to fasting. *Am. J. Physiol.* **1992**, *262*, E631–E636. [CrossRef] [PubMed]
17. Welton, S.; Minty, R.; O'Driscoll, T.; Willms, H.; Poirier, D.; Madden, S.; Len, K. Intermittent fasting and weight loss: Systematic review. *Can. Fam. Phys.* **2020**, *66*, 117–125.
18. Moro, T.; Tinsley, G.; Bianco, A.; Marcolin, G.; Pacelli, Q.F.; Battaglia, G.; Palma, A.; Gentil, P.; Neri, M.; Paoli, A. Effects of eight weeks of time-restricted feeding (16/8) on basal metabolism, maximal strength, body composition, inflammation, and cardiovascular risk factors in resistance-trained males. *J. Transl. Med.* **2016**, *14*, 290. [CrossRef]
19. Carlson, O.; Martin, B.; Stote, K.S.; Golden, E.; Maudsley, S.; Najjar, S.N.; Ferrucci, L.; Ingram, D.K.; Longo, D.L.; Rumpler, W.V.; et al. Impact of reduced meal frequency without caloric restriction on glucose regulation in healthy, normal-weight middle-aged men and women. *Metabolism* **2007**, *56*, 1729–1734. [CrossRef]
20. Stote, K.S.; Baer, D.J.; Spears, K.; Paul, D.R.; Harris, G.K.; Rumpler, W.V.; Strycula, P.; Najjar, S.S.; Ferrucci, L.; Ingram, D.K. A controlled trial of reduced meal frequency without caloric restriction in healthy, normal-weight, middle-aged adults. *Am. J. Clin. Nutr.* **2007**, *85*, 981–988. [CrossRef]
21. Tinsley, G.M.; Forsse, J.S.; Butler, N.K.; Paoli, A.; Bane, A.A.; Bounty, P.M.L.; Morgan, G.B.; Grandjean, P.W. Time-restricted feeding in young men performing resistance training: A randomized controlled trial. *Eur. J. Sport Sci.* **2017**, *17*, 200–207. [CrossRef]
22. Anton, S.D.; LEE, S.A.; Donahoo, W.T.; McLaren, C.; Manini, T.; Leeuwenburgh, C.; Pahor, M. The effects of time restricted feeding on overweight, older adults: A pilot study. *Nutrients* **2019**, *11*, 1500. [CrossRef]
23. Anderson, A.R.; Jack, S.L. An introduction to the constant comparative technique. In *Hallbook of Qualitative Research Techniques and Analyses in Entrepreneurships*; Edward Elgar Publishing: Troutham, UK, 2015.
24. Jackson, S.E.; Steptoe, A.; Wardle, J. The influence of partner's behavior on health behavior change: The english longitudinal study of ageing. *JAMA Intern. Med.* **2015**, *175*, 385–392. [CrossRef] [PubMed]
25. Verplanken, B.; Wood, W. Intervention to break and create consumer habits. *J. Public Policy Market.* **2006**, *25*, 90–103. [CrossRef]
26. Marshall, D.W.; Anderson, A.S. Proper meals in transition: Young married couples on the nature of eating together. *Appetite* **2002**, *39*, 193–206. [CrossRef] [PubMed]
27. Burgess, E.; Hassmen, P.; Pumpa, K.L. Determinants of adherence to lifestyle intervention in adults with obesity: A systematic review. *Clin. Obes.* **2017**, *7*, 123–135. [CrossRef] [PubMed]
28. Venditti, E.M.; Wylie-Rosett, J.; Delahanty, L.M.; Mele, L.; Hoskin, M.A.; Edelstein, S.L. Short and long-term lifestyle coaching approaches used to address diverse participant barriers to weight loss and physical activity adherence. *Int. J. Behav. Nutr. Phys. Act.* **2014**, *11*, 16. [CrossRef]
29. Leone, L.A.; Ward, D.S. A mixed methods comparison of perceived benefits and barriers to exercise between obese and nonobese women. *J. Phys. Act. Health* **2013**, *10*, 461–469. [CrossRef]
30. Middleton, K.R.; Anton, S.D.; Perri, M.G. Long-term adherence to health behavior change. *Am. J. Lifestyle Med.* **2013**, *7*, 395–404. [CrossRef]

16

Role of Citrate in Pathophysiology and Medical Management of Bone Diseases

Donatella Granchi [1,*], Nicola Baldini [1,2], Fabio Massimo Ulivieri [3] and Renata Caudarella [4]

[1] Laboratory for Orthopedic Pathophysiology and Regenerative Medicine, IRCCS Istituto Ortopedico Rizzoli, via di Barbiano 1/10, 40136 Bologna, Italy; nicola.baldini@ior.it

[2] Department of Biomedical and Neuromotor Sciences, Via Pupilli 1, University of Bologna, 40136 Bologna, Italy

[3] Nuclear Medicine, Bone Metabolic Unit, IRCCS Ca' Granda Ospedale Maggiore Policlinico, Via F.Sforza 35, 20122 Milano, Italy; ulivieri@gmail.com

[4] Maria Cecilia Hospital, GVM Care and Research, Via Corriera 1, 48033 Cotignola (RA), Italy; renata.caudarella@gmail.com

* Correspondence: donatella.granchi@ior.it

Abstract: Citrate is an intermediate in the "Tricarboxylic Acid Cycle" and is used by all aerobic organisms to produce usable chemical energy. It is a derivative of citric acid, a weak organic acid which can be introduced with diet since it naturally exists in a variety of fruits and vegetables, and can be consumed as a dietary supplement. The close association between this compound and bone was pointed out for the first time by Dickens in 1941, who showed that approximately 90% of the citrate bulk of the human body resides in mineralised tissues. Since then, the number of published articles has increased exponentially, and considerable progress in understanding how citrate is involved in bone metabolism has been made. This review summarises current knowledge regarding the role of citrate in the pathophysiology and medical management of bone disorders.

Keywords: bone metabolism; bone mineral density; bone remodelling; citrate supplement; osteopenia; osteoporosis; kidney diseases

---

1. Introduction

Citrate is an intermediate in the tricarboxylic acid cycle (TCA cycle, Krebs cycle), a central metabolic pathway for all aerobic organisms, including animals, plants, and bacteria [1,2]. In humans, citrate is produced in the mitochondria after the condensation of acetyl coenzyme A (acetylCoA) and oxaloacetate, which are catalysed by citrate synthase; it then enters the TCA cycle, thus becoming the primary adenosine 5′-triphosphate (ATP) provider by which living cells harvest the energy they need to accomplish essential and specific functions [1].

The intracellular citrate level reflects the energy status of the cell and acts as a regulator. When the cellular ATP is abundant and the energy demand of the cells is low, the excess citrate can be exported to the cytosol by means of a mitochondrial citrate carrier [3]. It can be used for the lipid biosynthesis of highly proliferating cells [4] or for supporting the tissue-related functions of specialised cells, including the mineralisation of the extracellular matrix by osteoblasts, the bone-forming cells [5]. In this regard, the close association between citrate and bone was pointed out for the first time by Dickens in 1941 [6]. Since then, the number of published articles dealing with this topic has increased exponentially (Figure 1), and considerable progress in understanding how citrate is involved in bone metabolism has been made. This review summarises the current knowledge regarding the relationship between citrate and bone pathophysiology, starting from the link with bone cells and the mineralised matrix, moving through the role of citrate in the onset of bone disorders, and concluding with a critical evaluation of the clinical use of citrate supplements for the medical management of bone diseases.

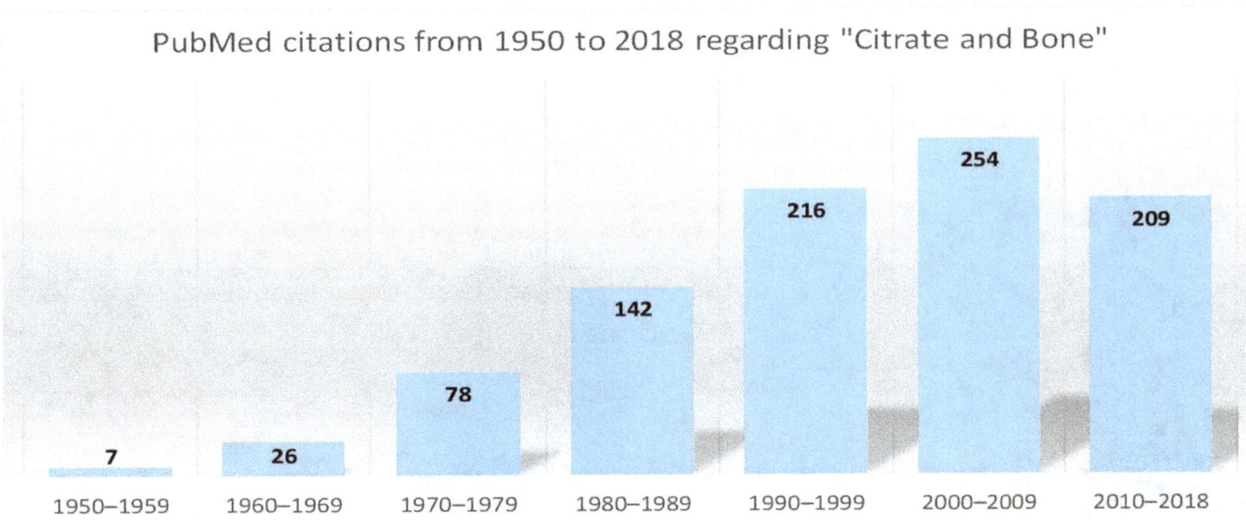

Figure 1. Distribution of the biomedical citations indexed by PubMed over seven decades (n = 949, from 1949 to 2018). The search query focused on "citrate" and "bone", with a search restricted to the terms "Title", "Abstract" or "Medical Subject Headings". Only citations related to studies on humans are included with the exception of those dealing with citrate as an anticoagulant.

2. Citrate Homeostasis: General Physiological Concepts

2.1. The Pillars of Citrate Homeostasis

There is a balance between citrate availability and elimination, depending on physiological requirements. Basically, citrate homeostasis depends on four domains, i.e., nutritional intake, renal clearance, cellular metabolism, and bone remodelling (Figure 2).

Citric acid is naturally contained in fruits and vegetables, particularly in citrus fruits, with concentrations ranging from 0.005 mol/L in oranges and grapefruit to 0.30 mol/L in lemons and limes [7,8]. Food citrate may also be produced biotechnologically by many microorganisms through a fermentation process, and of these, Aspergillum Niger has been recognised as the most efficient producer [9]. Industrial-scale citric acid is employed instead of fresh lemon juice in a variety of pre-prepared meals, and it is also used as an additive in foods and beverages since it acts as a preservative, acidity regulator, flavoring substance and emulsifying agent. In fact, due to the variety of applications, citric acid is the most consumed organic acid in the world, leading to high commercial interest as well as motivating scientists to discover new super-producing techniques [10].

The usual nutritional intake of citrate is approximately 4 grams per day [11] and more than 95% of it is absorbed in the small intestine [12] by means of the sodium-dicarboxylate (NaDC) cotransporter similar to that described in the kidney [13]. The total daily consumption of citric acid may exceed 500 mg/kg of body weight, but considering the low citrate amount in foods, both those in which it is naturally contained and those in which it is added in artificial form, the ingestion of excessive doses is very unlikely [14].

The dietary ingestion of citrate is able to enhance the plasma level within thirty minutes; it is then filtered at the glomerular level just as quickly, and eventually reabsorbed according to physiological needs [15]. In healthy individuals, the serum concentration of circulating citrate is relatively constant, ranging from 19 to 50 mg/L with an average of 20 mg/L [16,17]. Citrate in plasma exists as ≈95% tricarboxylate, ≈4% dicarboxylate, and 1% monocarboxylate, and the majority is complexed to divalent ions, such as calcium and magnesium. The high impermeability of the plasma membrane precludes the cellular uptake of citrate from the extracellular fluid. Under special conditions, some cells (i.e., intestinal enterocytes and kidney tubular cells) express a plasma membrane citrate transporter belonging to the "solute carrier" 13 family (Slc13, NaDC), which is essential for uptake from the gastrointestinal tract and tubular fluid.

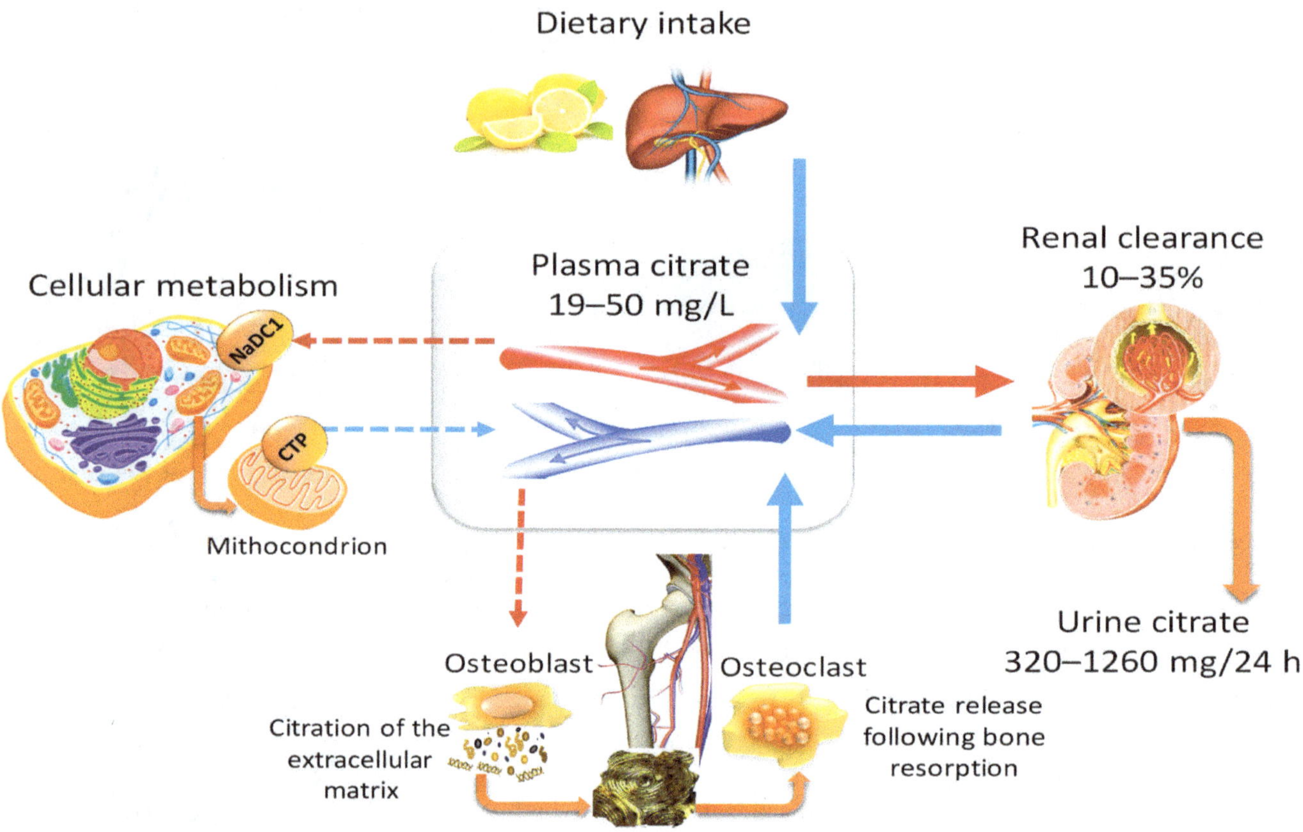

Figure 2. The four domains of citrate homeostasis. The plasma level of citrate mainly depends on four sources, i.e., nutritional intake, renal clearance, cellular metabolism, and bone remodelling. Food citrate is rapidly introduced into the circulation, filtered at the glomerular level, and eventually reabsorbed according to physiological needs. The citrate uptake from the extracellular milieu may occur only when specific transporter proteins are expressed, i.e., sodium-dicarboxylate (NaDC)1 belonging to the "solute carrier" 13 (Slc13) family. The citrate produced by mitochondria only marginally contributes to citrate homeostasis, since it is almost all used by cells as an energy source, or for the synthesis of lipids and other specific functions, i.e., citration of the extracellular matrix by the osteoblasts. In fact, the bulk stored in bone is the main endogenous source of citrate which becomes available following the resorption of the mineralised matrix by the osteoclasts. The mitochondrial citrate-transport protein (CTP) is essential for the release of citrate from the mitochondria to cytosol.

However, the net balance between gastrointestinal absorption and the urinary excretion of citrate suggests that nutritional intake cannot be solely responsible for the maintenance of plasma homeostasis [15,17]. The cellular metabolism also has a scarce impact on citrate availability since almost all the mitochondrial production is consumed by cells as an energy source or for supporting specific cell functions [4,5]. Nowadays, it is well known that the main endogenous bulk of citrate is stored in bone and is mobilised following the resorption of the mineralised matrix by the osteoclasts [17].

2.2. *Citraturia as A Marker of Citrate Homeostasis and Bone Health Status*

As circulating citrate is freely filtered in the glomerulus, 24-h excretion is considered to be a valid marker for highlighting alterations of citrate homeostasis [11]. The reference values for urinary citrate levels range from 320 to 1260 mg/24 h, with an average in males of 550 mg/24 h and in females of 680 mg/24 h [18,19]. The higher excretion of citrate in females is in relation to the estrogenic rate [20] and explains the lower incidence of nephrolithiasis in premenopausal women, considering that citrate-calcium binding is one of the main mechanisms for inhibiting stone formation [21]. Based on the reference values for lithogenic risk, the threshold for the diagnosis of hypocitraturia is usually fixed as less than 320 mg per day. However, hypocitraturia may be severe (citrate excretion of less than 100 mg per day) or mild-moderate (from 100 to 320 mg), but low excretion (less than 640 mg per day) could also be a significant sign and should be monitored [18]. In general, elevated citrate excretion may be considered a non-pathological condition which reflects the restoration of the acid-base balance and occurs, for instance, after chronic alkali intake [22]. Low citrate excretion is a relatively common finding, and even though the majority of patients have idiopathic hypocitraturia, there are several medical and physiological conditions associated with this abnormality. All the conditions listed in Table 1 may be potentially associated with skeletal disorders or, more broadly, with bone metabolism alterations, even when there are no obvious symptoms.

Table 1. Causes of low citrate excretion.

Cause	Annotation
Acid-base status [16,23]	• Acidosis increases citrate utilization by the mitochondria in the tricarboxylic acid cycle (TCA cycle), thus decreasing intra- and extracellular availability. As a consequence, citrate reabsorption is enhanced and urine excretion is reduced. On the contrary, alkalosis increases citrate elimination.
Hypokalemia [16,23]	• Low potassium levels cause intracellular acidosis (see above).
Diet [24,25]	• Low intake of high-citrate content food (fruit/vegetables). • A diet rich in animal proteins contains sulfate and phosphate moieties which are not metabolised and are excreted as acids which decrease urinary pH and citrate excretion. • High sodium intake, ketosis-promoting diet, and starvation.
Distal renal tubular acidosis (dRTA) [26]	• Complete form (hyperchloremic metabolic acidosis, hypokalemia, elevated urine pH). • Incomplete form (normal serum electrolytes, inability to acidify urine following an ammonium chloride load).
Chronic diarrheal syndrome [16,23]	• The fluid loss and intestinal alkali wasting alter the acid-base status, with low urinary pH and citrate retention.
Medications [16,23,27,28]	• Thiazide diuretics induce hypokalemia with resultant intracellular acidosis. • Acetazolamide (carbonic anhydrase inhibitor) produces changes in urine composition which are similar to those found in dRTA. • Angiotensin-converting enzyme inhibitors cause a reduction in urinary citrate by increasing the adenosine triphosphate (ATP) citrate lyase activity. • Topiramate (carbonic anhydrase inhibitor) exerts a dose-dependent effect on the renal excretion of citrate.
Strenuous physical exercise [23]	• It causes lactic acidosis, producing hypocitraturia.
Hyperuricosuria [23]	• With normouricemia, generally caused by dietary excess of purines (animal proteins). • With hyperuricemia (gouty diathesis), the urinary pH is typically low, with increased citrate reabsorption.

Table 1. *Cont.*

Cause	Annotation
Active urinary tract infection [23]	• Bacteria which degrade citrate lower the urinary citrate concentration.
Chronic kidney disease (CKD) [29]	• The decrease in the glomerular filtration rate causes a stepwise reduction in the amount of filtered citrate. Overt hypocitraturia is usually observed in advanced stages of CKD.
Primary hyperaldosteronism [30]	• Hypocitraturia (and hypercalciuria) occurs via Na-dependent volume expansion and chronic hypokalemia.
Menopause [31–34]	• Estrogen deficiency induces metabolic alteration related to the lowering of estrogen-induced signaling onto the mitochondria which promotes glycolysis and glycolytic-coupled TCA cycle function. Hormone replacement therapy restores the citrate level which is decreased in postmenopausal women.
Genetic defects [16]	• All inheritable diseases, gene defects, and polymorphisms associated with the above mentioned conditions (additional details in Table 2).

Modulation of citrate excretion in the kidney is influenced by multiple factors, but pH regulation, particularly in the proximal tubule, has the strongest impact, and even a small decrease in tubular pH significantly increases tubular reabsorption [16]. Therefore, in response to the elevated acid load occurring in metabolic acidosis, there is a notable increase in citrate recovery with subsequent hypocitraturia; urinary citrate excretion may be used as a laboratory parameter for monitoring the diet- and metabolism-dependent systemic acid-base status, even in subjects without overt metabolic acidosis [29,35,36].

The detrimental effect of acid-base imbalance on bone metabolism has been proven without a doubt [36,37], thus suggesting that citraturia could be a noninvasive and indirect view of bone health status. Actually, the relationship among urinary citrate excretion, bone quality parameters, and circulating levels of bone turnover markers has been demonstrated [34,36], even if its clinical usefulness is still controversial [37].

3. Citrate and Bone Tissue

In 1941 Dickens stated that approximately 90% of the total citrate found in the body of "osteovertebrates" resides in mineralised tissues, but the most valuable insight was that, due to its high binding affinity to calcium stored in the hard tissue, citrate could play a pivotal role in regulating metabolic functions and in maintaining the structural integrity of bone [6]. Moreover, Dickens postulated that the presence of citrate in bone is crucial for preventing calcium precipitation, either when bone tissue is resorbed in response to lowered serum calcium or when the biomineralisation process starts. Over time, data in the literature regarding the relationship between citrate and bone physiology have been increasing exponentially (Figure 1), but the role of citrate in driving the structural and functional properties of healthy bone in humans has only been partially elucidated. Early studies were mainly aimed at searching for the origin and the role of calciotropic hormones (calcitonin, parathyroid hormone (PTH), and vitamin D) in the regulation of its metabolism. However, these issues have remained largely unresolved and/or highly speculative, due to the absence of necessary research methodology and technology. Nowadays, there is adequate knowledge regarding the role of bone cells in producing citrate, how citrate enters the crystalline structure of bone, and how it controls the size and morphology of apatite nanocrystals.

3.1. Citrate and Mineral Structure

Citrate is abundant in bone, representing 1–5 weight percent (wt%) of the organic components with a density of approximately 1 molecule per 2 nm^2, which implies that more than 15% of the apatite surface area available in bone is covered by citrate molecules [38]. Before the introduction of modern analytical techniques, the testing methods to evaluate bone tissue composition were entirely limited to classic wet-chemical analyses. At that time, the evidence of a higher amount of the citrate metabolic activity in bone as compared to other tissues, such as kidney or liver, was a significant breakthrough. These findings allowed hypothesising that bone tissue was endowed with the special capacity of producing and storing a high concentration of citric acid, and suggested the role of citrate in regulating the mineralisation process [39]. On the one hand, citrate may influence the amount of mineral deposition by complexing calcium-phosphate (CaP) and favouring its precipitation; on the other hand, if citrate exceeds the amount incorporated in the bone matrix, it could even reverse the mineralisation phase, thus functioning as a solubilising agent which recalls calcium ions. Hu et al. (2010) have proven that citrate is not a dissolved solubilising agent but is firmly bound to apatite as an integral part of the nanocrystal structure. This could be explained by the fact that the elevated amount of citrate in the organic fraction (5.5 wt%) provides more COO- groups than all the noncollagenous proteins in bone, and therefore, the chances of the binding between citrate and calcium of apatite are proportionally increased [40]. Simultaneously, Xie and Nancollas (2010) proposed a three-phase model to explain how citrate may influence the size, longitudinal growth and thickness of apatite nanocrystals [38]. The biomineralisation process initiates with the formation of the amorphous CaP phase starting from an oversaturated CaP solution [41] (Figure 3A). At the early stage, few citrate molecules can bind with the surface of small-size amorphous CaP clusters, but even so, they are sufficient to slow down particle aggregation (Figure 3B). In the next phase, the noncollagenous proteins released from bone cells promote the amorphous CaP cluster clumping, and apatite nucleation starts within these larger amorphous aggregates. Moreover, the presence of collagen fibrils promotes the self-assembly of the small amorphous CaP clusters and guides their direction on the collagen surface [42] (Figure 3C). At the final stage, the surface of mature apatite nanocrystals is fully covered by citrate, so that the increase in thickness is inhibited whilst the growth may continue in a longitudinal direction, thus explaining the plate-like morphology which apatite crystals exhibit in bone [38]. The final apatite structure has a unique geometry since it does not exceed 30–50 nm in length and maintains 2–6 nm thickness [43].

By using a combination of solid-state Nuclear Magnetic Resonance spectroscopy, powder X-ray diffraction, and the principles of electronic structure calculations, Davies et al. (2014) postulated that citrate anions could be incorporated in a hydrated layer of the CaP structure. This binding configuration favours the growth of the mineral crystals in a plate-like morphology and explains their propensity to form stacks [44,45] (Figure 3D). More recently, Delgado-Lopez et al. (2017) focused on the early mineralisation phase, taking into account the interaction between citrate and collagen [46]. By means of an in-depth characterisation based on X-ray scattering and imaging techniques, they found that collagen and citrate work synergically to favour the platy morphology, since both contributed to maintaining the transient amorphous phase. The amorphous CaP clusters are figured as spherulites or globules which gradually occupy the gap zones of the aligned collagen fibrils [43].

The results of the above-mentioned studies confirmed that citrate is an integral part of the apatite-collagen nanocomposite, and the degree of incorporation into bone mineral, as well as the spatial orientation in the mineral structure, play a key role in maintaining the biomechanic properties of bone, i.e., stability, strength, and resistance to fracture. In light of its structural role, citrate has been used to explain the changes in the bone microarchitecture typical of some diseases [47]. In addition, a series of citrate-based materials for orthopaedic applications have been developed to favour the osteoinductive and osteoconductive properties of scaffolds for bone tissue engineering [48,49], as well as to promote bone healing in other surgical procedures [50–52].

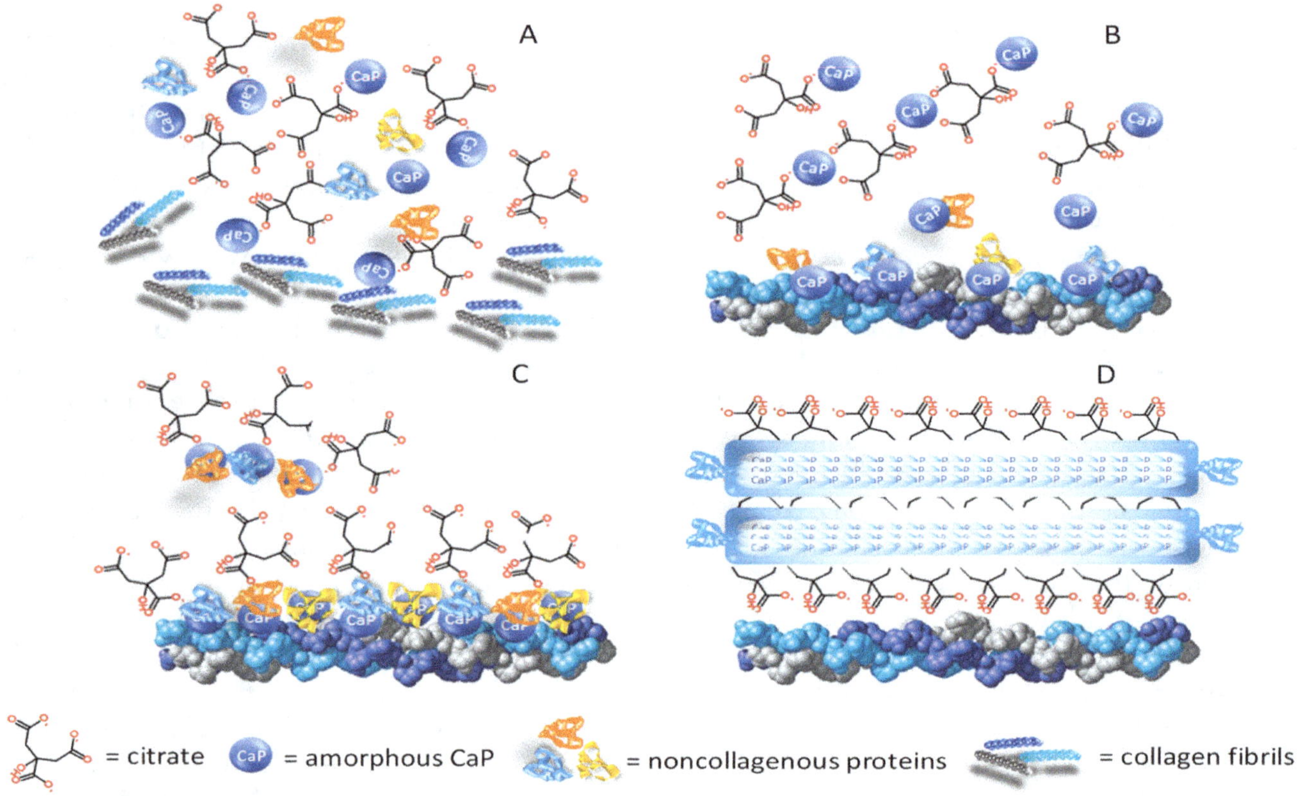

Figure 3. Citrate in the formation of the mineral matrix. The figure combines the theories proposed by different authors regarding the role of citrate in the mineralisation process [38,40,43–45]. (**A**) The amorphous calcium-phosphate (CaP) phase originates from an oversaturated CaP solution, and the mineralisation process starts when the organic phase (citrate, collagen fibrils, and noncollagenous proteins) is available in the bone microenvironment. (**B**) At the early stage, few citrate molecules bind with the amorphous CaP and the particle aggregation is slowed down. (**C**) In the next phase, the noncollagenous proteins released from bone cells favour CaP aggregation and apatite nucleation while the collagen promotes the self-assembly of CaP and guides the aggregate deposition on the collagen surface. (**D**) When the surface is fully covered by citrate, the thickness increase is inhibited (2–6 nm), while longitudinal growth continues up to 30–50 nm, thus explaining the flat morphology of bone mineral platelets. In addition, citrate forms bridges between the mineral platelets which can explain the stacked arrangement which is relevant to the mechanical properties of bone.

3.2. Citrate and Bone Cells

Once the presence of high concentrations of citrate in bone tissue was proven and the role of citrate in the mineralisation process clarified, the main goal of research in this field was to understand what the source of citrate in bone tissue was. Costello et al. (2012) demonstrated that murine osteoblasts were able to secrete citrate [53], thus laying the groundwork for additional studies which elucidated the metabolic process. Basically, the mechanisms were similar to those demonstrated in the prostatic cell, which is the other highly specialised cell capable of releasing high levels of citrate into the extracellular fluid. The elevated level of citrate production is due to the low activity of mitochondrial aconitase. This enzyme activity is suppressed by the zinc (Zn^{2+}) that is accumulated by cells through the solute carrier 39A (SLC39A1), also known as "zinc importer protein 1" (ZIP1) [54–56].

Additional studies have confirmed that human osteoblasts were citrate-producing cells, that ZIP1 expression and intracellular zinc increased during the differentiation of the osteogenic precursors into bone-forming cells, that ZIP1 knockdown prevented the intracellular accumulation of citrate [5], and that ZIP1 expression was promoted by bone morphogenetic protein 2 during the mineralisation process [57]. In addition, the upregulation of the mitochondrial solute carrier 25A (SLC25A1), the citrate transport protein (CTP), was essential for the release of citrate from the mitochondria [56]. In order to define the gene expression patterns underlying the differentiation of mesenchymal stem cells (MSCs) into mature osteoblasts, a large-scale transcriptome analysis starting from the bone-marrow MSCs maintained in osteogenic medium up to deposition of mineral nodules was carried out [58]. While the role of ZIP1 was already described [5,56,59], the microarray analysis showed that solute carrier 13A (SLC39A13), or ZIP13, was upregulated throughout osteogenic differentiation and was also detectable during the mineralisation process [60].

As shown in Figure 4A–E, changes in the citrate metabolism occur during the whole process of differentiation of the MSCs into mature osteoblasts. After the osteogenic commitment of resting MSCs, a highly proliferative phase is expected, and the exportation of citrate into cytosol provides the acetylCoA for the synthesis of the new lipids required for the assembly of the new plasma membranes during cell duplication. Mitochondrial citrate seems to be the preferential source of acetylCoA, since the alternative sources pose some limitations. In fact, extracellular citrate could be used for lipogenesis; however, cellular uptake is subordinated to the expression of the specific transporter, i.e., "sodium-dependent citrate transporter" (NaCT; SLC13A5) [61]. AcetyilCoA could also be obtained from plasma acetate passing through the cell membrane by means of the monocarboxylate transporter (MCT/SLC16A). In order to use this source, the upregulation of acetylCoA synthetase is required, but it is not highly expressed in mammalian cells [56]. Moreover, aconitase inhibition and the lack of mitochondrial citrate affect the energy supply via the Krebs cycle, so that the bioenergetic demand for proliferating/differentiating cells has to be satisfied by alternative sources. For instance, cytosol malate may enter the mitochondrion by CTP in exchange for citrate and may be converted into oxalacetic acid, which in turn may originate new citrate [56].

On the basis of recent studies, citrate released during the bone resorption phase could be considered a matrix-derived signal which contributes to the overall process of bone remodelling within the "basic multicellular unit" [62]. In this regard, Ma et al. have demonstrated that extracellular citrate played a pivotal role regarding the osteogenic differentiation of MSCs [63]. This "metabonegenic" regulation started with citrate uptake through the sodium-citrate transporter SLC13A5 followed by the activation of energy-producing pathways leading to an elevated cell energy status, which in turn fueled the high metabolic demands of MSCs differentiating into osteoblasts. In vitro experiments have shown that the timing and dosage of the citrate supply were critical factors. In fact, the effects were dose-dependent and more evident at the early stages of osteogenic differentiation, with higher proliferation and increased expression of bone-related genes, i.e., alkaline phosphatase and alpha 1 chain of type I collagen [63]. Identical effects have also been observed in a microenvironment hostile to bone cells, for instance using culture conditions which simulated low-grade acidosis [64]. In fact, citrate supplementation opposed the detrimental effects resulting from extracellular acidosis, which inhibited the synthesis of collagen and non-collagen proteins, the activity of alkaline phosphatase, and the formation of mineral nodules [65].

Taken together, studies regarding the role of citrate in the nanocrystal structure and those showing that osteoblasts were the specialised citrate-producing cells in bone have led to a new concept of bone formation related to "citration". Briefly, Costello et al. (2012) stated that . . . ."when considering the mineralisation role of osteoblasts in bone formation, it now becomes evident that 'citration' must be included in the process. Mineralisation without 'citration' will not result in the formation of normal bone, i.e., bone that exhibits its important properties, such as stability, strength, and resistance to fracture" [53].

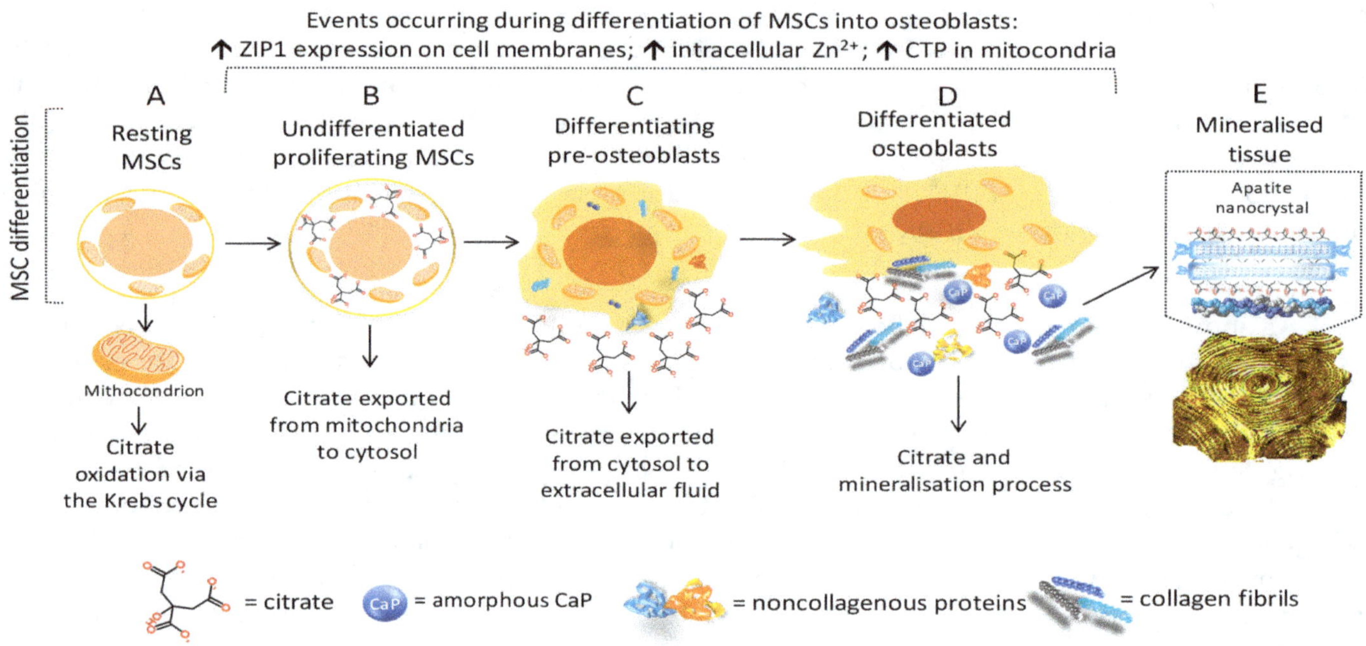

Figure 4. Citrate metabolism, osteoblast differentiation, and mineralisation process. The figure combines the concept of "osteoblast citration" with the main steps of the differentiation of mesenchymal stem cells (MSCs) into bone-forming cells (osteoblasts) [5,53,56]. (**A**) Resting MSCs are quiescent, nonproliferating cells which exhibit the typical mitochondrial metabolism with the oxidation of citrate via the Krebs cycle. (**B**) In the presence of proper stimuli, the undifferentiated MSCs are committed to osteogenic differentiation and, at the early phase, high proliferation is required. To accomplish this goal, the following events are necessary: (1) the upregulation of ZIP1 which promotes the zinc intake, (2) the accumulation of mitochondrial citrate due to the zinc-dependent inhibition of the mitochondrial aconitase, (3) the exportation of citrate into cytosol by means of the "citrate transport protein" (CTP/SLC25A1), (4) the use of cytosol citrate for the lipogenesis process which is essential for cell duplication. (**C**,**D**) The citrate exportation from cytosol to extracellular fluid starts during cell differentiation, and it is simultaneous for the synthesis and the release of amorphous CaP, collagen, and noncollagenous proteins. (**E**) The "osteoblast citration" is completed when the mineralised matrix is assembled. The role of citrate in growing the apatite nanocrystals and driving the mineralisation process is explained in Figure 3.

4. Citrate Pathophysiology and Bone Diseases

The role of citrate in mineralised tissues poses several questions regarding the consequences of a low bioavailability at the systemic level. For the most part, published data linking citrate alteration with bone metabolism refer to renal diseases, acid-base imbalance or also physiological conditions such as menopause, but there are also inheritable genetic defects which affect the TCA cycle in mitochondria or the citrate transport. In the following paragraphs, the medical conditions in which the association between citrate and bone health status has been implied are discussed.

4.1. Bone Health Status and Alterations of Citrate Homeostasis in Kidney Diseases

With the progressive aging of the population, epidemiological studies have shown a higher rate of elderly-related illnesses, including the impairment of bone quality leading to osteoporosis and decreased renal function with chronic kidney disease (CKD), which in turn may influence bone health status [66–68]. The decrease in renal function may be mild, moderate or severe on the basis of estimated-glomerular filtration rate (GFR) equations and is associated with the simultaneous impairment of mineral homeostasis, including serum and tissue concentrations of phosphorus and calcium, circulating levels of calciotropic hormones (PTH, 25-hydroxyvitamin D, 1,25-dihydroxyvitamin

D), fibroblast growth factor-23, and growth hormone. The modifications of mineral homeostasis may promote a loss of bone mass and an increase in bone fragility [69]. As observed by Malmgren et al. (2015), approximately 95% of women over 75 years of age showed a mild-moderate decrease in renal function (CKD stages 2–3) which may have had a harmful effect on bone health [70]. In a 10-year longitudinal study, the authors evaluated the long-term influence of impaired renal function on bone mineral density (BMD) [71]. They analysed 1044 Caucasian women from the "Osteoporosis Prospective Risk Assessment" (OPRA) cohort and found that renal function was positively correlated with femoral neck BMD in elderly women, although the association attenuated as aging progressed. Women with poor renal function had a higher annual rate of bone loss over 5 years compared to those with normal function, and markers of mineral homeostasis were more frequently altered.

High-throughput "omics" approaches, including metabolomics, have been proposed to identify new biomarkers which could help the management of CKD patients, and TCA cycle-metabolites are emerging as potential candidates [72]. A significantly reduced urinary excretion of citrate (–68%) has been observed in non-diabetic patients with CKD as compared to subjects with normal renal function. The renal expression of genes regulating the TCA cycle was decreased in subjects who had impaired renal function, thus suggesting that mitochondrial dysfunction could be involved in the pathogenesis of CKD [73]. Moreover, GFR positively correlated with citrate excretion, and kidney stone formers with CKD had significantly lower urinary citrate excretion than subjects with kidney stone disease and normal renal function [74].

To the authors' knowledge, the link between CKD, urinary citrate and bone health status has still not been elucidated but, taking into account the information emerging from the previous paragraphs, it is reasonable to assume that the link exists. Some indications have derived from the data regarding kidney stone disease, which is the paradigmatic expression of a relationship between citrate alterations, BMD decrease and fracture risk that has been investigated since the 1970s [75]. In fact, several studies have shown that osteoporotic fractures occurred more frequently in patients with kidney stones than in the general population [76–79].

The connection between kidney stones and bone metabolism is related to several factors. Briefly, kidney stones form when urine becomes supersaturated with respect to its specific components. Since 80% of kidney stones are composed of calcium-oxalate (CaOx) or CaP, the regulation of calcium excretion plays a pivotal role in the etiopathogenesis of nephrolithiasis [80]. As urinary citrate is able to bind calcium and prevent the growth and agglomeration of CaOx and CaP crystals, the close relationship between low citrate excretion and kidney stone formation has been fully established [11]. The incidence of hypocitraturia varies from 20% to 60% in people who have a propensity to form stones, either as a single abnormality or in conjunction with other metabolic disorders [16]. Hypercalciuria may occur either when filtered calcium is abnormally increased or when its reabsorption is abnormally decreased. The former may be associated with enhanced bone resorption which raises calcium bioavailability at the systemic level, while the latter may be the consequence of decreased renal function as occurs in CKD. Theoretically, reduced GFR in CKD should lead to decreased urinary calcium concentration, but the consequences of defective tubular reabsorption are more relevant and are responsible for the supersaturation of calcium salts. In addition, in the distal nephron, calcium reabsorption is a PTH-dependent process, PTH being the hormone capable of stimulating the resorption of the bone matrix in response to low, systemic calcium availability [81]. Therefore, as the decrease in the renal function progresses, PTH levels and bone loss gradually increase, thus explaining why kidney stones are a significant predictor of osteoporotic fracture in patients with CKD [82]. Moreover, when nephrolithiasis occurs, patients are frequently advised to reduce calcium intake, thus favouring a negative calcium balance which is an additional risk factor promoting a decrease in BMD [11].

Recent findings have demonstrated that lithogenic risk factors, including hypocitraturia, are also detectable in patients without kidney stones who exhibit osteoporosis or osteopenia, thus leading to the hypothesis that the evaluation of lithogenic risk could have significant implications for monitoring bone health status [34,83].

4.2. Postmenopausal Osteopenia and "Net Citrate Loss"

Estrogen deficiency and aging are the main factors responsible for the depletion of bone mass [84], but they are also associated with changes in urine composition which are similar to those of subjects having an increased risk of kidney stones [11]. The circulating citrate levels and the citrate content in bone are markedly reduced in animals with age-related or ovariectomy-induced bone loss [85]. A low citrate excretion, less severe than true hypocitraturia fixed at less than 320 mg per day, has been described in postmenopausal women [11,33] and in subjects with a low bone mass [34,83]. Nurses' Health Study II considered an ongoing cohort of 108,639 participants from whom information on menopause and kidney stones was obtained. In general, postmenopausal status was associated with lower BMD and a higher incidence of kidney stones in this cohort. Moreover, small but significant differences in urine composition were found in 658 participants who had pre- and postmenopausal 24-h urine analyses, including a lower citrate excretion [86].

The postmenopausal decline in estrogen concentration influences the activation rate of basic multicellular units composed of bone-resorbing osteoclasts and bone-forming osteoblasts. However, according to Drake et al., resorption increased by 90% while formation increased by only 45% [87] and the final result was a "net bone loss". This imbalanced bone remodelling depends on the effects that the lack of estrogen has on bone cells. On the one hand, the activity of the receptor activator of the nuclear factor-κ B ligand (RANKL) is promoted, a key factor in osteoclast differentiation; on the other hand, the osteogenic precursors are destined to differentiate into adipocytes, and the survival of mature osteoblasts is suppressed [88]. The result is the reduction of mature osteoblasts, and since they are the cells capable of synthesising citrate [5], the consequence is lower citrate production which impairs the quality and the stability of the bone microarchitecture [38,40]. Moreover, osteoclast differentiation and bone resorption are energy-demanding processes, and the citrate which is synthesised cannot be accumulated because it is essentially utilised through the citric acid cycle [89,90]. Similarly, the MSC differentiation towards adipocytes requires more citrate as a source of cytosolic acetylCoA for lipid biosynthesis [85]. In conclusion, according to Granchi et al., estrogen deficiency leads to a "net citrate loss" which could explain the diminished citrate excretion observed in postmenopausal women [91].

4.3. Genetic Variations Influencing Citrate Homeostasis and Skeletal Development

The "Online Mendelian Inheritance in Man®" database (OMIM®) is a comprehensive repository of information on the relationship between genetic variation and phenotypic expression [92]. The annotations connecting citrate homeostasis with skeletal defects are listed in Table 2, and many of these concern Slc proteins, which are a family of solute transporters through the membranes.

Mutations of the Cl2/HCO3·2 exchanger AE1, encoded by SLC4A1 which is expressed in red blood cells and in type A intercalated cells of the renal collecting tubule, may be responsible for distal renal tubular acidosis (dRTA), with or without haemolytic anemia. The corresponding phenotype displays defective urine acidification, nephrocalcinosis, nephrolithiasis, hypercalciuria, and hypocitraturia [93]. The clinical phenotype in patients with inherited dRTA is characterised by stunted growth with bone abnormalities in children, as well as nephrocalcinosis and nephrolithiasis which develop as the consequence of hypercalciuria, hypocitraturia, and relatively alkaline urine.

The same cytogenetic location of SLC4A1 (17q21.31) is involved in Glycogen storage disease Ia which is caused by a deficiency in glucose-6-phosphatase activity that catalyses the synthesis of glucose from glucose-6-phosphate. This enzymopathy results in a failure to maintain normal glucose control with glycogen accumulation in the liver, kidney, and intestine. Low citrate excretion and hypercalciuria have been described by Weinstein et al. (2001), and the combination of these metabolic alterations correlated with the onset of nephrocalcinosis and nephrolithiasis [94]. Furthermore, there is increasing evidence that poor metabolic control, including chronic acidosis (lactic), low muscle mass and delayed puberty, may negatively affect BMD in half of the patients [95].

NaCT is the sodium-coupled tricarboxylate transporter predominantly expressed in the liver, at several-fold lower levels in the testis and the brain, and at weak levels in the kidney and the heart.

The association between the mutations of the SLC13a5 gene on chromosome 17p13 and early infantile epileptic encephalopathy-25 with amelogenesis imperfecta has been clearly recognised [96]. More recently, Irizarry et al. have shown that SLC13a5 deficiency led to decreased BMD and impaired bone formation in homozygote (Slc13a5-/-) and heterozygote (Slc13a5+/-) mice [97]. As shown by Diaz et al. (2017), the epigenetic modulation of SLC13a5 gene may also influence skeletal development, since DNA hypermethylation and low gene expression have been found in the placenta and cord blood of infants born small-for-gestational-age and correlated with low height and weight at birth, low BMD, and low mineral content [98].

Bartter syndrome refers to a group of autosomal recessive disorders characterised by impaired salt reabsorption in the thick ascending limb of the loop of Henle with pronounced salt wasting, e.g., potassium and calcium, and hypokalemic metabolic alkalosis [99]. The antenatal variant or Bartter syndrome type I is caused by a homozygous or compound heterozygous mutation in the sodium-potassium-chloride cotransporter-2 gene [100]. The affected infants develop marked hypercalciuria and, as a secondary consequence, nephrocalcinosis and osteopenia [101]. To the best of the authors' knowledge, low citrate excretion in patients affected by Bartter syndrome has not been described, but citrate potassium administration is able to correct biochemical alterations [102,103].

Familial hypomagnesemia with hypercalciuria and nephrocalcinosis is an autosomal-recessive renal tubular disorder caused by mutations in claudin-16 and claudin-19, which are members of the transmembrane family proteins regulating calcium and magnesium reabsorption in the kidney [104]. Thorleifsson et al. have also identified claudin-14 as a major risk gene of hypercalciuric nephrolithiasis associated with a decrease in BMD [105]. Patients can develop hypomagnesaemia, hypercalciuria, and nephrocalcinosis, and their clinical course is often complicated by the progressive loss of kidney function. Other biochemical anomalies consist of elevated serum PTH levels before the onset of CKD, incomplete distal tubular acidosis, hyperuricemia and hypocitraturia [106]. Additional symptoms may be recurrent urinary tract infections, nephrolithiasis, polyuria, polydipsia and/or failure to thrive [106]. Amelogenesis imperfecta has also been described in some patients [107].

The human gene SLC13A2 encodes the sodium-dicarboxylate cotransporter (NaDC1) which is highly expressed in the brush-border membranes of the renal proximal tubule and intestinal cells, and reabsorbs Krebs cycle intermediates, i.e., succinate and citrate [108]. Although to date no distinctive phenotype has been linked with SLC13A2 variation in the OMIM database, Okamoto et al. (2006) have hypothesised that NaDC1 alterations could play a role in the development of kidney stones by affecting the citrate concentration in the urine [109]. The functional properties and protein expression of eight coding region variants of NaDC1 have recently been characterised; the majority of them appeared to decrease transport activity and were predicted to result in decreased citrate absorption in the intestine and kidney [110]. Even if not investigated, it is reasonable to assume that effects on bone mass may occur since these conditions influence citrate metabolism and predispose to renal stone formation as well.

The mitochondrial CTP, coded by the SLC25A1 gene located on chromosome 22q11.21, is embedded in the inner membrane and determines the efflux of tricarboxylic citrate from the mitochondria to cytosol in exchange for dicarboxylic malate [111]. The high citrate concentration into cytoplasm modulates the lipid synthesis and affects glycolysis by inhibiting phosphofructokinase-1 [112]. Genetic variations of SLC25A1 mainly lead to inheritable diseases featured by alterations of the central nervous system (combined D-2- and L-2-hydroxyglutaric aciduria; OMIM ID: 615182) and skeletal muscle (congenital myasthenic syndrome-23; OMIM ID: 618197) while the presence of bone defects is less relevant. However, SLC25A1 impairment also occurs in the 22q11.2 deletion syndrome which is characterised by congenital absence of the thymus and parathyroid glands as well as cardiac, renal and eye anomalies, developmental delay, and also skeletal defects. As additional evidence of a relationship between citrate transport and bone pathophysiology, it has been shown that SLC25A1 knockout in mice causes a notable decrease in the number of osteoblasts and the amount of osteoid [113].

As mentioned above, zinc plays a crucial role in regulating the extracellular bioavailability of citrate in the formation of new mineralised matrix and, therefore, gene defects involving a zinc transporter may be involved in alterations of the citrate metabolism and bone diseases. Of these, the solute carrier 39A family (SLC39A or ZIP) controls the influx of zinc into the cytoplasm [56]. In a previous study, the authors found that SLC39A13 (ZIP13) is upregulated throughout osteogenic differentiation, and no changes were recorded during the mineralisation process [58]. SLC39A13 gene defects have been associated with low bone mass in knockout mice [56] and spondylodysplastic Ehlers-Danlos syndrome, type 3 (Phenotype MIM number 612350).

Table 2. Genes involved in the regulation of citrate homeostasis with a genotype/phenotype relationship regarding skeletal development and/or bone metabolism (retrieved from the OMIM®database, last access 25 May 2019).

Gene/Locus Name	Gene/Locus	Cytogenetic Location	MIM Number: Phenotype	Inheritance
Solute carrier family 4, anion exchanger, member 1 (erythrocyte membrane protein band 3, Diego blood group)	SLC4A1, AE1, EPB3, SPH4, SAO, CHC	17q21.31	179800: Distal renal tubular acidosis	Autosomal dominant
Solute carrier family 4, anion exchanger, member 1 (erythrocyte membrane protein band 3, Diego blood group)	SLC4A1, AE1, EPB3, SPH4, SAO, CHC	17q21.31	611590: Distal renal tubular acidosis	Autosomal recessive
Glucose-6-phosphatase, catalytic	G6PC, G6PT	17q21.31	232200: Glycogen storage disease Ia	Autosomal recessive
Solute carrier family 13 (sodium-dependent citrate transporter), member 5	SLC13A5, NACT, INDY	17p13.1	615905: Early infantile, epileptic encephalopathy, 25	Autosomal recessive
Solute carrier family 12 (sodium/potassium/chloride transporters), member 1	SLC12A1, NKCC2	15q21.1	60167: Bartter syndrome, type 1	Autosomal recessive
Claudin 16 (paracellin 1)	CLDN16, PCLN1, HOMG3	3q28	248250: Renal hypomagnesemia 3	Autosomal recessive

5. Medical Management of Patients with Metabolic Bone Diseases Associated with Citrate Alterations

5.1. Clinical Work-Up

At present, the guidelines dealing with the clinical management of metabolic bone diseases do not highlight the role of citrate in maintaining bone integrity. Nevertheless, based on research findings, the causes of hypocitraturia should be considered in carrying out a complete evaluation of patients who present BMD alterations; vice versa, the accurate monitoring of BMD is advisable in subjects who have reduced urinary citrate excretion.

Regarding laboratory investigations, citrate homeostasis should be evaluated together with all factors which influence mineral metabolism. Although citrate excretion must be measured over a 24-h period and referred to the 24 h-urine volume, the detection of citrate levels in fasting-morning urine (expressed as creatinine ratios) may be an addional element to complete the metabolic profile. Urine pH can be a valid and simple indicator of acid-base balance. Laboratory testings for evaluation of mineral metabolism have to be carried out on plasma and urine by considering renal function, calcium-phosphorus balance, other electrolytes (in particular, potassium and magnesium), and calciotropic hormones. In addition, bone turnover markers (BTMs), including bone-resorption and bone formation indicators, are considered a useful and inexpensive tool for evaluating turnover rate (high or low) and response to any treatment [114].

Quantitative assessment of BMD is mandatory for evaluating bone health status and for calculating fracture risk [115]. Dual-energy X-ray absorptiometry (DXA), the T score (the number of standard deviations above or below the mean for a healthy 30-year-old adult of the same sex and ethnicity), or the Z-score (the number of standard deviations above or below the mean for the patients of the same age, sex and ethnicity) are employed for measuring areal density (g·cm^{-2}) at any skeletal site. The assesment of bone quality may be additionally explored by evaluating the trabecular bone score which reflects bone microarchitecture [116]. "High-resolution peripheral quantitative computed-tomography" allows an accurate assessment of bone strength; however, due to its elevated cost, the diffusion of this technology is still limited.

Even though noninvasive techniques are preferred, bone biopsy remains a valid tool for assessing the tissue quality in metabolic bone diseases, and it is the gold standard for estimating bone impairment in kidney disease and for guiding the clinician in deciding proper treatment [117]. In fact, according to the Kidney Disease Improving Global Outcomes (KDIGO) guidelines, the term renal osteodystrophy may be used exclusively to define the histological alterations in bone morphology associated with CKD, which can be additionally assessed using histomorphometry. Instead, without histological confirmation, the clinical syndrome which develops as a systemic disorder of the mineral and the bone metabolisms is generally called "CKD-Mineral and Bone Disorder" [69,118]. However, bone biopsies in a routine work-up present some drawbacks, which are foremost the availability limited to specialised centres, discomfort for the patients, and the length of time required to process and analyse bone tissue.

Whenever instrumental and laboratory investigations show a significant bone loss, pharmacological treatment has to be planned according to the indications of the current guidelines, eventually adding specific drugs in case of secondary osteoporosis. Moreover, all recommendations related to lifestyle and dietary modifications should be explained to the patient [115]. In the presence of low urine citrate excretion, citrate-based supplements could be recommended to prevent progressive damage to bone and a progressive reduction in BMD.

5.2. *Dietary Modification*

Since hypocitraturia may depend on food habits (Table 1), dietary modifications should be considered as a first level intervention for the medical management of citrate deficiencies. Diet is aimed at correcting the excessive acid load and, as a consequence, the negative effects that acidosis has on bone metabolism [119]. The acid-ash hypothesis emphasises the role of the skeleton in maintaining the acid-base balance since the hydroxyapatite of the mineral matrix is a reservoir of alkali groups which may be released to neutralise proton excess [120]. Acute and chronic acid loading show distinct effects, with acute acidity first eroding the bone surface to release sodium, potassium and bicarbonate into the circulation, while chronic acidity leads to the release of calcium and phosphate [121]. Moreover, acidosis directly influences the activity of bone cells within the bone remodelling unit by promoting osteoclast-mediated resorption and inhibiting bone formation by osteoblasts [65]. Hypocitraturia is a response to the elevated acid load occurring in metabolic acidosis, since there is a notable increase in citrate reabsorption in the renal proximal tubule when the tubular pH decreases [16]. In this regard, there is consensus in considering citraturia as a biomarker for monitoring diet and the metabolism-dependent systemic acid-base status, even in subjects without overt metabolic acidosis [33–35].

Under physiological conditions, the acid-base balance is strictly controlled by net endogenous acid production related to acid and alkali dietary intake, and incomplete metabolism of organic acids. By using proper methods, such as "net endogenous acid production" (NEAP) [122] and "potential renal acid load" (PRAL) [123], it is possible to determine the production of acids and characterise foods according to their ability to release acids and bases into the bloodstream. The prolonged and excessive consumption of acid precursor foods leads to chronic low-grade metabolic acidosis which reduces the excretion of citrate and predisposes to diseases [124], including alteration of bone health status, especially in older subjects with diminished renal function [125]. Some authors have discarded the acid-ash hypothesis, claiming that the increase in the diet acid load did not promote skeletal bone mineral loss or osteoporosis [126], and the main role in regulating acid-base homeostasis should be attributed to the kidney [127]. However, the above studies did not consider the role played by citrate in preserving the mineralised matrix and it would be interesting to know whether the relationship between acid dietary intake and alterations in the bone metabolism varied according to low or normal urine citrate excretion. As supporting evidence for the link between citrate and bone health, previous studies have demonstrated a positive correlation between citrate excretion and radius densitometric values in pre- and postmenopause, as well as a significant relationship between citraturia and the prevalence of vertebral fracture in postmenopausal women [11].

The general dietary approach to counteract elevated acid load is to limit the intake of foods with a high acidifying potential, i.e., meat (beef, pork, poultry), fish and seafood, eggs, beans and oilseeds, in favour of foods which contribute the most to the release of bases, i.e., fruits and vegetables [128]. However, dietary modifications cannot disregard the medical history of the patients, and the best nutritional approach should be evaluated on a case-by-case basis. For instance, in the elderly, inadequate protein intake could be a greater problem for bone health than protein excess [129], and the intake of high amounts of fruits and vegetables could be contraindicated in patients with CKD due to their high potassium content [130].

The intake of foods with a high citrate content may be a valid approach to compensate for the high demand due to acidosis or other causes of hypocitraturia [24,124]. The daily citrate intake is approximately 4 grams, and almost all citrate introduced by exogenous sources is absorbed into the gastrointestinal tract, arrives in the liver and is metabolised to bicarbonate [11].

Prezioso et al. (2015) examined the relationship between a diet rich in vegetables and urinary citrate excretion [24]. Fruits and vegetables (except for those with high oxalate content) favour citrate excretion; consequently, they decrease urinary saturation for CaOx and CaP, thus having a protective effect on the formation of kidney stones [24]. In general, fruit intake is lower in hypocitraturic than in normocitraturic subjects [131].

In order to provide dietary recommendations aimed at correcting hypocitraturia, Haleblian et al. (2008) carried out an exhaustive analysis of citrate concentrations in citrus juices, noncitrus juices, and commercially available beverages. The highest concentration was found in grapefruit juice (35% more than in lemon juice), and a glass corresponded approximately to a 40 mEq tablet of potassium citrate. In general, commercial beverages had lower amounts of citrate [7].

Several authors have studied the possible influence of the consumption of fruit juices (both citrus and noncitrus) on urinary citrate excretion. Orange juice increased the excretion of urinary oxalate, and therefore, its consumption could result in the biochemical modification of stone risk factors [132]. It should also be noted that grapefruit juice significantly increased urinary oxalate levels, but it was not associated with an increased lithogenic risk probably due to the protective effect of the high citrate content [133]. Regarding noncitrus juices, cranberry juice had a controversial effect on urine citrate (no effect or an increase of 31%), but resulted in a significantly increased concentration of urinary calcium and oxalate. In addition, diluted blackcurrant juice and melon had a positive effect in increasing citraturia [24]. In a recent meta-analysis, Pachaly et al. aimed at systematically investigating the effects of dietary measures on urinary citrate and nephrolithiasis [124]. They searched for randomised controlled and crossover studies which evaluated urine citrate excretion after the intake of citrus-based beverages, including fruit juices and soft drinks, calcium/magnesium rich mineral water, a high-fibre diet, a low-animal-protein diet, and plant extracts. The authors identified thirteen studies involving 358 participants, the majority of whom were stone formers. Summarised estimates showed a significant increase in citraturia levels only in subjects who consumed fruit juice and other beverages while the other dietary modifications did not determine significant changes [7,8].

Clinical trials aimed at evaluating whether an increase in dietary citrate preserved the bone health status are lacking. In a clinical trial, postmenopausal women were randomised into four groups, i.e., a diet (additional daily portion of 300 g of self-selected fruit and vegetables), two doses of potassium citrate (12.5 and 55.5 mEq/day) and a placebo (control group). The participants were followed for two years, and the effects on bone turnover were determined by measuring BTMs and BMD. The authors concluded that neither potassium citrate nor fruit and vegetables influenced bone turnover or prevented BMD loss over 2 years in healthy postmenopausal women (Table 3) [134].

In summary, natural sources of dietary citrate should be considered as a first option for preventing kidney stone recurrence as an alternative to medical treatment [24]. From a theoretical point of view, published data have suggested that dietary modifications could also be effective in preserving bone health. However, at present, there is insufficient evidence supporting the use of natural sources of citrate as the sole treatment for preventing bone loss.

5.3. Citrate-Based Supplements

Nephrolithiasis was the first clinical condition in which oral citrate supplementation showed therapeutic efficacy, particularly in lowering high stone recurrence rate which is more prevalent in people with low urinary citrate levels [11]. The rationale for using citrate salts in kidney stone disease was explained in previous paragraphs and was based on four main issues: (1) citrate salts are rapidly absorbed through the intestine and equally rapidly filtered in the urine; (2) citrate forms calcium citrate complexes, which in turn increase solubility and decrease the amount of free calcium in urine; (3) citrate acts as an inhibitor of CaOx and CaP crystal growth and aggregation, and (4) in the intestine, the complexation between calcium and citrate reduces enteric absorption of calcium, and therefore renal excretion. A recent systematic review has demonstrated that citrate-based therapy reduced recurrent calcium urinary stone formation compared to controls (placebo, usual care) [135]; however, evidence was limited in children [136].

There have also been interventional clinical trials concerning the effect of citrate supplements in preserving bone health status. As stated for dietary modifications, the rationale of the published trials was based on the assumption that citrate-based supplements may be useful as alkalising agents which neutralise the effects of an excessive acid load [16,65,119–121]. Other than diets rich in salt and animal protein [128], several conditions may induce low-grade acidosis, and the majority of them are age-related, such as menopause [33], subclinical inflammatory status [137], and decreased renal function [68]. On the basis of this assumption, Lambert et al. (2015) carried out a meta-analysis aimed at determining whether alkaline potassium salts, including potassium citrate and potassium bicarbonate, had some effect on calcium metabolism and bone health [138]. The seven eligible studies dealing with potassium citrate supplementation did not include subjects with nephrolithiasis and/or other relevant comorbidities in order to avoid confounding factors potentially leading to overestimation or underestimation of the intervention. Citrate salts significantly reduced calcium and acid excretion similarly to potassium bicarbonate, but they seemed to be more effective in preventing collagen resorption. However, insufficient data were available regarding changes in BMD, since it was investigated in only two studies. The authors found major differences in terms of study design, inclusion/exclusion criteria, doses, timing of supplement administration and outcome measures; this heterogeneity represented a notable limitation for translation into a clinical setting.

In the current review, the interventional clinical trials which were primarily aimed at evaluating the effect of citrate supplements on mineral metabolism and bone turnover were reviewed. Sixteen eligible studies were identified which (1) recruited more than 10 subjects, (2) excluded nephrolithiasis and other significant comorbidities and (3) reported the results related to bone health status, including BMD and/or BTMs. Data regarding study design, population, intervention, follow-up, additional supplementation or controlled dietary intake, as well as a summary of results and conclusions, are shown in Table 3.

Table 3. Interventional clinical trials based on the use of citrate supplements with primary or secondary outcomes related to bone health status.

Reference	Study Design; Population	Intervention (Dose/Day) (I) Control (C)	Other Supplements (Dose/Day) and/or Controlled Dietary Intake	Follow Up and Outcomes	BTM Changes (Intragroup)	Changes in BTM and BMD Induced by Intervention (Intergroup)	Conclusion
Dawson-Hughes, 1990 [141]	RCT, controlled vs placebo, double-blind; ≥6 months postmenopausal women (early, <5 years: *n* = 67; late, >5 years: *n* = 169); age ≥ 65 years	I 1: Ca citrate malate (500 mg Ca), *n* = 78 I 2: Ca carbonate (500 mg Ca), *n* = 78 C: Placebo (*n* = 80)	Controlled Ca intake	Baseline, 18, 24, 36 months; BTM (BAP) and BMD	I 1: 24 months ↓ BAP I 2: 24 months ↓ BAP C: 24 months ↓ BAP	BTM I 1 vs. C: 36 months ↓ BAP, related to the Ca intake I 2 vs. C: 36 months ↓ BAP, related to the Ca intake BMD I 1 vs. C: 12, 24 months ↑ only in late postmenopause and Ca intake ≤400 mg/day I 2 vs C: ↓ in both groups	Adequate Ca intake is essential in preventing postmenopausal bone loss; Ca citrate is more effective than Ca carbonate.
Dawson-Hughes, 1997 [142]	RCT, controlled vs. placebo, double-blind; healthy subjects living in a community (176 M/ 213 F); age ≥ 65 years	I: Ca citrate malate (500 mg Ca) & Vit D3 (700 IU), *n* = 187 C: Placebo, *n* = 202	Controlled Ca intake	Baseline, 6, 12, 18, 24, 30, 36 months; BTM (OC, u-NTX) and BMD	I: n.s C: n.s.	BTM I vs. C: 36 months ↓ OC BMD I vs. C: 36 months ↑	Ca and vitamin D supplementation leads to a moderate reduction in bone loss and may substantially reduce the risk of nonvertebral fractures among elderly subjects who live in the community.
* Ruml, 1999 [143]	RCT, controlled vs. placebo; postmenopausal women (90% ≤5 years)	I: Ca citrate (800 mg Ca), *n* = 25 C: Placebo, *n* = 31		Baseline, 12, 24 months BTM (BAP, OC, u-NTX, u- OH proline) and BMD	I: all BTMs are ↓, at unspecified time points	BMD I: 24 months, stable	Ca citrate supplementation averted bone loss and stabilised bone density in early postmenopausal women.
Sellmeyer, 2002 [144]	RCT, controlled vs. placebo, double-blind; ≥2 years postmenopausal women; age I: 65 ± 8 years; C: 63 ± 8 years	I: K citrate (90 mmol), *n* = 26 C: Placebo, *n* = 26	Ca carbonate (500 mg); controlled salt intake	Baseline, 1 months; BTM (OC, u-NTX)	I: n.s. C: 1 month ↓ OC, ↑ u-NTX	BTM I vs. C: 1 month, ↓ u-NTX	K citrate prevents increased bone resorption due to high salt intake.
Dawson-Hughes, 2002 [145]	RCT, controlled vs. placebo, double-blind; healthy subjects (161 M/ 181F); normal BMD; age ≥ 65 years	I: Ca citrate malate (500 mg Ca), *n* = 158 C: Placebo, *n* = 184	Vitamin D3 (700 IU); controlled protein intake	Baseline, 18, 36 months; BTM (OC, u-NTX) and BMD	I: 36 months ↓ u-NTX, related to the protein intake; C: n.s.	BTM I vs C: 36 months, ↓ u-NTX BMD I vs C: 36 month, ↑ related to the protein intake	BMD may be improved by increasing protein intake as long as an adequate intake of Ca and vitamin D is assumed.

Table 3. *Cont.*

Reference	Study Design; Population	Intervention (Dose/Day) (I) Control (C)	Other Supplements (Dose/Day) and/or Controlled Dietary Intake	Follow Up and Outcomes	BTM Changes (Intragroup)	Changes in BTM and BMD Induced by Intervention (Intergroup)	Conclusion
Marangella, 2004 [146]	Controlled vs. untreated; postmenopausal women; T score: <−1.0; age: 43–72 years	I: K citrate 37-74 mEq (≈1 mEq/kg), n = 30 C: No treatment, n = 24	Controlled Ca intake	Baseline, 3 months BTM (BAP, OC, u-OH proline, u-DPD)	I: 3 months ↓ OC, u-OH proline, u-DPD; C: 3 months ↑ OC	not shown	K citrate decreases bone resorption thereby contrasting the potential adverse effects caused by chronic acidemia. The implication for the prevention and treatment of postmenopausal osteoporosis has to be confirmed.
Kenny, 2004 [147]	RCT, crossover, open label, 2 phases; 3 months/phase with a washout period of 2 weeks between phases; postmenopausal women; T score: <−1.0 and >−3.5; age: 73 ± 5 years	I 1: Ca citrate (1000 mg Ca), n = 20; I 2: Ca carbonate (1000 mg Ca), n = 20	Vitamin D3 (900 IU); controlled Ca intake	Baseline, 1, 3 months (each phase) BTM (BAP, OC, NTX, u-CTX, u-NTX, u-DPD)	I 1: 3 months ↓ NTX, u-CTX, u-NTX, u-DPD I 2: n.s		Ca citrate inhibits bone resorption more than Ca carbonate.
Sakhae, 2005 [139]	RCT, crossover, placebo controlled, double-blind, 4 phases; 2 weeks/phase with a washout period of 2 weeks between phases; postmenopausal women; age: 48–76 years	I 1: K citrate (40 mEq), n = 18 I 2: Ca citrate (800 mg), n = 18 I 3: K citrate (40 mEq) and Ca citrate (800 mg), n = 18 C (1st phase): Placebo, n = 18	Rigid diet with fixed content of protein, Ca, P, Na, K and fluids	Baseline and at the end of each phase; BTM (BAP, CTX, OC, u-NTX, u-OH proline)	I 1: n.s I 2: ↓ CTX, u-OH proline I 3: I: ↓ CTX, u-OH proline, u NTX	I 3 vs I 1: ↓ u NTX	In postmenopausal women, combined treatment with K citrate and Ca citrate decreases bone resorption by providing an alkali load and increasing absorbed Ca.
Jehle, 2006 [148]	RCT, controlled; ≥5 years postmenopausal women; T score −1/−4; age: ≤70 years	I: K citrate (30 mEq), n = 82 C: KCl (30 mmol), n = 79	Ca carbonate (500 mg), Vitamin D3 (400 IU); free, nonvegetarian diet	Baseline, 3, 6, 9, 12 months; BTM (BAP, CTX, OC, u-DPD, u-PD) and BMD	I: 3 months, ↓ u-DPD, u-PD; 6 months, ↑ BAP and ↓ OC, u-DPD, u-PD; 9 months, ↓ u-DPD, u-PD; 12 months, ↑ BAP and ↓ OC, u-DPD, u-PD; C: 3 months, ↓ OC, u-DPD, u-PD; 6 months, ↑ BAP, u-DPD, u-PD and ↓ OC; 9 months, ↑ u-DPD, u-PD and ↓ OC; 12 months, ↑ BAP, u-DPD, u-PD and ↓ OC	BTM I vs C: 3 months, ↓ u-DPD BMD I vs C: 12 months ↑	In postmenopausal women, bone mass can be increased significantly by K citrate. The effect on bone resorption seems to be unrelated to K intake.

Table 3. *Cont.*

Reference	Study Design; Population	Intervention (Dose/Day) (I) Control (C)	Other Supplements (Dose/Day) and/or Controlled Dietary Intake	Follow Up and Outcomes	BTM Changes (Intragroup)	Changes in BTM and BMD Induced by Intervention (Intergroup)	Conclusion
Macdonald, 2008 [134]	RCT, controlled vs. placebo, double-blind for I1 e I2; ≥5 years postmenopausal women; age: 49–54 years	I 1: K citrate (55.5 mEq), $n = 70$ I 2: K citrate (18.5 mEq), $n = 70$ I 3: Diet (300 g fruit = 18.5 mEq alkali), $n = 66$ C: Placebo, $n = 70$	Food diary (free nonvegetarian diet)	Baseline, 3, 6, 12, 18, 24 months; BTM (CTX, P1NP, u-DPD) and BMD	I 1: n.s. I 2: n.s. I 3: n.s. C: n.s	BTM I 1, I 2, I 3 vs. C: n.s BMD I 1, I 2, I 3 vs. C: n.s	In healthy postmenopausal women, neither K citrate at 18.5 or 55.6 mEq/d, nor 300 g self-selected fruit and vegetables influenced bone turnover or prevented BMD loss over 2 years.
Thomas, 2008 [149]	RCT, crossover, double-blind, 2 phases; postmenopausal women for 2 to 6 years; age: 50–60 years	I 1: Ca carbonate (1000 mg Ca), $n = 12$ I 2: 2) Ca citrate (500 mg Ca), $n = 13$	Controlled Ca intake	Baseline, 7 days; BTM (CTX)	I 1: 7 days, ↓ CTX I 2: 7 days, ↓ CTX		Ca citrate is at least as effective as Ca carbonate in decreasing PTH and CTX cross-links, at half the dose. All changes are numerically superior after Ca citrate supplementation.
Karp, 2009 [140]	RCT, controlled, 24 h study sessions; women of child-bearing age: 22–30 years	I 1: Ca carbonate (1000 mg Ca), $n = 12$ I 2: Ca citrate (Ca: 1000 mg; citrate: 3145 mg), $n = 12$ I 3: K citrate (K: 57 mEq; citrate: 3145 mg), $n = 12$	4-day diary to estimate food habits before starting the study session; the meals served during each study session were identical	Baseline, 2, 4, 6, 8, 20, 24 h; BTM (BAP, u-NTX) and BMD	I 1: 24 h, ↓ u-NTX I 2: n.s I 3: 24 h, ↓ u-NTX		K citrate supplementation decreases urinary Ca excretion and reduces bone resorption even when the diet is not acidogenic, and reduces the bone resorption marker despite low Ca intake.
Jehle, 2013 [150]	RCT, controlled vs. placebo, double-blind; healthy subjects (79 M/122 F); T score > −2.5; age 65–80 years; women were past the perimenopausal peak turnover	I: K citrate (60 mEq), $n = 101$ C: Placebo, $n = 100$	Ca carbonate (500 mg), Vitamin D3 (400 IU); free nonvegetarian diet	Baseline, 6, 12, 18, 24; BTM (BAP, P1NP, u-NTX) and BMD	I: 6, 12 months, ↓ u-NTX; 18, 24 months, ↑ P1NP C: n.s.	BTM I vs. C: 6 months, ↓ u-NTX BMD I vs. C: 12, 18, 24 months ↑	K citrate administered in a background of vitamin D and Ca supplementation is well tolerated and constitutes an inexpensive intervention to improve BMD and bone microarchitecture in healthy elderly people.
Moseley, 2013 [151]	RCT, controlled vs. placebo, double blind; healthy subjects (17 M/35 F); age ≥ 55 years; women were ≥5 years postmenopause	I 1: K citrate (60 mmol), $n = 17$ I 2: K citrate (90 mmol), $n = 17$ C: Placebo, $n = 18$	Ca citrate (630 mg), Vitamin D3 (400 IU); controlled Ca, Na, P, protein, fat intake	Baseline, 6 months; BTM, (BAP, CTX)		BTM I 1, I2 vs. C: 6 months, ↓ CTX	K citrate decreases markers of bone resorption over 6 months, but a significant improvement in Ca balance is obtained with 90 mmol/day. This dose is well tolerated.

Table 3. *Cont.*

Reference	Study Design; Population	Intervention (Dose/Day) (I) Control (C)	Other Supplements (Dose/Day) and/or Controlled Dietary Intake	Follow Up and Outcomes	BTM Changes (Intragroup)	Changes in BTM and BMD Induced by Intervention (Intergroup)	Conclusion
Gregory, 2015 [152]	RCT, controlled vs. placebo, double-blind; ≥2 year postmenopausal women s; T score: <−1.0 > −2.5, or <−2.5 unable to take any other medication; age I: 65.1 ± 5.9 years; C: 66.1 ± 7.1 years	I: K citrate (40 mEq), $n = 42$ C: Placebo, $n = 41$	Ca citrate (630 mg), Vitamin D3 (400 IU); free nonvegetarian diet	Baseline, 1, 3, 6, 12 months; BTM (BAP, OC, P1NP, u-NTX) and BMD	I: 1 month, ↓ P1NP; 3, 6, 12 months, ↓ P1NP, u-NTX C. I: 6 months, ↓ P1NP u-NTX; 12 months, ↓ P1NP	BTM I vs. C: n.s BMD I: 12 months, stable	In postmenopausal osteopenia, K citrate improves the effect of supplementation with Ca citrate and Vitamin D, as proven by the more rapid decrease in BTM levels.
Granchi, 2018 [91]	RCT, controlled vs. placebo, double-blind; ≥5 years postmenopausal women; T score: <−1.0 and >−2.5; age I: 60.8 ± 1.0 years; C: 58.2 ± 1.1 years	I: K citrate (30 mEq), $n = 20$ C: Placebo, $n = 20$	Ca carbonate (500 mg), Vitamin D3 (400 IU); free nonvegetarian diet	Baseline, 3, 6 months; BTM (BAP, CTX, P1NP, TRAcP)	I: 6 months, ↓ BAP, CTX C: 3, 6 months, ↓ BAP, CTX	BTM I vs. C: 6 months ↓ BAP, CTX in subjects with low excretion of K and/or citrate, and/or low urine pH	In postmenopausal osteopenia, K citrate improves the effects of supplementation with Ca carbonate and vitamin D, but only in women with low K and/or citrate excretion and/or low urine pH.

C: control; I: Intervention; RCT: randomised clinical trial; K citrate: potassium citrate; Ca carbonate: calcium carbonate; Ca citrate: calcium citrate; KCl: potassium chloride; Na: sodium; P: phosporus; BMD: bone mineral density; BTM: bone turnover markers; n.a.: not applicable; n.s.: not significant; BAP: bone-specific alkaline phosphatase; BMD: bone mineral density; K: tpotassium; Ca: calcium; u-DPD: urinary deoxypyridinoline; u-PYR: urinary pyridinoline; u-OH proline: urinary hydroxyproline; OC: osteocalcin; P1NP: amino-terminal propeptide of type 1 procollagen; u-NTX: urinary N-telopeptide of collagen type 1; M: male; F: female; IU: International Units; PTH: parathyroid hormone; ↓ and ↑ show significant decreases and increases, respectively, according to the criteria indicated by the authors. * Partial data collected from the abstract.

The authors investigated the effect of potassium citrate (one clinical trial, seven randomised clinical trials (RCTs)) [92,134,139–144], calcium citrate (four RCTs and two crossover studies) [145–150], and two studies compared the above-mentioned treatments (one RCT, one crossover study) [139,140]. Regarding the intervention under investigation, doses, timing of administration, and follow-up varied greatly among the trials and, in thirteen studies, the co-administration of additional supplements was planned, i.e., calcium carbonate and/or vitamin D3. The majority of the studies included postmenopausal women (n = 11) while, in one study, the participants were of childbearing age. The other trials were designed to recruit healthy individuals, i.e., males and females at least 55 years of age. The dietary intake of calcium and/or protein and/or salts was controlled in ten studies; in five studies, the subject consumed a free nonvegetarian diet; in one study, the management of food habits was not described.

Overall, the studies selected provided more than 1000 experimental cases and more than 900 controls. As Lambert et al. reported previously, very high heterogeneity among the studies was observed, and therefore the meta-analysis lost its inferential value while the descriptive overview was more informative. By examining the conclusions reported by various authors, two recurring key points emerged: (1) an adequate calcium intake was essential in preventing bone loss in elderly subjects and in postmenopausal women, and calcium citrate seemed to be more effective than calcium carbonate [145–150] and (2) potassium citrate prevented the increased bone resorption caused by menopause, chronic acidemia and high salt intake [139–144].

Additional findings regarding potassiun citrate can be summarised as follows: effectiveness may be enhanced by combined treatment with calcium citrate [139]; positive effects have also been observed in young women and in the absence of an excessive acid load [140]. Moreover, supplementation with alkalising potassium citrate improved the beneficial effects of calcium and vitamin D only in osteopenic postmenopausal women who exhibited the target conditions, namely low potassium and/or citrate excretion and/or low urine pH [91]. Finally, one study questioned the beneficial effects of potassium citrate since, at 24 months, no significant modifications in BTMs and BMD were recorded [134]. It should be noted that compliance may decrease by 25% over time, mainly due to gastrointestinal side effects (approximately 10%) and costs [24].

Despite the encouraging results, a consensus statement regarding the use of citrate supplementation for the management of metabolic bone diseases is still lacking since the heterogeneity of the current evidence is a major limitation for identifying the best practice. Interestingly, the identification of subjects who better respond to exogenous citrate supplementation could be the correct way to maximise the beneficial effect of the treatment.

6. Conclusions

Since citrate is a ubiquitous metabolite with a multidimensional role in the human organism, it is not surprising that it is involved in the pathophysiology of tissues, organs and systems. In fact, recent data in the literature have highlighted the relationship between citrate defects and various medical conditions with considerable financial and social impact, e.g., cancer [153], dyslipidemia [154], vascular calcifications [155], and visual disabilities [156].

Overall, this review has highlighted the main functions of citrate, and, more specifically, focused on the role of citrate in the pathophysiology and medical management of metabolic bone diseases, thus identifying some key points which are summarised in Table 4.

Although interest in the role of citrate is spreading, a consensus statement regarding the use of citrate supplementation for the management of metabolic bone diseases is still lacking, since the heterogeneity of the current evidence is a major limitation in identifying the best practice. Even when the study design is well planned, there are some reasons which may explain the difficulty in obtaining unique and compelling results from clinical trials.

First, dietary supplementation cannot be regarded as a pharmacological treatment, and therefore the effects on measurable clinical outcomes are expected to be less prominent. Hence, baseline differences between participants which are beyond the investigator's control become selection biases that attenuate the strength of randomisation and interfere with the interpretation of the results. On the other hand, current scientific knowledge provides a sufficient background, leading the clinician and the researcher to further investigate the beneficial effects of citrate-based treatment in depth, as proven by multiple studies which have dealt with this matter.

At present, it can be argued that the use of citrate supplementation should be considered in the medical management of bone diseases, but it is also reasonable to assume that the effects could be maximised in a personalised approach in which the scientific knowledge and the clinical judgement of practitioners are essential in identifying patients who could reap real benefits.

Table 4. The role of citrate in the pathophysiology and medical management of bone diseases.

Highlights
• Citrate is an essential metabolite and plays a pivotal role in maintaining the acid-base balance. • Citrate is an essential component of bone, and serves to maintain the integrity of the skeletal nano- and microstructures.
• Citrate is produced by osteoblasts but, at the same time, it influences their differentiation and functionality. • Bone tissue is the main source of citrate and is therefore a leading actor in maintaining citrate homeostasis. • Citrate excretion is a significant biomarker of citrate homeostasis.
• Genetic and acquired diseases characterised by an alteration in citrate homeostasis are often accompanied by alterations in the development and/or metabolism of bone tissue. • Exogenous supplementation may be a useful tool in treating medical conditions related to poor citrate bioavailability, including bone diseases.

Author Contributions: All the authors (D.G., N.B., F.M.U., and R.C.) participated in the development of the ideas for this review, contributed to reading the articles, and to the writing and editing the manuscript.

Acknowledgments: We acknowledge Gerald Goldsmith for his valuable assistance in revising the English language.

Abbreviations

acetylCoA: Acetyl Coenzyme A; ATP: Adenosine 5′-Triphosphate; BMD: Bone Mineral Density; BTM: Bone Turnover Marker; CaOx: Calcium-Oxalate; CaP: Calcium-Phosphate; CKD: Chronic Kidney Disease; CTP: mitochondrial Citrate Transport Protein; dRTA: distal Renal Tubular Acidosis; DXA: Dual-energy X-ray Absorptiometry; GFR: Glomerular Filtration Rate; KDIGO: Kidney Disease Improving Global Outcomes; MSC: Mesenchymal Stem Cell; NaCT: Sodium-dependent Citrate Transporter; NaDC: Sodium-Dicarboxylate; NEAP: Net Endogenous Acid Production; OMIM: Online Mendelian Inheritance in Man; OPRA: Osteoporosis Prospective Risk Assessment; PRAL: Potential Renal Acid Load; PTH: Parathyroid Hormone; RCT: Randomised Clinical Trial; Slc: Solute Carrier; TCA cycle: Tricarboxylic Acid Cycle or Krebs cycle; ZIP1: Zinc Importer Protein 1.

References

1. Krebs, H.A.; Johnson, W.A. The role of citric acid in intermediate metabolism in animal tissues. *FEBS Lett.* **1980**, *117* (Suppl. 1), K1–K10. [CrossRef]
2. Available online: https://www.genome.jp/kegg-bin/show_pathway?map00020 (accessed on 4 July 2019).
3. Iacobazzi, V.; Infantino, V. Citrate—New functions for an old metabolite. *Biol. Chem.* **2014**, *395*, 387–399. [CrossRef] [PubMed]
4. Mycielska, M.E.; Milenkovic, V.M.; Wetzel, C.H.; Rümmele, P.; Geissler, E.K. Extracellular Citrate in Health and Disease. *Curr. Mol. Med.* **2015**, *15*, 884–891. [CrossRef] [PubMed]
5. Franklin, R.B.; Chellaiah, M.; Zou, J.; Reynolds, M.A.; Costello, L.C. Evidence that Osteoblasts are Specialized Citrate-producing Cells that Provide the Citrate for Incorporation into the Structure of Bone. *Open Bone J.* **2014**, *6*, 1–7. [CrossRef] [PubMed]

6. Dickens, F. The citric acid content of animal tissues, with reference to its occurrence in bone and tumour. *Biochem. J.* **1941**, *35*, 1011–1023. [CrossRef] [PubMed]
7. Haleblian, G.E.; Leitao, V.A.; Pierre, S.A.; Robinson, M.R.; Albala, D.M.; Ribeiro, A.A.; Preminger, G.M. Assessment of citrate concentrations in citrus fruit-based juices and beverages: Implications for management of hypocitraturic nephrolithiasis. *J. Endourol.* **2008**, *22*, 1359–1366. [CrossRef] [PubMed]
8. Penniston, K.L.; Nakada, S.Y.; Holmes, R.P.; Assimos, D.G. Quantitative assessment of citric acid in lemon juice, lime juice, and commercially-available fruit juice products. *J. Endourol.* **2008**, *22*, 567–570. [CrossRef] [PubMed]
9. Schuster, E.; Dunn-Coleman, N.; Frisvad, J.C.; Van Dijck, P.W. On the safety of *Aspergillus niger*—A review. *Appl. Microbiol. Biotechnol.* **2002**, *59*, 426–435. [CrossRef]
10. Hu, W.; Li, W.J.; Yang, H.Q.; Chen, J.H. Current strategies and future prospects for enhancing microbial production of citric acid. *Appl. Microbiol. Biotechnol.* **2019**, *103*, 201–209. [CrossRef]
11. Caudarella, R.; Vescini, F.; Buffa, A.; Stefoni, S. Citrate and mineral metabolism, kidney stones and bone disease. *Front. Biosci.* **2003**, *8*, s1084–s1106.
12. Fegan, J.; Khan, R.; Poindexter, J.; Pak, C.Y. Gastrointestinal citrate absorption in nephrolithiasis. *J. Urol.* **1992**, *147*, 1212–1214. [CrossRef]
13. Pajor, A.M. Sodium-coupled transporters for Krebs cycle intermediates. *Annu. Rev. Physiol.* **1999**, *61*, 663–682. [CrossRef] [PubMed]
14. Poerwono, H.; Higashiyama, K.; Kubo, H.; Poernomo, A.T.; Suharjono, I.; Sudiana, I.K.; Indrayanto, G.; Brittain, H.G. Citric acid. In *Analytical Profiles of Drug Substances and Excipients*, 1st ed.; Brittain, H.G., Ed.; Academic Press: San Diego, CA, USA, 2001; Volume 28, pp. 1–76.
15. Sakhaee, K.; Alpern, R.; Poindexter, J.; Pak, C.Y. Citraturic response to oral citric acid load. *J. Urol.* **1992**, *147*, 975–976. [CrossRef]
16. Zuckerman, J.M.; Assimos, D.G. Hypocitraturia: Pathophysiology and medical management. *Rev. Urol.* **2009**, *11*, 134–144. [CrossRef]
17. Costello, L.C.; Franklin, R.B. Plasma citrate homeostasis, how it is regulated, and its physiological and clinical implications. An important, but neglected, relationship in medicine. *HSOA J. Hum. Endocrinol.* **2016**, *1*, 5. [CrossRef]
18. Pak, C.Y.; Resnick, M. Medical therapy and new approaches to management of urolithiasis. *Urol. Clin. N. Am.* **2000**, *27*, 243–253. [CrossRef]
19. Mayo Clinic Medical Laboratories. Endocrinology Catalog Bone/Minerals. Available online: https//endocrinology.testcatalog.org/show/CITR (accessed on 30 May 2019).
20. Heller, H.J.; Sakhaee, K.; Moe, O.W.; Pak, C.Y. Etiological role of estrogen status in renal stone formation. *J. Urol.* **2002**, *168*, 1923–1927. [CrossRef]
21. Caudarella, R.; Vescini, F. Urinary citrate and renal stone disease: The preventive role of alkali citrate treatment. *Arch. Ital. Urol.* **2009**, *81*, 182–187.
22. Melnick, J.Z.; Preisig, P.A.; Moe, O.W.; Srere, P.; Alpern, R.J. Renal cortical mitochondrial aconitase is regulated in hypo- and hypercitraturia. *Kidney Int.* **1998**, *54*, 160–165. [CrossRef]
23. Lerma, E.V. Hypocitraturia. Updated 5 October 2015. Available online: https://emedicine.medscape.com/article/444968-overview (accessed on 29 July 2019).
24. Prezioso, D.; Strazzullo, P.; Lotti, T.; Bianchi, G.; Borghi, L.; Caione, P.; Carini, M.; Caudarella, R.; Ferraro, M.; Gambaro, G.; et al. Dietary treatment of urinary risk factors for renal stone formation. A review of CLU Working Group. *Arch. Ital. Urol.* **2015**, *87*, 105–120. [CrossRef]
25. Dolan, E.; Sale, C. Protein and bone health across the lifespan. *Proc. Nutr. Soc.* **2019**, *78*, 45–55. [CrossRef] [PubMed]
26. Vallés, P.G.; Batlle, D. Hypokalemic Distal Renal Tubular Acidosis. *Adv. Chronic Kidney Dis.* **2018**, *25*, 303–320. [CrossRef] [PubMed]
27. Melnick, J.Z.; Preisig, P.A.; Haynes, S.; Pak, C.Y.; Sakhaee, K.; Alpern, R.J. Converting enzyme inhibition causes hypocitraturia independent of acidosis or hypokalemia. *Kidney Int.* **1998**, *54*, 1670–1674. [CrossRef]
28. Warner, B.W.; LaGrange, C.A.; Tucker, T.; Bensalem-Owen, M.; Pais, V.M., Jr. Induction of progressive profound hypocitraturia with increasing doses of topiramate. *Urology* **2008**, *72*, 29–32. [CrossRef] [PubMed]

29. Goraya, N.; Simoni, J.; Sager, L.N.; Madias, N.E.; Wesson, D.E. Urine citrate excretion as a marker of acid retention in patients with chronic kidney disease without overt metabolic acidosis. *Kidney Int.* **2019**, *95*, 1190–1196. [CrossRef] [PubMed]
30. Shey, J.; Cameron, M.A.; Sakhaee, K.; Moe, O.W. Recurrent calcium nephrolithiasis associated with primary aldosteronism. *Am. J. Kidney Dis.* **2004**, *44*, e7–e12. [CrossRef]
31. Dey, J.; Creighton, A.; Lindberg, J.S.; Fuselier, H.A.; Kok, D.J.; Cole, F.E.; Hamm, L. Estrogen replacement increased the citrate and calcium excretion rates in postmenopausal women with recurrent urolithiasis. *J. Urol.* **2002**, *167*, 169–171. [CrossRef]
32. Brinton, R.D. The healthy cell bias of estrogen action, mitochondrial bioenergetics and neurological implications. *Trends Neurosci.* **2008**, *31*, 529–537. [CrossRef]
33. Mai, Z.; Li, X.; Jiang, C.; Liu, Y.; Chen, Y.; Wu, W.; Zeng, G. Comparison of metabolic changes for stone risks in 24-hour urine between non- and postmenopausal women. *PLoS ONE* **2019**, *14*, e0208893. [CrossRef]
34. Granchi, D.; Caudarella, R.; Ripamonti, C.; Spinnato, P.; Bazzocchi, A.; Torreggiani, E.; Massa, A.; Baldini, N. Association between markers of bone loss and urinary lithogenic risk factors in osteopenic postmenopausal women. *J. Biol. Regul. Homeost. Agents* **2016**, *30*, S145–S151.
35. Adeva, M.M.; Souto, G. Diet-induced metabolic acidosis. *Clin. Nutr.* **2011**, *30*, 416–421. [CrossRef] [PubMed]
36. Esche, J.; Johner, S.; Shi, L.; Schönau, E.; Remer, T. Urinary Citrate, an Index of Acid-Base Status, Predicts Bone Strength in Youths and Fracture Risk in Adult Females. *J. Clin. Endocrinol. Metab.* **2016**, *101*, 4914–4921. [CrossRef] [PubMed]
37. Shea, M.K.; Dawson-Hughes, B. Association of Urinary Citrate With Acid-Base Status, Bone Resorption, and Calcium Excretion in Older Men and Women. *J. Clin. Endocrinol. Metab.* **2018**, *103*, 452–459. [CrossRef] [PubMed]
38. Xie, B.; Nancollas, G.H. How to control the size and morphology of apatite nanocrystals in bone. *Proc. Natl. Acad. Sci. USA* **2010**, *107*, 22369–22370. [CrossRef]
39. Dixon, T.F.; Perkins, H.R. Citric acid and bone metabolism. *Biochem. J.* **1952**, *52*, 260–265. [CrossRef]
40. Hu, Y.Y.; Rawal, A.; Schmidt-Rohr, K. Strongly bound citrate stabilizes the apatite nanocrystals in bone. *Proc. Natl. Acad. Sci. USA* **2010**, *107*, 22425–22429. [CrossRef]
41. Mahamid, J.; Sharir, A.; Addadi, L.; Weiner, S. Amorphous calcium phosphate is major component of the forming fin bones of zebrafish. Indications for an amorphous precursor phase. *Proc. Natl. Acad. Sci. USA* **2008**, *105*, 12748–12753. [CrossRef]
42. Bradt, J.H.; Mertig, M.; Teresiak, A.; Pompe, W. Biomimetic mineralization of collagen by combined fibril assembly and calcium phosphate formation. *Chem. Mater.* **1999**, *11*, 2694–2701. [CrossRef]
43. Lotsari, A.; Rajasekharan, A.K.; Halvarsson, M.; Andersson, M. Transformation of amorphous calcium phosphate to bone-like apatite. *Nat. Commun.* **2018**, *9*, 4170. [CrossRef]
44. Davies, E.; Müller, K.H.; Wong, W.C.; Pickard, C.J.; Reid, D.G.; Skepper, J.N.; Duer, M.J. Citrate bridges between mineral platelets in bone. *Proc. Natl. Acad. Sci. USA* **2014**, *111*, E1354–E1363. [CrossRef]
45. Costello, L.C.; Chellaiah, M.; Zou, J.; Franklin, R.B.; Reynolds, M.A. The status of citrate in the hydroxyapatite/collagen complex of bone, and Its role in bone formation. *J. Regen. Med. Tissue Eng.* **2014**, *3*, 4. [CrossRef] [PubMed]
46. Delgado-López, J.M.; Bertolotti, F.; Lyngsø, J.; Pedersen, J.S.; Cervellino, A.; Masciocchi, N.; Guagliardi, A. The synergic role of collagen and citrate in stabilizing amorphous calcium phosphate precursors with platy morphology. *Acta Biomater.* **2017**, *49*, 555–562. [CrossRef] [PubMed]
47. Einhorn, T.A.; Boskey, A.L.; Gundberg, C.M.; Vigorita, V.J.; Devlin, V.J.; Beyer, M.M. The mineral and mechanical properties of bone in chronic experimental diabetes. *J. Orthop. Res.* **1988**, *6*, 317–323. [CrossRef] [PubMed]
48. Tran, R.T.; Yang, J.; Ameer, G.A. Citrate-Based Biomaterials and Their Applications in Regenerative Engineering. *Annu. Rev. Mater. Res.* **2015**, *45*, 277–310. [CrossRef]
49. Ma, C.; Gerhard, E.; Lu, D.; Yang, J. Citrate chemistry and biology for biomaterials design. *Biomaterials* **2018**, *178*, 383–400. [CrossRef]
50. Qiu, H.; Yang, J.; Kodali, P.; Koh, J.; Ameer, G.A. A citric acid-based hydroxyapatite composite for orthopedic implants. *Biomaterials* **2006**, *27*, 5845–5854. [CrossRef]
51. Xie, D.; Guo, J.; Mehdizadeh, M.; Tran, R.T.; Chen, R.; Sun, D.; Qian, G.; Jin, D.; Bai, X.; Yang, J. Development of Injectable Citrate-Based Bioadhesive Bone Implants. *J. Mater. Chem. B* **2015**, *3*, 387–398. [CrossRef]

52. Chung, E.J.; Sugimoto, M.J.; Koh, J.L.; Ameer, G.A. A biodegradable tri-component graft for anterior cruciate ligament reconstruction. *J. Tissue Eng. Regen. Med.* **2017**, *11*, 704–712. [CrossRef]
53. Costello, L.C.; Franklin, R.B.; Reynolds, M.A.; Chellaiah, M. The Important Role of Osteoblasts and Citrate Production in Bone Formation: "Osteoblast Citration" as a New Concept for an Old Relationship. *Open Bone J.* **2012**, *4*. [CrossRef]
54. Costello, L.C.; Liu, Y.; Franklin, R.B.; Kennedy, M.C. Zinc inhibition of mitochondrial aconitase and its importance in citrate metabolism of prostate epithelial cells. *J. Biol. Chem.* **1997**, *272*, 28875–28881. [CrossRef]
55. Franklin, R.B.; Ma, J.; Zou, J.; Guan, Z.; Kukoyi, B.I.; Feng, P.; Costello, L.C. Human ZIP1 is a major zinc uptake transporter for the accumulation of zinc in prostate cells. *J. Inorg. Biochem.* **2003**, *96*, 435–442. [CrossRef]
56. Costello, L.C.; Franklin, R.B. A review of the important central role of altered citrate metabolism during the process of stem cell differentiation. *J. Regen. Med. Tissue Eng.* **2013**, *2*, 1. [CrossRef] [PubMed]
57. Costello, L.C.; Chellaiah, M.A.; Zou, J.; Reynolds, M.A.; Franklin, R.B. In vitro BMP2 stimulation of osteoblast citrate production in concert with mineralized bone nodule formation. *J. Regen Med. Tissue Eng.* **2015**, *4*, 2. [CrossRef] [PubMed]
58. Granchi, D.; Ochoa, G.; Leonardi, E.; Devescovi, V.; Baglìo, S.R.; Osaba, L.; Baldini, N.; Ciapetti, G. Gene expression patterns related to osteogenic differentiation of bone marrow-derived mesenchymal stem cells during ex vivo expansion. *Tissue Eng. Part C Methods* **2010**, *16*, 511–524. [CrossRef]
59. Fu, X.; Li, Y.; Huang, T.; Yu, Z.; Ma, K.; Yang, M.; Liu, Q.; Pan, H.; Wang, H.; Wang, J.; et al. Runx2/Osterix and Zinc Uptake Synergize to Orchestrate Osteogenic Differentiation and Citrate Containing Bone Apatite Formation. *Adv. Sci.* **2018**, *5*, 1700755. [CrossRef]
60. Accession Number GSE12267. Available online: https://www.ncbi.nlm.nih.gov/geo (accessed on 4 July 2019).
61. Inoue, K.; Zhuang, L.; Ganapathy, V. Human Na+ -coupled citrate transporter: Primary structure, genomic organization, and transport function. *Biochem. Biophys. Res. Commun.* **2002**, *299*, 465–471. [CrossRef]
62. Sims, N.A.; Martin, T.J. Coupling the activities of bone formation and resorption: A multitude of signals within the basic multicellular unit. *Bonekey Rep.* **2014**, *3*, 481. [CrossRef]
63. Ma, C.; Tian, X.; Kim, J.P.; Xie, D.; Ao, X.; Shan, D.; Lin, Q.; Hudock, M.R.; Bai, X.; Yang, J. Citrate-based materials fuel human stem cells by metabonegenic regulation. *Proc. Natl. Acad. Sci. USA* **2018**, *115*, E11741–E11750. [CrossRef]
64. Granchi, D.; Torreggiani, E.; Massa, A.; Caudarella, R.; Di Pompo, G.; Baldini, N. Potassium citrate prevents increased osteoclastogenesis resulting from acidic conditions: Implication for the treatment of postmenopausal bone loss. *PLoS ONE* **2017**, *12*, e0181230. [CrossRef]
65. Arnett, T.R. Acidosis, hypoxia and bone. *Arch. Biochem. Biophys.* **2010**, *503*, 103–109. [CrossRef]
66. Lindeman, R.D.; Tobin, J.D.; Shock, N.W. Association between blood pressure and the rate of decline in renal function with age. *Kidney Int.* **1984**, *26*, 861–868. [CrossRef] [PubMed]
67. Kanis, J.A.; Johnell, O.; Oden, A.; Sembo, I.; Redlund-Johnell, I.; Dawson, A.; De Laet, C.; Jonsson, B. Long-term risk of osteoporotic fracture in Malmo. *Osteoporos Int.* **2000**, *11*, 669–674. [CrossRef] [PubMed]
68. Jassal, S.K.; von Muhlen, D.; Barrett-Connor, E. Measures of renal function, BMD, bone loss, and osteoporotic fracture in older adults: The Rancho Bernardo study. *J. Bone Min. Res.* **2007**, *22*, 203–210. [CrossRef] [PubMed]
69. Kidney Disease: Improving Global Outcomes (KDIGO) CKD-MBD Update Work Group. KDIGO 2017 Clinical Practice Guideline Update for the Diagnosis, Evaluation, Prevention, and Treatment of Chronic Kidney Disease-Mineral and Bone Disorder (CKD-MBD). *Kidney Int.* **2017**, *7*, 1–59. [CrossRef] [PubMed]
70. Malmgren, L.; McGuigan, F.E.; Berglundh, S.; Westman, K.; Christensson, A.; Akesson, K. Declining estimated glomerular filtration rate and its association with mortality and comorbidity over 10 years in elderly women. *Nephron* **2015**, *130*, 245–255. [CrossRef]
71. Malmgren, L.; McGuigan, F.E.; Christensson, A.; Akesson, K. Reduced kidney function is associated with BMD, bone loss and markers of mineral homeostasis in older women: A 10-year longitudinal study. *Osteoporos. Int.* **2017**, *28*, 3463–3473. [CrossRef]
72. Hocher, B.; Adamski, J. Metabolomics for clinical use and research in chronic kidney disease. *Nat. Rev. Nephrol.* **2017**, *13*, 269–284. [CrossRef]

73. Hallan, S.; Afkarian, M.; Zelnick, L.R.; Kestenbaum, B.; Sharma, S.; Saito, R.; Darshi, M.; Barding, G.; Raftery, D.; Ju, W.; et al. Metabolomics and Gene Expression Analysis Reveal Down-regulation of the Citric Acid (TCA) Cycle in Non-diabetic CKD Patients. *Ebiomedicine* **2017**, *26*, 68–77. [CrossRef]
74. Kang, H.W.; Seo, S.P.; Kim, W.T.; Kim, Y.J.; Yun, S.J.; Lee, S.C.; Kim, W.J. Effect of renal insufficiency on stone recurrence in patients with urolithiasis. *J. Korean Med. Sci.* **2014**, *29*, 1132–1137. [CrossRef]
75. Krieger, N.S.; Bushinsky, D.A. The relation between bone and stone formation. *Calcif. Tissue Int.* **2013**, *93*, 374–381. [CrossRef]
76. Sakhaee, K.; Maalouf, N.M.; Kumar, R.; Pasch, A.; Moe, O.W. Nephrolithiasis-associated bone disease: Pathogenesis and treatment options. *Kidney Int.* **2011**, *79*, 393–403. [CrossRef] [PubMed]
77. Denburg, M.R.; Leonard, M.B.; Haynes, K.; Tuchman, S.; Tasian, G.; Shults, J.; Copelovitch, L. Risk of fracture in urolithiasis: A population-based cohort study using thehealth improvement network. *Clin. J. Am. Soc. Nephrol.* **2014**, *9*, 2133–2140. [CrossRef] [PubMed]
78. Taylor, E.N.; Feskanich, D.; Paik, J.M.; Curhan, G.C. Nephrolithiasis and Risk of Incident Bone Fracture. *J. Urol.* **2016**, *195*, 1482–1486. [CrossRef] [PubMed]
79. Lucato, P.; Trevisan, C.; Stubbs, B.; Zanforlini, B.M.; Solmi, M.; Luchini, C.; Girotti, G.; Pizzato, S.; Manzato, E.; Sergi, G.; et al. Nephrolithiasis, bone mineral density, osteoporosis, and fractures: A systematic review and comparative meta-analysis. *Osteoporos. Int.* **2016**, *27*, 3155–3164. [CrossRef] [PubMed]
80. Khan, S.R.; Pearle, M.S.; Robertson, W.G.; Gambaro, G.; Canales, B.K.; Doizi, S.; Traxer, O.; Tiselius, H.G. Kidney stones. *Nat. Rev. Dis. Primers* **2016**, *2*, 16008. [CrossRef] [PubMed]
81. Muntner, P.; Jones, T.M.; Hyre, A.D.; Melamed, M.L.; Alper, A.; Raggi, P.; Leonard, M.B. Association of serum intact parathyroid hormone with lower estimated glomerular filtration rate. *Clin. J. Am. Soc. Nephrol.* **2009**, *4*, 186–194. [CrossRef] [PubMed]
82. Han, S.G.; Oh, J.; Jeon, H.J.; Park, C.; Cho, J.; Shin, D.H. Kidney Stones and Risk of Osteoporotic Fracture in Chronic Kidney Disease. *Sci. Rep.* **2019**, *9*, 1929. [CrossRef]
83. Arrabal-Polo, M.A.; Girón-Prieto, M.S.; Cano-García Mdel, C.; Poyatos-Andujar, A.; Quesada Charneco, M.; Abad-Menor, F.; Arias-Santiago, S.; Zuluaga-Gomez, A.; Arrabal-Martin, M. Retrospective review of serum and urinary lithogenic risk factors in patients with osteoporosis and osteopenia. *Urology* **2015**, *85*, 782–785. [CrossRef]
84. Khosla, S.; Oursler, M.J.; Monroe, D.G. Estrogen and the skeleton. *Trends Endocrinol. Metab.* **2012**, *23*, 576–581. [CrossRef]
85. Chen, H.; Wang, Y.; Dai, H.; Tian, X.; Cui, Z.K.; Chen, Z.; Hu, L.; Song, Q.; Liu, A.; Zhang, Z.; et al. Bone and plasma citrate is reduced in osteoporosis. *Bone* **2018**, *114*, 189–197. [CrossRef]
86. Prochaska, M.; Taylor, E.N.; Curhan, G. Menopause and Risk of Kidney Stones. *J. Urol.* **2018**, *200*, 823–828. [CrossRef] [PubMed]
87. Drake, M.T.; Clarke, B.L.; Lewiecki, E.M. The Pathophysiology and Treatment of Osteoporosis. *Clin. Ther.* **2015**, *37*, 1837–1850. [CrossRef] [PubMed]
88. Rharass, T.; Lucas, S. Mechanisms in endocrinology: Bone marrow adiposity and bone, a bad romance? *Eur. J. Endocrinol.* **2018**, *179*, R165–R182. [CrossRef] [PubMed]
89. Kim, J.M.; Jeong, D.; Kang, H.K.; Jung, S.Y.; Kang, S.S.; Min, B.M. Osteoclast precursors display dynamic metabolic shifts toward accelerated glucose metabolism at an early stage of RANKL-stimulated osteoclast differentiation. *Cell. Physiol. Biochem.* **2007**, *20*, 935–946. [CrossRef] [PubMed]
90. Lemma, S.; Sboarina, M.; Porporato, P.E.; Zini, N.; Sonveaux, P.; Di Pompo, G.; Baldini, N.; Avnet, S. Energy metabolism in osteoclast formation and activity. *Int. J. Biochem. Cell Biol.* **2016**, *79*, 168–180. [CrossRef] [PubMed]
91. Granchi, D.; Caudarella, R.; Ripamonti, C.; Spinnato, P.; Bazzocchi, A.; Massa, A.; Baldini, N. Potassium Citrate Supplementation Decreases the Biochemical Markers of Bone Loss in a Group of Osteopenic Women: The Results of a Randomized, Double-Blind, Placebo-Controlled Pilot Study. *Nutrients* **2018**, *10*, 1293. [CrossRef]
92. Available online: https://www.omim.org/ (accessed on 4 July 2019).
93. Watanabe, T. Improving outcomes for patients with distal renal tubular acidosis: Recent advances and challenges ahead. *Pediatr. Health Med. Ther.* **2018**, *9*, 181–190. [CrossRef]

94. Weinstein, D.A.; Somers, M.J.; Wolfsdorf, J.I. Decreased urinary citrate excretion in type 1a glycogen storage disease. *J. Pediatr.* **2001**, *138*, 378–382. [CrossRef]
95. Kaiser, N.; Gautschi, M.; Bosanska, L.; Meienberg, F.; Baumgartner, M.R.; Spinas, G.A.; Hochuli, M. Glycemic control and complications in glycogen storage disease type I: Results from the Swiss registry. *Mol. Genet. Metab.* **2019**, *126*, 355–361. [CrossRef]
96. Thevenon, J.; Milh, M.; Feillet, F.; St-Onge, J.; Duffourd, Y.; Jugé, C.; Roubertie, A.; Héron, D.; Mignot, C.; Raffo, E.; et al. Mutations in SLC13A5 cause autosomal-recessive epileptic encephalopathy with seizure onset in the first days of life. *Am. J. Hum. Genet.* **2014**, *95*, 113–120. [CrossRef]
97. Irizarry, A.R.; Yan, G.; Zeng, Q.; Lucchesi, J.; Hamang, M.J.; Ma, Y.L.; Rong, J.X. Defective enamel and bone development in sodium-dependent citrate transporter (NaCT) Slc13a5 deficient mice. *PLoS ONE* **2017**, *12*, e0175465. [CrossRef] [PubMed]
98. Díaz, M.; García, C.; Sebastiani, G.; de Zegher, F.; López-Bermejo, A.; Ibáñez, L. Placental and cord blood methylation of genes involved in energy homeostasis: Association with fetal growth and neonatal body composition. *Diabetes* **2017**, *66*, 779–784. [CrossRef] [PubMed]
99. Cunha, T.D.S.; Heilberg, I.P. Bartter syndrome: Causes, diagnosis, and treatment. *Int. J. Nephrol. Renov. Dis.* **2018**, *11*, 291–301. [CrossRef] [PubMed]
100. Simon, D.B.; Karet, F.E.; Hamdan, J.M.; DiPietro, A.; Sanjad, S.A.; Lifton, R.P. Bartter's syndrome, hypokalaemic alkalosis with hypercalciuria, is caused by mutations in the Na-K-2Cl cotransporter NKCC2. *Nat. Genet.* **1996**, *13*, 183–188. [CrossRef]
101. International Collaborative Study Group for Bartter-like Syndromes. Mutations in the gene encoding the inwardly-rectifying renal potassium channel, ROMK, cause the antenatal variant of Bartter syndrome: Evidence for genetic heterogeneity. *Hum. Molec. Genet.* **1997**, *6*, 17–26.
102. Gross, I.; Siedner-Weintraub, Y.; Simckes, A.; Gillis, D. Antenatal Bartter syndrome presenting as hyperparathyroidism with hypercalcemia and hypercalciuria: A case report and review. *J. Pediatr. Endocrinol. Metab.* **2015**, *28*, 943–946. [CrossRef]
103. Li, D.; Tian, L.; Hou, C.; Kim, C.E.; Hakonarson, H.; Levine, M.A. Association of Mutations in SLC12A1 Encoding the NKCC2 Cotransporter with Neonatal Primary Hyperparathyroidism. *J. Clin. Endocrinol. Metab.* **2016**, *101*, 2196–2200. [CrossRef]
104. Hou, J. Claudins and mineral metabolism. *Curr. Opin. Nephrol. Hypertens.* **2016**, *25*, 308–313. [CrossRef]
105. Thorleifsson, G.; Holm, H.; Edvardsson, V.; Walters, G.B.; Styrkarsdottir, U.; Gudbjartsson, D.F.; Sulem, P.; Halldorsson, B.V.; de Vegt, F.; d'Ancona, F.C.; et al. Sequence variants in the CLDN14 gene associate with kidney stones and bone mineral density. *Nat. Genet.* **2009**, *41*, 926–930. [CrossRef]
106. Claverie-Martin, F. Familial hypomagnesaemia with hypercalciuria and nephrocalcinosis, clinical and molecular characteristics. *Clin. Kidney J.* **2015**, *8*, 656–664. [CrossRef]
107. Bardet, C.; Courson, F.; Wu, Y.; Khaddam, M.; Salmon, B.; Ribes, S.; Thumfart, J.; Yamaguti, P.M.; Rochefort, G.Y.; Figueres, M.L.; et al. Claudin-16 Deficiency Impairs Tight Junction Function in Ameloblasts, Leading to Abnormal Enamel Formation. *J. Bone Min. Res.* **2016**, *31*, 498–513. [CrossRef] [PubMed]
108. Pajor, A.M. Sodium-coupled dicarboxylate and citrate transporters from the SLC13 family. *Pflug. Arch* **2014**, *466*, 119–130. [CrossRef] [PubMed]
109. Okamoto, N.; Aruga, S.; Matsuzaki, S.; Takahashi, S.; Matsushita, K.; Kitamura, T. Associations between renal sodium-citrate cotransporter (hNaDC-1) gene polymorphism and urinary citrate excretion in recurrent renal calcium stone formers and normal controls. *Int. J. Urol.* **2007**, *14*, 344–349. [CrossRef] [PubMed]
110. Pajor, A.M.; Sun, N.N. Single nucleotide polymorphisms in the human Na+-dicarboxylate cotransporter affect transport activity and protein expression. *Am. J. Physiol. Ren. Physiol.* **2010**, *299*, F704–F711. [CrossRef]
111. Catalina-Rodriguez, O.; Kolukula, V.K.; Tomita, Y.; Preet, A.; Palmieri, F.; Wellstein, A.; Byers, S.; Giaccia, A.J.; Glasgow, E.; Albanese, C.; et al. The mitochondrial citrate transporter, CIC, is essential for mitochondrial homeostasis. *Oncotarget* **2012**, *3*, 1220–1235. [CrossRef]
112. Cosso, R.; Falchetti, A. Mitochondriopathies and bone health. *J. Tre. Biol. Res.* **2018**, *1*, 1–7. [CrossRef]
113. Brommage, R.; Liu, J.; Hansen, G.M.; Kirkpatrick, L.L.; Potter, D.G.; Sands, A.T.; Zambrowicz, B.; Powell, D.R.; Vogel, P. High-throughput screening of mouse gene knockouts identifies established and novel skeletal phenotypes. *Bone Res.* **2014**, *2*, 14034. [CrossRef]

114. Lorentzon, M.; Branco, J.; Brandi, M.L.; Bruyère, O.; Chapurlat, R.; Cooper, C.; Cortet, B.; Diez-Perez, A.; Ferrari, S.; Gasparik, A.; et al. Algorithm for the Use of Biochemical Markers of Bone Turnover in the Diagnosis, Assessment and Follow-Up of Treatment for Osteoporosis. *Adv. Ther.* **2019**. [CrossRef]
115. Kanis, J.A.; Cooper, C.; Rizzoli, R.; Reginster, J.Y.; Scientific Advisory Board of the European Society for Clinical and Economic Aspects of Osteoporosis (ESCEO) and the Committees of Scientific Advisors and National Societies of the International Osteoporosis Foundation (IOF). European guidance for the diagnosis and management of osteoporosis in postmenopausal women. *Osteoporos. Int.* **2019**, *30*, 3–44. [CrossRef]
116. Ripamonti, C.; Lisi, L.; Buffa, A.; Gnudi, S.; Caudarella, R. The Trabecular Bone Score Predicts Spine Fragility Fractures in Postmenopausal Caucasian Women Without Osteoporosis Independently of Bone Mineral Density. *Med. Arch.* **2018**, *72*, 46–50. [CrossRef]
117. Damasiewicz, M.J.; Nickolas, T.L. Rethinking Bone Disease in Kidney Disease. *JBMR Plus* **2018**, *2*, 309–322. [CrossRef] [PubMed]
118. Moe, S.; Drüeke, T.; Cunningham, J.; Goodman, W.; Martin, K.; Olgaard, K.; Ott, S.; Sprague, S.; Lameire, N.; Eknoyan, G. Kidney Disease: Improving Global Outcomes (KDIGO). Definition, evaluation, and classification of renal osteodystrophy: A position statement from Kidney Disease: Improving Global Outcomes (KDIGO). *Kidney Int.* **2006**, *69*, 1945–1953. [CrossRef] [PubMed]
119. Jorgetti, V.; Drüeke, T.B.; Ott, S.M. Role of proton receptor OGR1 in bone response to metabolic acidosis? *Kidney Int.* **2016**, *89*, 529–531. [CrossRef] [PubMed]
120. Wachman, A.; Bernstein, D.S. Diet and osteoporosis. *Lancet* **1968**, *1*, 958–959. [CrossRef]
121. Nicoll, R.; McLaren Howard, J. The acid-ash hypothesis revisited: A reassessment of the impact of dietary acidity on bone. *J. Bone Min. Metab.* **2014**, *32*, 469–475. [CrossRef] [PubMed]
122. Frassetto, L.A.; Todd, K.M.; Morris, R.C., Jr.; Sebastian, A. Estimation of net endogenous noncarbonic acidproduction in humans from diet potassium and protein contents. *Am. J. Clin. Nutr.* **1998**, *68*, 576–583. [CrossRef]
123. Remer, T.; Manz, F. Estimation of the renal net acid excretion by adults consuming diets containing variable amounts of protein. *Am. J. Clin. Nutr.* **1994**, *59*, 1356–1361. [CrossRef]
124. Pachaly, M.A.; Baena, C.P.; Buiar, A.C.; de Fraga, F.S.; Carvalho, M. Effects of non-pharmacological interventions on urinary citrate levels: A systematic review and meta-analysis. *Nephrol. Dial. Transpl.* **2016**, *31*, 1203–1211. [CrossRef]
125. Frassetto, L.; Banerjee, T.; Powe, N.; Sebastian, A. Acid Balance, Dietary Acid Load, and Bone Effects-A Controversial Subject. *Nutrients* **2018**, *10*, 517. [CrossRef]
126. Fenton, T.R.; Lyon, A.W.; Eliasziw, M.; Tough, S.C.; Hanley, D.A. Meta-analysis of the effect of the acid-ash hypothesis of osteoporosis on calcium balance. *J. Bone Min. Res.* **2009**, *24*, 1835–1840. [CrossRef]
127. Bonjour, J.P. Nutritional disturbance in acid-base balance and osteoporosis: A hypothesis that disregards the essential homeostatic role of the kidney. *Br. J. Nutr.* **2013**, *110*, 1168–1177. [CrossRef] [PubMed]
128. Carnauba, R.A.; Baptistella, A.B.; Paschoal, V.; Hübscher, G.H. Diet-Induced Low-Grade Metabolic Acidosis and Clinical Outcomes: A Review. *Nutrients* **2017**, *9*, 538. [CrossRef] [PubMed]
129. Hirschfeld, H.P.; Kinsella, R.; Duque, G. Osteosarcopenia: Where bone, muscle, and fat collide. *Osteoporos. Int.* **2017**, *28*, 2781–2790. [CrossRef] [PubMed]
130. Cases, A.; Cigarrán-Guldrís, S.; Mas, S.; Gonzalez-Parra, E. Vegetable-Based Diets for Chronic Kidney Disease? It Is Time to Reconsider. *Nutrients* **2019**, *11*, 1263. [CrossRef] [PubMed]
131. Domrongkitchaiporn, S.; Stitchantrakul, W.; Kochakarn, W. Causes of hypocitraturia in recurrent calcium stone formers: Focusing on urinary potassium excretion. *Am. J. Kidney Dis.* **2006**, *48*, 546–554. [CrossRef]
132. Odvina, C.V. Comparative value of orange juice versus lemonade in reducing stone-forming risk. *Clin. J. Am. Soc. Nephrol.* **2006**, *1*, 1269–1274. [CrossRef]
133. Goldfarb, D.S.; Asplin, J.R. Effect of grapefruit juice on urinary lithogenicity. *J. Urol.* **2001**, *166*, 263–267. [CrossRef]
134. Macdonald, H.M.; Black, A.J.; Aucott, L.; Duthie, G.; Duthie, S.; Sandison, R.; Hardcastle, A.C.; Lanham New, S.A.; Fraser, W.D.; Reid, D.M. Effect of potassium citrate supplementation or increased fruit and vegetable intake on bone metabolism in healthy postmenopausal women: A randomized controlled trial. *Am. J. Clin. Nutr.* **2008**, *88*, 465–474. [CrossRef]

135. Phillips, R.; Hanchanale, V.S.; Myatt, A.; Somani, B.; Nabi, G.; Biyani, C.S. Citrate salts for preventing and treating calcium containing kidney stones in adults. *Cochrane Database Syst. Rev.* **2015**, *10*, CD010057. [CrossRef]
136. Kern, A.; Grimsby, G.; Mayo, H.; Baker, L.A. Medical and dietary interventions for preventing recurrent urinary stones in children. *Cochrane Database Syst. Rev.* **2017**, *11*, CD011252. [CrossRef]
137. Lencel, P.; Magne, D. Inflammaging: The driving force in osteoporosis? *Med. Hypotheses* **2011**, *76*, 317–321. [CrossRef] [PubMed]
138. Lambert, H.; Frassetto, L.; Moore, J.B.; Torgerson, D.; Gannon, R.; Burckhardt, P.; Lanham-New, S. The effect of supplementation with alkaline potassium salts on bone metabolism: A meta-analysis. *Osteoporos. Int.* **2015**, *26*, 1311–1318. [CrossRef] [PubMed]
139. Sakhaee, K.; Maalouf, N.M.; Abrams, S.A.; Pak, C.Y. Effects of potassium alkali and calcium supplementation on bone turnover in postmenopausal women. *J. Clin. Endocrinol. Metab.* **2005**, *90*, 3528–3533. [CrossRef] [PubMed]
140. Karp, H.J.; Ketola, M.E.; Lamberg-Allardt, C.J. Acute effects of calcium carbonate, calcium citrate and potassium citrate on markers of calcium and bone metabolism in young women. *Br. J. Nutr.* **2009**, *102*, 1341–1347. [CrossRef]
141. Dawson-Hughes, B.; Dallal, G.E.; Krall, E.A.; Sadowski, L.; Sahyoun, N.; Tannenbaum, S. A Controlled Trial of the Effect of Calcium Supplementation on Bone Density in Postmenopausal Women. *N. Engl. J. Med.* **1990**, *323*, 878–883. [CrossRef]
142. Dawson-Hughes, B.; Harris, S.S.; Krall, E.A.; Dallal, G.E. Effect of Calcium and Vitamin D Supplementation on Bone Density in Men and Women 65 Years of Age Or Older. *N. Engl. J. Med.* **1997**, *337*, 670–676. [CrossRef]
143. Ruml, L.A.; Sakhaee, K.; Peterson, R.; Adams-Huet, B.; Pak, C.Y. The Effect of Calcium Citrate on Bone Density in the Early and Mid-Postmenopausal Period: A Randomized Placebo-Controlled Study. *Am. J. Ther.* **1999**, *6*, 303–311. [CrossRef]
144. Sellmeyer, D.E.; Schloetter, M.; Sebastian, A. Potassium Citrate Prevents Increased Urine Calcium Excretion and Bone Resorption Induced by a High Sodium Chloride Diet. *J. Clin. Endocrinol. Metab.* **2002**, *87*, 2008–2012. [CrossRef]
145. Dawson-Hughes, B.; Harris, S.S. Calcium Intake Influences the Association of Protein Intake with Rates of Bone Loss in Elderly Men and Women. *Am. J. Clin. Nutr.* **2002**, *75*, 773–779. [CrossRef]
146. Marangella, M.; Di Stefano, M.; Casalis, S.; Berutti, S.; D'Amelio, P.; Isaia, G.C. Effects of potassium citrate supplementation on bone metabolism. *Calcif. Tissue Int.* **2004**, *74*, 330–335. [CrossRef]
147. Kenny, A.M.; Prestwood, K.M.; Biskup, B.; Robbins, B.; Zayas, E.; Kleppinger, A.; Burleson, J.A.; Raisz, L.G. Comparison of the Effects of Calcium Loading with Calcium Citrate Or Calcium Carbonate on Bone Turnover in Postmenopausal Women. *Osteoporos. Int.* **2004**, *15*, 290–294. [CrossRef] [PubMed]
148. Jehle, S.; Zanetti, A.; Muser, J.; Hulter, H.N.; Krapf, R. Partial Neutralization of the Acidogenic Western Diet with Potassium Citrate Increases Bone Mass in Postmenopausal Women with Osteopenia. *J. Am. Soc. Nephrol.* **2006**, *17*, 3213–3222. [CrossRef] [PubMed]
149. Thomas, S.D.; Need, A.G.; Tucker, G.; Slobodian, P.; O'Loughlin, P.D.; Nordin, B.E. Suppression of parathyroid hormone and bone resorption by calcium carbonate and calcium citrate in postmenopausal women. *Calcif. Tissue Int.* **2008**, *83*, 81–84. [CrossRef] [PubMed]
150. Jehle, S.; Hulter, H.N.; Krapf, R. Effect of potassium citrate on bone density, microarchitecture, and fracture risk in healthy older adults without osteoporosis: A randomized controlled trial. *J. Clin. Endocrinol. Metab.* **2013**, *98*, 207–217. [CrossRef] [PubMed]
151. Moseley, K.F.; Weaver, C.M.; Appel, L.; Sebastian, A.; Sellmeyer, D.E. Potassium Citrate Supplementation Results in Sustained Improvement in Calcium Balance in Older Men and Women. *J. Bone Min. Res.* **2013**, *28*, 497–504. [CrossRef] [PubMed]
152. Gregory, N.S.; Kumar, R.; Stein, E.M.; Alexander, E.; Christos, P.; Bockman, R.S.; Rodman, J.S. Potassium Citrate Decreases Bone Resorption in Postmenopausal Women with Osteopenia: A Randomized, Double-Blind Clinical Trial. *Endocr. Pr.* **2015**, *21*, 1380–1386. [CrossRef] [PubMed]
153. Anderson, N.M.; Mucka, P.; Kern, J.G.; Feng, H. The emerging role and targetability of the TCA cycle in cancer metabolism. *Protein Cell* **2018**, *9*, 216–237. [CrossRef]
154. Sathiyakumar, V.; Kapoor, K.; Jones, S.R.; Banach, M.; Martin, S.S.; Toth, P.P. Novel Therapeutic Targets for Managing Dyslipidemia. *Trends Pharm. Sci.* **2018**, *39*, 733–747. [CrossRef] [PubMed]

Permissions

All chapters in this book were first published by MDPI; hereby published with permission under the Creative Commons Attribution License or equivalent. Every chapter published in this book has been scrutinized by our experts. Their significance has been extensively debated. The topics covered herein carry significant findings which will fuel the growth of the discipline. They may even be implemented as practical applications or may be referred to as a beginning point for another development.

The contributors of this book come from diverse backgrounds, making this book a truly international effort. This book will bring forth new frontiers with its revolutionizing research information and detailed analysis of the nascent developments around the world.

We would like to thank all the contributing authors for lending their expertise to make the book truly unique. They have played a crucial role in the development of this book. Without their invaluable contributions this book wouldn't have been possible. They have made vital efforts to compile up to date information on the varied aspects of this subject to make this book a valuable addition to the collection of many professionals and students.

This book was conceptualized with the vision of imparting up-to-date information and advanced data in this field. To ensure the same, a matchless editorial board was set up. Every individual on the board went through rigorous rounds of assessment to prove their worth. After which they invested a large part of their time researching and compiling the most relevant data for our readers.

The editorial board has been involved in producing this book since its inception. They have spent rigorous hours researching and exploring the diverse topics which have resulted in the successful publishing of this book. They have passed on their knowledge of decades through this book. To expedite this challenging task, the publisher supported the team at every step. A small team of assistant editors was also appointed to further simplify the editing procedure and attain best results for the readers.

Apart from the editorial board, the designing team has also invested a significant amount of their time in understanding the subject and creating the most relevant covers. They scrutinized every image to scout for the most suitable representation of the subject and create an appropriate cover for the book.

The publishing team has been an ardent support to the editorial, designing and production team. Their endless efforts to recruit the best for this project, has resulted in the accomplishment of this book. They are a veteran in the field of academics and their pool of knowledge is as vast as their experience in printing. Their expertise and guidance has proved useful at every step. Their uncompromising quality standards have made this book an exceptional effort. Their encouragement from time to time has been an inspiration for everyone.

The publisher and the editorial board hope that this book will prove to be a valuable piece of knowledge for researchers, students, practitioners and scholars across the globe.

List of Contributors

Melanie Mülek and Petra Högger
Institut für Pharmazie und Lebensmittelchemie, Universität Würzburg, 97074 Würzburg, Germany

Lothar Seefried and Franca Genest
Department of Orthopedics, Orthopedic Center for Musculoskeletal Research, 97074 Würzburg, Germany

Anna Picca, Riccardo Calvani, Jacopo Gervasoni, Aniello Primiano, Antonio Gasbarrini, Francesco Landi, Roberto Bernabei and Emanuele Marzetti
Institute of Internal Medicine and Geriatrics, Università Cattolica del Sacro Cuore, 00168 Rome, Italy
Fondazione Policlinico Universitario "Agostino Gemelli" IRCCS, 00168 Rome, Italy

Francesca Romana Ponziani
Fondazione Policlinico Universitario "Agostino Gemelli" IRCCS, 00168 Rome, Italy

Federico Marini
Department of Chemistry, Sapienza Università di Roma, 00185 Rome, Italy

Alessandra Biancolillo
Department of Chemistry, Sapienza Università di Roma, 00185 Rome, Italy
Department of Physical and Chemical Sciences, Università degli Studi dell'Aquila, 67100 L'Aquila, Italy

Hélio José Coelho-Júnior
Applied Kinesiology Laboratory–LCA, School of Physical Education, University of Campinas, 13.083-851 Campinas-SP, Brazil

Lorenza Putignani
Unit of Parasitology and Unit of Human Microbiome, Bambino Gesù Children's Hospital IRCCS, 00168 Rome, Italy

Federica Del Chierico and Sofia Reddel
Unit of Human Microbiome, Bambino Gesù Children's Hospital IRCCS, 00168 Rome, Italy

Claudia Romano and Giovanni Corsetti
Division of Human Anatomy and Physiopathology, Department of Clinical and Experimental Sciences, University of Brescia, 25124 Brescia, Italy

Vincenzo Flati
Department of Biotechnological and Applied Clinical Sciences, University of L'Aquila, 67100 L'Aquila, Italy

Evasio Pasini
Istituti Clinici Scientifici Maugeri - IRCCS Lumezzane - Cardiac Rehabilitation Division, 25065 Lumezzane (Brescia), Italy

Emanuele Marzetti
Fondazione Policlinico Universitario "Agostino Gemelli" IRCCS, 00168 Rome, Italy

Anna Picca and Riccardo Calvani
Fondazione Policlinico Universitario "Agostino Gemelli" IRCCS, 00168 Rome, Italy
Institute of Internal Medicine and Geriatrics, Università Cattolica del Sacro Cuore, 00168 Rome, Italy

Francesco Saverio Dioguardi
Department of Internal Medicine, University of Cagliari, 09042 Monserrato (Cagliari), Italy

Soo Im Chung and Mi Young Kang
Department of Food Science and Nutrition, Brain Korea 21 Plus, Kyungpook National University, Daegu 41566, Korea

Su Noh Ryu
Department of Agricultural Science, Korea National Open University, Seoul 03087, Korea

Bahram H. Arjmandi, Shirin Pourafshar, Kelli S. George and Neda S. Akhavan
Department of Nutrition, Food and Exercise Sciences, College of Human Sciences, Florida State University, Tallahassee, FL 32306, USA
Center for Advancing Exercise and Nutrition Research on Aging (CAENRA), College of Human Sciences, Florida State University, Tallahassee, FL 32306, USA

Sarah A. Johnson
Department of Food Science and Human Nutrition, College of Health and Human Sciences, Colorado State University, Fort Collins, CO 80523, USA

Negin Navaei
Department of Nutrition, Food and Exercise Sciences, College of Human Sciences, Florida State University, Tallahassee, FL 32306, USA
Center for Advancing Exercise and Nutrition Research on Aging (CAENRA), College of Human Sciences, Florida State University, Tallahassee, FL 32306, USA
Department of Nutrition, College of Graduate and Undergraduate Studies, Life University, Marietta, GA 30060, USA

Shirin Hooshmand
School of Exercise and Nutritional Sciences, College of Health & Human Services, San Diego State University, San Diego, CA 92182, USA

Sheau C. Chai
Department of Behavioral Health and Nutrition, College of Health Sciences, University of Delaware, Newark, DE 19716, USA

Melissa M. Melough, Xin Sun and Ock K. Chun
Department of Nutritional Sciences, University of Connecticut, Storrs, CT 06269, USA

Riccardo Calvani, Anna Picca, Jacopo Gervasoni, Aniello Primiano, Roberto Bernabei, Emanuele Marzetti and Giovanni Gambassi
Università Cattolica del Sacro Cuore, 00168 Rome, Italy
Fondazione Policlinico Universitario "Agostino Gemelli" IRCCS, 00168 Rome, Italy

Leocadio Rodriguez-Mañas
Servicio de Geriatría, Hospital Universitario de Getafe, 28905 Madrid, Spain

Federico Marini and Giorgia Conta
Department of Chemistry, Sapienza Università di Roma, 00185 Rome, Italy

Olga Laosa and Laura Pedraza
Foundation for Biomedical Research, Hospital Universitario de Getafe, 28905 Madrid, Spain

Isabelle Bourdel-Marchasson and Sophie C. Regueme
Centre Hospitalier Universitaire de Bordeaux, 33000 Bordeaux, France

Alan J. Sinclair
Foundation for Diabetes Research in Older People, Diabetes Frail Ltd., Luton LU1 3UA, UK

Yoshitaka Ohno, Koki Ando, Takafumi Ito, Yohei Suda, Yuki Matsui, Akiko Oyama, Hikari Kaneko and Shingo Yokoyama
Laboratory of Physiology, School of Health Sciences, Toyohashi SOZO University, Toyohashi 440-8511, Japan

Tatsuro Egawa
Laboratory of Sports and Exercise Medicine, Graduate School of Human and Environmental Studies, Kyoto University, Kyoto 606-8501, Japan

Katsumasa Goto
Laboratory of Physiology, School of Health Sciences, Toyohashi SOZO University, Toyohashi 440-8511, Japan
Department of Physiology, Graduate School of Health Sciences, Toyohashi SOZO University, Toyohashi 440-8511, Japan

Dorin Dragos
Medical Semiology Department, Faculty of General Medicine, "Carol Davila" University of Medicine and Pharmacy, B-dul "Eroilor Sanitari" nr. 8, Sector 6, 76241 Bucharest, Romania
Nephrology Clinic, University Emergency Hospital Bucharest, 050098 Bucharest, Romania

Marilena Gilca and Laura Gaman
Biochemistry Department, Faculty of General Medicine, "Carol Davila" University of Medicine and Pharmacy, B-dul "Eroilor Sanitari" nr. 8, Sector 6, 76241 Bucharest, Romania

Irina Stoian
Biochemistry Department, Faculty of General Medicine, "Carol Davila" University of Medicine and Pharmacy, B-dul "Eroilor Sanitari" nr. 8, Sector 6, 76241 Bucharest, Romania
R&D IRIST LABMED SRL, Str. Miraslau, nr. 24, Sector 3, 031235 Bucharest, Romania

Adelina Vlad
Physiology Department, Faculty of General Medicine, "Carol Davila" University of Medicine and Pharmacy, B-dul "Eroilor Sanitari" nr. 8, Sector 6, 76241 Bucharest, Romania

Liviu Iosif
R&D IRIST LABMED SRL, Str. Miraslau, nr. 24, Sector 3, 031235 Bucharest, Romania

Olivera Lupescu
Orthopaedic and Trauma Clinic 2, Faculty of General Medicine, "Carol Davila" University of Medicine and Pharmacy, 020022 Bucharest, Romania
Clinical Emergency Hospital Bucharest, 014461 Bucharest, Romania

Małgorzata M. Brzóska, Alicja Roszczenko, Joanna Rogalska, Małgorzata Gałażyn-Sidorczuk and Magdalena Mężyńska
Department of Toxicology, Medical University of Bialystok, Adama Mickiewicza 2C street, 15-222 Bialystok, Poland

Joey S.J. Smeets and Luc J.C. van Loon
Department of Human Biology, NUTRIM School of Nutrition and Translational Research in Metabolism, Maastricht University Medical Centre+, 6200 MD Maastricht, The Netherlands

Floris K. Hendriks
Department of Human Biology, NUTRIM School of Nutrition and Translational Research in Metabolism, Maastricht University Medical Centre+, 6200 MD Maastricht, The Netherlands
Department of Internal Medicine, NUTRIM School of Nutrition and Translational Research in Metabolism, Maastricht University Medical Centre+, 6200 MD Maastricht, The Netherlands

Jeroen P. Kooman
Department of Internal Medicine, NUTRIM School of Nutrition and Translational Research in Metabolism, Maastricht University Medical Centre+, 6200 MD Maastricht, The Netherlands
Division of Nephrology, Department of Internal Medicine, Maastricht University Medical Centre+, 6202 AZ Maastricht, The Netherlands

Frank M. van der Sande
Division of Nephrology, Department of Internal Medicine, Maastricht University Medical Centre+, 6202 AZ Maastricht, The Netherlands

Domenico Azzolino and Matteo Cesari
Geriatric Unit, Fondazione IRCCS Ca' Granda Ospedale Maggiore Policlinico, 20122 Milan, Italy
Department of Clinical Sciences and Community Health, University of Milan, 20122 Milan, Italy

Pier Carmine Passarelli, Paolo De Angelis, Giovan Battista Piccirillo and Antonio D'Addona
Department of Head and Neck, Oral Surgery and Implantology Unit, Institute of Clinical Dentistry, Catholic University of Sacred Hearth, Fondazione Policlinico Universitario Gemelli, 00168 Rome, Italy

Vincenzo Arcoraci, Marco Atteritano, Francesco Squadrito, Herbert Marini, Domenico Santoro, Letteria Minutoli and Alessandra Bitto
Department of Clinical and Experimental Medicine, University of Messina, 98100 Messina, Italy

Rosario D'Anna and Sonia Messina
Department of Neurosciences and Nemo Sud Clinical Center, University of Messina, 98100 Messina, Italy

Domenica Altavilla
Department of Paediatric, Gynaecological, Microbiological and Biomedical Sciences, University of Messina, 98100 Messina, Italy

Sandra M. Sacco
Department of Kinesiology, Faculty of Applied Health Sciences, Brock University, St. Catharines, ON L2S 3A1, Canada
Centre for Bone and Muscle Health, Brock University, St. Catharines, ON L2S 3A1, Canada

Caitlin Saint and Paul J. LeBlanc
Centre for Bone and Muscle Health, Brock University, St. Catharines, ON L2S 3A1, Canada
Department of Health Sciences, Faculty of Applied Health Sciences, Brock University, St. Catharines, ON L2S 3A1, Canada

Wendy E. Ward
Department of Kinesiology, Faculty of Applied Health Sciences, Brock University, St. Catharines, ON L2S 3A1, Canada
Centre for Bone and Muscle Health, Brock University, St. Catharines, ON L2S 3A1, Canada
Department of Health Sciences, Faculty of Applied Health Sciences, Brock University, St. Catharines, ON L2S 3A1, Canada

Stephanie A. Lee, Caroline Sypniewski, Benjamin A. Bensadon, Christian McLaren and Kimberly T. Sibille
Department of Aging and Geriatric Research, Institute on Aging, University of Florida, Gainesville, FL 32610, USA

William T. Donahoo
Department of Medicine, University of Florida, Gainesville, FL 32610, USA

Stephen Anton
Department of Aging and Geriatric Research, Institute on Aging, University of Florida, Gainesville, FL 32610, USA
Department of Clinical and Health Psychology, University of Florida, Gainesville, FL 32610, USA

Donatella Granchi
Laboratory for Orthopedic Pathophysiology and Regenerative Medicine, IRCCS Istituto Ortopedico Rizzoli, via di Barbiano 1/10, 40136 Bologna, Italy

Nicola Baldini
Laboratory for Orthopedic Pathophysiology and Regenerative Medicine, IRCCS Istituto Ortopedico Rizzoli, via di Barbiano 1/10, 40136 Bologna, Italy
Department of Biomedical and Neuromotor Sciences, Via Pupilli 1, University of Bologna, 40136 Bologna, Italy

Fabio Massimo Ulivieri
Nuclear Medicine, Bone Metabolic Unit, IRCCS Ca' Granda Ospedale Maggiore Policlinico, Via F. Sforza 35, 20122 Milano, Italy

Renata Caudarella
Maria Cecilia Hospital, GVM Care and Research, Via Corriera 1, 48033 Cotignola (RA), Italy

Index

www.ingramcontent.com/pod-product-compliance
Lightning Source LLC
LaVergne TN
LVHW081029210926
848485LV00004B/980